European Respiratory M

Antibiotics and the Lung

Edited by

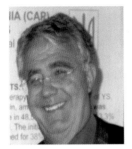
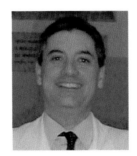
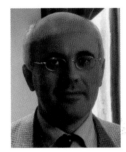

M. Cazzola   F. Blasi   S. Ewig

M. Cazzola is presently Consultant of Respiratory Medicine and Chief of the Respiratory Clinical Pharmacology at the Dept of Respiratory Medicine, at A. Cardarelli Hospital, Naples, Italy. He is also Visiting Senior Lecturer at the Sackler Institute of Pulmonary Pharmacology, GKT School of Biomedical Sciences, London, UK. He is the author and co-author of more that 320 peer-reviewed publications and scientific contributions to books and journals. He currently serves as the Editor for *Pulmonary Pharmacology & Therapeutics*, and is an Editorial Board Member for *Respiratory Medicine, Respiration*, and *Monaldi Archives for Chest Diseases*. He is also the Chairman of the Airway Pharmacology and Treatment Group of the European Respiratory Society. His research has focused on pharmacology of airway diseases, particularly with the use of bronchodilators in chronic obstructive pulmonary disease and respiratory infections, particularly pharmacokinetics of antimicrobial drugs.

F. Blasi is currently Professor of Respiratory Medicine at the Institute of Respiratory Diseases at the university of Milan, Italy. He is presently the Secretary for the Respiratory Infection Assembly within the European Respsiratory Society and is Officer of the Italian Respiratory Society (SiMER). His ongoing research interests include investigations into *Chlamydia pneumoniae* with respect to its infection incidences and prevalence in chronic bronchitis and HIV infected patients as well as its role in the onset of asthma. Other areas of research include the use of molecular methods in the diagnosis of viral and bacterial infections and antibiotic-resistance detection. He is also working on the role of antibiotics in asthma and chronic obstructive pulmonary disease exacerbations and the role of antibiotic-resistant strains in the outcome of pneumonia.

S. Ewig is professor of medicine and presently Chief of the Dept for Respiratory Medicine and Infectious Diseases at the Augusta-Kranken-Anstalt tertiary care and teaching hospital in Germany. Moreover, he is Lecturer of Respiratory Medicine at the University of Bonn, Germany. He is author and co-author of more than 250 publications and scientific contributions to journals and authoritative books. He has contributed to numerous national and international guidelines for the treatment of adult pulmonary infections. He currently serves as Associate Editor for the *European Respiratory Journal*. His primary scientific interest includes lower respiratory tract infections (acute exacerbations of chronic obstructive pulmonary disease and community-acquired pneumonia), nosocomial pneumonia as well as pulmonary infections in the immunocompromised host. Ethics in medicine is another important area of his activity.

The European Respiratory Monograph

Number 28 April 2004

CONTENTS

Preface

To serve its primary function of gas exchange, the lung is the organ with the largest epithelial surface area in continuous contact with the external environment. The upper and lower airways of humans are repeatedly exposed to airborne particles and microorganisms. Infectious respiratory disorders are therefore an important part of our daily activities as practising physicians. Furthermore, the management of these infectious diseases continues to evolve. Physicians are continuously confronted with new challenges in the cost-effective management of these infectious diseases.

Antibiotic treatment is a key factor in the treatment schedules of these diseases. Optimal treatment would be an antibiotic regimen specifically suited for a specific patient, the type of infection and the infecting pathogen to assure an optimal therapeutic outcome. The present issue of the Monograph not only covers basic knowledge about treatment with antibiotics but also provides state of the art information about a variety of different classes of antibiotics. Indeed, the efficacy of antibiotics traditionally used in the treatment of respiratory infections is increasingly compromised by the emerge of resistant bacteria. Furthermore, state of the art treatment of specific infectious respiratory problems is reviewed in different chapters. This issue of the Monograph also focuses attention on the health economical aspects of antibiotic treatment andon the epidemiological consequences of antibiotic use in the community. State of the art information regarding the management of these diseases is indeed crucial to solve future resistance problems. This issue of the Monograph offers the physician the essential information for state of the art management of infectious problems in daily clinical practice.

E.F.M. Wouters
Editor in Chief

Eur Respir Mon, 2004, 28, a. Printed in UK - all rights reserved. Copyright ERS Journals Ltd 2004; European Respiratory Monograph; ISSN 1025-448x. ISBN 1-904097-32-4.

INTRODUCTION

Lower respiratory tract infections (LRTIs) are a major healthcare and economical problem due to their high morbidity and to the direct and indirect costs that their management engenders. However, the dimension of the public health problem is not the only reason for the great interest in LRTIs. They are usually treated by antimicrobial agents. Actually, once a diagnosis of LRTI has been made, empirical antibiotic therapy may be justified. When it is, the selection of antimicrobial treatment should be based on a careful clinical assessment of severity, the expected general microbial and resistance pattern and the assessment of the presence of individual risk factors for infection with resistant pathogens. Also having this concept in mind, traditional agents such as β-lactams and macrolides remain those most frequently used, although they have been compromised by bacterial resistance in the common pathogens *e.g. Streptococcus pneumoniae, Haemophilus influenzae* and *Moraxella catarrhalis*. In recent years, there have been worldwide efforts to reduce inappropriate antimicrobial prescribing in response to mounting concerns about the emergence of microbial resistance.

Several guidelines for the management of LRTIs have been published worldwide in response to the move towards evidence-based practice, concern over the misuse of antimicrobial agents and the changes in susceptibility to some of these. However, although the rational use of antibiotics can limit the development of resistances, it is not sufficient to abate the resistant bacteria. The spread of penicillin- and macrolide-resistant *S. pneumoniae*, the increasing emergence of erythromycin-resistant strains of *Streptococcus pyogenes*, the growing problem with methicillin-resistant staphylococci (MRSA) as well as the emergence of glycopeptide-resistant staphylococci underline the need for therapeutic alternatives. Therefore, new drugs must be designed with emerging needs in mind *i.e.* specific resistant and hard-to-treat organisms.

The focus of this monograph is on antimicrobial agents and their impact on lungs. For this reason, the readers will find detailed descriptions not only of the advancements in the different classes of antimicrobial agents that are usually prescribed for treating LRTIs, but also of the pulmonary distribution of these agents, the interrelationship between their pharmacokinetic profile and pharmacodynamic action, the interactions between antimicrobial agents and host defences, and the interactions between antimicrobial agents and other drugs. We are confident that consolidated and also novel information on the correct approach to the different forms of LRTI, with particular emphasis on the position of these agents in the new guidelines for the treatment of LRTIs, will add scientific value to these basic findings.

Finally, the description of the therapeutic perspectives in development will confer to this monograph a well-founded hope for an always more effective therapeutic approach to LRTIs and will provide us the opportunity to speculate on the treatment of these infectious conditions in the coming years.

Eur Respir Mon, 2004, 28, b. Printed in UK - all rights reserved. Copyright ERS Journals Ltd 2004; European Respiratory Monograph; ISSN 1025-448x. ISBN 1-904097-32-4.

CHAPTER 1

Interrelationship of pharmacokinetics/ pharmacodynamics: antibiotic dosing for the future

G.W. Amsden

Correspondence: G.W. Amsden, Clinical Pharmacology Research Center, Bassett Healthcare, One Atwell Road, Cooperstown, NY 13326, USA.

Choosing an antibiotic and its regimen for lower respiratory tract infections, let alone any infection, used to be a rote process. Based on an individual's age, end-organ clearance capabilities and sometimes weight, it was a *fait accompli* that whatever drug was chosen to treat the patient's infection, its dosing regimen would be the same as for anyone else. Although this "one dose for all" mentality still exists to a point in the present day prescribing of antibiotics, a shift away from this method towards the desire for individualised dosing has started to be observed. Ideally, individualised dosing would assure better clinical and bacteriological efficacy, even against resistant pathogens, and minimise resistance development, adverse effects and potentially cost.

Knowing the basics

To talk about this type of dosing there has to be a level playing field and a clear understanding of the scientific terminology used. One of the most common and important phrases used in this scientific area is pharmacokinetics. In simple terms, pharmacokinetics refers to how the body handles a drug. It involves all of the processes that the body will put a drug through and can be summed up by the acronym ADME; absorption, distribution, metabolism, and elimination.

The term absorption is usually used in reference to how the body dissolves an oral-drug dose and how the dissolved drug moves from the gastrointestinal tract into the circulatory system. However, depending on the drug and where in the world the patient is being treated, absorption can also refer to how the body absorbs the drug from a rectal formulation of a drug or from an intramuscular injection site. Key absorption pharmacokinetic parameters come from attempts to characterise: 1) How long it takes until absorption of the drug is detectable (lag time or t_{lag}); 2) How long it takes before peak-serum or plasma concentrations are achieved (t_{max}); 3) What the peak serum or plasma concentration (C_{max}) that can be achieved using a certain dose of the drug; and 4) How the drug is distributed throughout the body, especially to the site of infection, as soon as the drug reaches the systemic circulation.

Distribution is a dynamic process as long as the drug is being passed through the circulation to the infection site and from the infection site back to the circulation, in and out of various cell types, eventually reaching the end-organ clearance system.

Metabolism does not necessarily occur with every administered drug, however, in the instances it does occur, the body is perceived to be reacting to a foreign substance and trying to change it to a compound more readily cleared from the body. When metabolism

Eur Respir Mon, 2004, 28, 1–12. Printed in UK - all rights reserved. Copyright ERS Journals Ltd 2004; European Respiratory Monograph; ISSN 1025-448x. ISBN 1-904097-32-4.

is discussed it normally refers to hepatic enzyme systems that are broken down to groups referred to as Phase I and Phase II. Phase-I metabolism involves the cytochrome P450 enzyme systems, the location for drug metabolism and the site where the majority of drug-to-drug interactions described in the literature involving metabolism-based systems occur. Phase-II metabolism involves other degradation/metabolic pathways *e.g.* the glucuronidation that occurs with zidovudine.

Elimination is the process in which the drug is expelled from the body and typically involves the kidneys, liver, or intestinal/biliary routes. Typical elimination pharmaco-kinetic parameters include: 1) clearance, which is described as total and/or predicated, dependent upon the route of clearance (*i.e.* renal *versus* nonrenal); and 2) elimination half-life ($t1/2$), which is the amount of time taken for the body to eliminate one-half of the total amount of drug at any given time point.

When all of the processes that the body puts a drug through are brought together, it becomes possible to estimate a patient's exposure to a drug for a given time period; this is normally calculated as the area under the curve (AUC) of a concentration/time curve for a set period of time [1].

The other key term in this scientific arena is pharmacodynamics. This term refers to the action of the drug on the body after the drug has encountered the organ and/or receptor type it was designed to interact with. With antibiotics, the effects on the body (*i.e.* normalisation of white-cell count and body temperature) are a secondary result of the interaction between the antibiotic and the infecting pathogen. The expected interaction between the two is typically measured outside of the body in laboratory procedures, in the guise of susceptibility-testing. Although the majority of institutions have only offered break-point testing in the past, due to the cumbersome nature of broth-microdilution susceptibility testing, the introduction of E-test strips has once again allowed clinicians to receive data on the actual minimal inhibitory concentration (MIC) that a pathogen has to an antibiotic [1]. The MIC is the concentration that is most typically used when calculating the pharmacokinetic-pharmacodynamic optimisation ratios discussed in this chapter.

The interrelationship between pharmacokinetics-pharmacodynamics

Although it seems that the use of a drug's pharmacokinetics and pharmacodynamics to optimise the outcome has been the most prevalent in the literature for the last decade, the idea is actually an old concept that was introduced some 50 yrs ago [2]. Significant progress on these concepts, for whatever reason, did not occur until more recent years [3]. Based on this progress, it is now common to break antibacterials into different groups based on the type of antibacterial activity that they demonstrate in relation to their pharmacokinetics [3, 4]. Antibiotics that demonstrate a higher rate and degree of antibacterial activity as their serum concentrations increase, are termed concentration-dependent killing drugs. Once it has been established that a drug meets this definition *e.g*, as was found with aminoglycosides and fluoroquinolones, the peak concentrations are varied in comparison with the MICs in an attempt to characterise a ratio value of the two, in which optimal clinical and bacteriological effects will be achieved. An example of this is a study by KASHUBA *et al.* [5], which analysed aminoglycoside treatment data for 78 patients with a diagnosis of nosocomial pneumonia to determine if optimisation of aminoglycoside-pharmacodynamic properties resulted in a more rapid therapeutic response.

Using patient-specific aminoglycoside pharmacokinetic data outcomes, and the number of days for the white blood cell count to reach normalisation and days to body temperature resolution as response variables, the treatment data was analysed. Cox proportional hazards, classification and regression tree (CART), and logistic regression analyses were all used to analyse the data. It was observed that from all the types of analyses used, it was the first measured peak serum concentration compared with the patient's pathogen MIC (C_{max}/MIC) that predicted the number of days to temperature resolution, and the second measured C_{max}/MIC that predicted the time to normalisation of white blood cell count. CART analysis predicted C_{max}/MIC ratio breakpoints for days to temperature and leukocyte normalisation with 89% and 86% success rates at 7 days of therapy with ratios >4.7 and >4.5, respectively. By logistic regression, there was a 90% probability of temperature and leukocyte normalisation by the seventh day of therapy if a C_{max}/MIC ratio of ≥ 10 was achieved within the first 48 h of treatment with the aminoglycoside [5]. In a second example, PRESTON et al. [6] attempted to prospectively quantitate the relationship between plasma concentrations of a fluoroquinolone, levofloxacin, and successful clinical and microbiological outcomes in infected patients. It was observed in this study that from the 313 patients, for which data had been collected, 134 patients had pharmacokinetic data sets available and clinical outcomes determined, and 116 had pharmacokinetic data sets as well as microbiological outcomes determined. Using logistic regression analysis, it was determined that optimal clinical and microbiological outcomes were obtained, regardless of infection site or organism, whenever patients achieved a C_{max}/MIC ratio ≥ 12.2. If this was achieved, positive clinical and microbiological outcomes were obtained in 99% and 100% of patients, respectively, as opposed to 83% and 81%, respectively, if the ratio was not achieved [6].

In contrast to concentration-dependent killing antibiotics, other antibiotics demonstrate minimal concentration dependence in their activity and appear to achieve peak activity when low multiples of a susceptible pathogen's MIC is achieved [3]. Typically, antibiotics that are concentration-independent, or time-dependent agents, achieve their full potential with concentrations that are approximately four to five times greater than that of a pathogen's MIC. Although logically it would seem necessary to maintain these concentrations above the MIC for the entire dosing interval, research in both animal models and in human patients has demonstrated otherwise. A neutropaenic mouse pneumonia model with *Klebsiella pneumoniae* demonstrated that cefotaxime achieved a bacteriostatic effect when serum concentrations were above the MIC for 30–40% of the dosing interval. When concentrations were maintained above the MIC for 60–70% of the dosing interval, the bacteriological activity increased from bacteriostasis to maximal killing [3, 7]. In humans, a clinical trial performed by PALLARES et al. [8] demonstrated that when higher doses of penicillins and cephalosporins were used, equal clinical outcomes were achieved in patients with severe pneumococcal pneumonia, regardless of whether isolates were susceptible or resistant to the treatment agents. Although overwhelming failures in the patients that had resistant isolates would be expected, the increase in doses of antibiotics maintained serum concentrations above the MIC for a longer period of time ($\geq 40\%$), thereby optimising the pharmacodynamics of the drugs [3, 8]. These concepts have been repeated and verified in other human trials, not only involving pneumococcal pneumonia in adults, but also in children as well as meningitis in adults [9–11].

Although the final pharmacokinetic/pharmacodynamic parameter that is most commonly referenced encompasses aspects taken from both other concepts, and is frequently grouped into discussions of concentration- or time-dependent activity, it is more appropriately discussed as a separate concept. The idea of comparing a patient's 24-h exposure (AUC_{24}) with an antibiotic and the MIC of their infecting pathogen, to adjust the dosage to assure that a break-point ratio was achieved for optimal activity, was first defined by SCHENTAG et al. [12] in the early 1990s. Despite the initial publication of this concept stating that the important pharmacokinetic variable of the ratio calculation was the amount of the AUC that was above the MIC, iterations since have evolved into the current concept that compares the full 24-h exposure to an antibiotic, regardless of the number of doses given in that 24-h period, with the MIC (AUC24/MIC) of the pathogen involved. Although some investigators have argued that this dosing paradigm is applicable to all classes of antibiotics, it is most commonly associated with research and discussions concerning the fluoroquinolones and macrolides [13, 14]. In contrast to concentration-dependent and time-dependent agents that all need to achieve relatively the same ratios for different types of pathogens and infections, this does not appear to hold true for drugs that are exposure-dependent active agents. As an example, in a retrospective study of exposure to intravenous (IV) ciprofloxacin for treatment of Gram-negative nosocomial pneumonia, it was determined that it was necessary to achieve an AUC24/MIC ratio of ≥125 serum inhibitory titer (SIT)·h^{-1} for optimal outcomes [13]. If a ratio of <125 was achieved, the probabilities of positive clinical and microbiological outcomes were 42% and 26%, respectively. In contrast, if a ratio of >125 was achieved, the probabilities increased to 80% and 82%, respectively. These ratios were also correlated with the time taken for bacterial eradication. These times varied between 32 days, when an AUC24/MIC ratio of <125 was achieved, and 6.6 and 1.9 days when ratios of 125–250 and >250 were achieved, respectively [13]. A separate *in vitro* study of different fluoroquinolones and their activities against three strains of *Pseudomonas aeruginosa* also demonstrated a similar AUC24/MIC ratio being necessary for optimal *in vitro* activity [15]. In contrast to the relatively high ratio needed for optimal activity against Gram-negative pathogens, it has been repeatedly demonstrated that an AUC24/MIC ratio of ≥30 SIT·h^{-1} necessary for optimal activity against Gram-positive pathogens including pneumococci [16–19]. This is shown in a study by AMBROSE *et al.* [19], which evaluated outcomes, pharmacokinetic and microbiological data from 58 patients with either pneumococcal community-acquired pneumonia (CAP) or an acute bacterial exacerbation of chronic bronchitis caused by *Streptococcus pneumoniae* [19]. Using univariate and multivariable logistic regression and CART analyses, not only was a significant (p=0.013) relationship between the microbiological response and the serum AUC24/MIC ratio detected, but also actual pharmacodynamic break points were detected. Regardless of whether patients were treated with levofloxacin or gatifloxacin, the probability of a positive microbiological response was only 64% if the serum AUC24/MIC ratio was <33.7 SIT·h^{-1}. In contrast, if the ratio was >33.7, positive microbiological responses occurred 100% of the time [19].

A summary of the different atibiotic classes and the pharmacokinetic/pharmacodynamic dosing optimisation concept(s) is given in table 1.

Optimisation at the bedside?

Although there is a plethora of literature to support the pharmacokinetic and pharmacodynamic optimisation theories that have been described above, the potential for prospective, individualised bedside use of them, is still some time in the future. Up-front exceptions to this statement are obvious and include the individualisation of aminoglycoside and vancomycin therapies which clinicians have done prospectively for many years to not only assure optimal clinical and microbiological outcomes, but also to decrease toxicities from them. However, the use of these concepts for the majority of mainstream antibiotics that are used in the treatment of lower respiratory tract infections, or any infection for that matter, are hampered due to a variety of issues. Sometimes these issues are resource or information inadequacies that cannot be

Table 1. – Antibiotic classes and the pharmacokinetic/pharmacodynamic dosing optimisation concept(s)# that have been demonstrated as relevant

Cmax/MIC	Time above MIC	AUC24/MIC
Aminoglycosides	All β-lactams	All macrolides
Fluoroquinolones	Vancomycin	Fluoroquinolones
Streptogramins	Linezolid	β-lactams
	Clindamycin	Aminoglycosides
	Erythromycin	Vancomycin
	Clarithromycin	Clindamycin
		Doxycycline
		Streptogramins
		All antibiotics

Cmax: peak serum or plasma concentration; MIC: minimum inhibitory concentration; AUC24: area under the curve in 24 h; #: drugs or classes that have conflicting data, demonstrating that more than one concept is relevant, have been listed in each of the relevant columns.

reasonably overcome. Other times questions arise regarding the appropriateness of the methods used or the application of the theories, which need to be answered prior to the widespread acceptance of these concepts.

In vitro *issues*

To appreciate fully the range of issues that still need to be overcome, enabling these theories to be used at the bedside, it is necessary to discuss all the types of research that are involved with developing them. Although *in vitro* models and studies provide valuable data, they also have inherent deficiencies that need to be taken into account prior to their data being extrapolated to a human system [20]. First, the various media used in the *in vitro* systems are nutritive ones, which are meant to help a cultured organism grow and be sustained. Therefore, any data produced involving the cultured organism and the antibiotic being tested against it, is a pure reflection of the inherent activity of the antibiotic in and of itself. Even though this data is important to assess, it lacks any study of the inter-relationship between the organism, antibiotic and the human immune system. An example of this is given by HARDY *et al.* [21]. When 50% human serum was added to *in vitro* media the pneumococcal MICs to clarithromycin and azithromycin were shown to fall a total of 1–2 and 2–6, two-fold dilutions respectively, from when they were tested without the addition of serum. Based on this information, standard (*i.e.* serum-free) *in vitro* results would overestimate the macrolide MICs of these pneumococci and not be reflective of the true activity that would occur in the 100% serum environment of the human body. Another example is provided in a study by MEYER *et al.* [22] that demonstrated that *Staphylococcus aureus* had a lower MIC to azithromycin after phagocytosis by an azithromycin-loaded monocyte compared with when it was exposed to the drug or a drug-free monocyte alone. These results suggest that the environment within the phagocyte is not only favourable for antibiotic activity, but also that there may be additive activity between the drug and the phagocyte. As *in vitro* systems are void of any immune system components, the beneficial relationship that may exist between the drug and immune system within a human body would fail to be identified or characterised *in vitro*.

Animal model issues

Like *in vitro* methods, animal models have also been a source of information that has been well accepted and relied upon for decades. Although an animal model may provide a better reflection of the penetration and activity of an antibiotic into a tissue-based infection site, this cannot always be true for all antibiotics, in all instances. First it is appropriate to assure that the tissue concentrations of the drug are being measured appropriately so that any break points developed from the data are truly reflective. A common method for determining tissue concentrations is harvesting the tissue of interest, homogenising it and then assaying the homogenate. Unfortunately, the resulting concentration from the assay is not a true reflection of the infection site penetration. Rather, the homogenate reflects the combined volume of interstitial (extracellular) fluid and intracellular fluid as well as any contributing volume from any nonlocal host cells e.g. responding phagocytes or infecting bacteria. As a mass of tissue is predominantly cells, the bulk of the homogenate volume represents intracellular fluid/components. As a result, any antibiotic that does not appreciably penetrate host cells, such as a β-lactam, would have a resulting assay concentration that is falsely low and not reflective of the concentration that actually existed in the extracellular space where it would be active. For aminoglycosides, the concentration may actually exceed serum concentrations since aminoglycosides do penetrate host cells. However, this penetration is not a therapeutic reservoir of drug and is usually associated with toxicity rather than efficacy. As a result, the concentration in the extracellular space where the drug is producing its effect is again not being reflected accurately in the assay results. Although this may still be done with an animal model of a respiratory infection, efforts in humans have been made to assess true extracellular/interstitial penetration of antibiotics in the lung by measuring such things as epithelial lining fluid concentrations or bronchial mucosa concentrations, to provide accurate data that is relevant for the infection types that would be treated [23].

Even if it was assured that an appropriate method (i.e. blister model, thread method) was utilised to measure peripheral interstitial fluid concentrations of drug in an animal model, the neutropaenic models that are frequently used would not provide accurate concentration amounts or efficacy results [24]. While they may be reflective of the penetration and activity of a drug in and of itself, this can be more easily established in an in vitro model of infection. Without the presence of the immune system and its response to an infection, it is impossible to get an accurate idea of the penetration by drugs that are dependent on inflammation for enhanced delivery via phagocytes to the infection site as can be seen with macrolides and fluoroquinolones, or the true activity of the antibiotic in conjunction with the activity of the immune system that would be present in any nonimmunocompromised human host [25–27]. KIEM AND CRAIG [26] compared the effects of gatifloxacin and levofloxacin in a murine thigh-infection model using S. pneumoniae as the test organism in two groups of mice; one neutropenic and one immunocompetent [26]. The results of the study not only indicated the growth rate of the bacterium was slower over the first 6 h after dosing in the immunocompetent mice, but that the extent of killing was enhanced and the length of the postantibiotic effect (PAE) increased almost 10-fold. The authors concluded that it was the persistent effects seen in the healthy mice that explained the six- to seven-fold decrease in 24-h AUC/MIC ratio that was necessary for efficacy in this model as compared with the neutropenic mouse model [26].

Human application and treatment issues

As the true test of a theory is the application of it and the outcome associated with it, when applied to a human host, the results from well-designed clinical trials are by far the most important results that should be taken into account when reviewing a topic. If this theorem proof were applied to the above described pharmacokinetic and pharmaco-dynamic optimisation concepts, the results would leave a clinician questioning their utility, since the results of such an analysis would be mixed. If the concepts were applied to the widely used β-lactams, there has been consistent literature support stating that when the serum concentrations are maintained above the MIC for ≥ 40–50% of the dosing interval, the clinical efficacy rates of these drugs against common respiratory pathogens such as pneumococci, including resistant isolates, have been maintained [8–11]. The proof associated with this application of optimization-dosing concepts is enhanced when one considers the infection types that have been investigated. Not only has the use of increased doses (which inherently improves the time period in which the serum concentration is above the MIC of the susceptible/resistant isolates) been associated with positive outcomes in tissue sites *i.e.* lungs (where interstitial concentrations are in relative equilibrium with serum concentrations), but also in physiological spaces that are difficult to penetrate such as the meninges. In a report by VILADRICH *et al.* [11], 10 episodes (nine patients) of pneumococcal meningitis caused by isolates with decreased susceptibilities to third-generation cephalosporins, all resolved promptly utilising doses of cefotaxime (300 mg·kg^{-1}·day^{-1}, max 24 g·day^{-1}) that far exceed those typically recommended (2 g every 4–6 h) [11, 28].

However, if the same concepts were applied to β-lactams against pathogens causing an infection at the site of clearance of the active drug, *e.g.* using a β-lactam to treat an uncomplicated urinary tract infection, it does not seem likely that they would apply equally, as local concentrations are log-folds higher than the corresponding serum concentrations. Evidence supporting this conclusion originates from data involving other drugs whose serum concentrations are inherently lower than those at an infection site, as is commonly seen with the macrolides and fluoroquinolones. In regards to the fluoroquinolones, a good example would involve the peak serum concentration to MIC ratio established by PRESTON *et al.* [6] for levofloxacin, the pharmacokinetics of levofloxacin and the current susceptibility pattern of pneumococcal clinical isolates. As the average steady-state peak concentration associated with daily, IV dosing of levofloxacin 500 mg is 8.0 mg·L^{-1}, the highest MIC that can be optimally treated by achieving a ratio of 12 is 0.67 mg·L^{-1} [6, 29]. As this MIC is below the average (1–2 mg·L^{-1}), which has been repeatedly documented for levofloxacin against pneumococci, the drug when dosed this way should be completely ineffective, both clinically and microbiologically [6, 30–32]. In contrast to the negative expected outcomes, patients continue to have positive clinical and microbiological efficacies that have resulted in levofloxacin being widely accepted as a first-line monotherapy treatment option for CAP [33–36].

When considering the macrolide class, including all its subclasses (azalides, ketolides, anhydrolides), evidence that the use of optimisation concepts in their current format cannot truly explain their activity is probably the most convincing. This is especially true for the azalide azithromycin, due to its unique pharmacokinetic profile. Azithromycin's pharmacokinetics is typified by very low serum concentrations that barely ever exceed the MIC of even susceptible isolates of Gram-positive and Gram-negative pathogens. As azithromycin has been stated to be dependent upon the optimisation of the 24-h serum AUC/MIC ratio, the fact that it has an activity against any typical respiratory pathogen should be a minor miracle [37]. For example, based on a goal AUC24/MIC ratio of 30 and an average 24-h AUC from a 500 mg oral dose of azithromycin of 2.1 mg·h^{-1}·L^{-1}, the highest MIC that azithromycin should be clinically active against is 0.07 mg·L^{-1} [38]. As the MIC where 90% of pneumococcal isolates were inhibited by azithromycin was 0.125 mg·L^{-1} in 1990 before the drug was widely marketed, the fact that it has demonstrated clinical and microbiological efficacy to date against pneumococcal respiratory infections means these theories are either wrong, or more likely, being applied to the wrong biological matrix [39, 40]. Although macrolides have interstitial infection-site concentrations that far exceed corresponding serum concentrations and interstitial concentrations of noninfected tissues, the concentrations and exposures achieved would not help explain how the macrolides have maintained their clinical efficacy rates despite widespread pneumococcal macrolide resistance [25, 40–42]. Since the macrolides, like the fluoroquinolones, are concentrated within the host cells clearing the bacteria from the human body, there is potential for the bacterial 24-h drug exposure after phagocytosis, being the appropriate matrices for the dosing optimisation calculations [38, 40]. For example after a 500 mg oral azithromycin dose, producing a 24-h serum exposure of 2.1 mg·h^{-1}·L^{-1}, the neutrophil and monocyte exposures are ~1,500 and ~12,000 mg·h^{-1}·L^{-1} [38]. If the same AUC24/MIC calculations are done to achieve a ratio of 30, the approximate MICs, at which azithromycin may have activity against the bacteria, would be on the order of 50 and 400 mg·L^{-1}, respectively. Despite rare clinical "failures" being reported in the literature, the wide and successful use of multiple macrolides internationally, even in areas with high incidences of pneumococcal macrolide resistance, lends credence to the concept that these phagocyte matrices may be the most appropriate for these dosing optimisation calculations [40, 43, 44].

Other general issues that represent major hurdles to these dosing concepts, which are receiving mass acceptance and being used readily at the bedside, include the ability to truly make these dosing concepts individualised and deciding how to apply them when combination therapy is desired. For the former issue, the use of these concepts at the bedside could be attempted one of two ways. The first possibility would be to develop population-based equations to calculate a person's AUC24 or Cmax based on a variety of demographic and laboratory data. After calculation of these parameters, they would be applied to the infecting pathogen's MIC or the institution's average encountered MIC for that pathogen and then the dosing regimen could be adjusted if necessary to achieve the optimal ratio. The second possibility would be to develop optimal sampling strategies so that a minimal number of serum samples could be collected and assayed and the results modelled so that they could be utilised to adjust the dose for dosing ratio achievement and optimal-clinical outcomes. While the second possibility would be the ideal method, not even the richest country or institution in the world could afford to have assay systems at the ready for all antibiotics so that the concept could be applied appropriately. As the first possibility is the most rational approach, that approach is more likely to be introduced in a mass market approach and it has already been used to treat respiratory tract infections in cystic fibrosis patients (*i.e.* continuous infusion β-lactams to optimise β-lactam pharmacodynamics) [45]. However, as most serum pharmacokinetic data for any given antibiotic is usually developed in healthy, young, nonobese adult volunteers, the equations may not take into account pharmacokinetic changes that may be present in any given disease state for which the drug would be used. Also, as each patient is an individual with their own inherent physiological abilities to absorb, distribute, metabolise and eliminate a drug, the use of population parameters, even if derived from a grouping of patients with the same disease as the patient in question, may not even come close to being representative of those of that patient. Therefore, any dose that is derived from the population parameters for the patient in question may be too low and result in clinical failure and resistance development, or, be too high and result in overt toxicity. In terms of the latter issue *i.e.* how to combine optimisation concepts or break points of all the antibiotics in a patient's regimen, research has already begun to address it.

Like other issues that have been discussed earlier, the findings from different researchers appear to be at odds with each other in their findings and conclusions. If it is assumed that all major classes of antibiotics have their efficacy optimised through the use of the AUC24/MIC break-point concept as SCHENTAG *et al.* [46] have suggested, it would be suspected that the individual drug ratio values may be able to be added to assess the overall antibiotic AUC24/MIC ratio being achieved in a patient. In the study, SCHENTAG *et al.* [46] dosed and sampled ciprofloxacin and piperacillin in healthy volunteers and conducted pharmacokinetic and pharmacodynamic modelling using the serum concentration exposures of each drug and the MICs of eight common Gram-positive and Gram-negative pathogens to each of the drugs. The results of their findings suggested that the individual AUC24/MIC ratios could be added and be reflective of an overall antibiotic therapy AUC24/MIC ratio that was predictive of bacterial killing rates. In a separate study by MOUTON et al. [47], 24-h efficacy data from various combinations of ceftazidime, ciprofloxacin, netilmicin, ticarcillin and tobramycin, and from when they were given singularly, were studied in a neutropaenic mouse-thigh infection model using P. aeruginosa as the test organism. Multiple logistic regression analysis was used to determine the most appropriate pharmacodynamic dosing indices for each drug given alone and in combination. In contrast to the results by SCHENTAG et al. [46] the investigators found that the appropriate dose optimisation method was class-dependent rather than one being all encompassing, and that this held true for the drugs not only when given as monotherapy, but also when they were used in combination. Even though combination therapy would involve two pharmacodynamic indices, the results of the study indicated that regardless of this, dosing optimisation of combination therapy should be approached as if attempting to optimise any single part of the combination as monotherapy [47]. Although the latter of these studies seems to be the most accepted to date, firm conclusions on how to interpret and optimise combination therapy regimens cannot be made without additional research.

Conclusion

There is no doubt that researchers have brought us closer to individualised dosing of antibiotics and to maintaining a drug's utility in the face of resistance trends than was ever thought possible. The ability to prescribe a dosing regimen for a patient that is specifically suited to that patient, their infection type and infecting pathogen so as to help assure optimal clinical and microbiological outcomes and potentially avoid unnecessary toxicities, would be a welcome addition to the armamentarium of any clinician. Instances when some of these dosing concepts have been applied, even in a general manner, have resulted in positive patient outcomes with drugs that otherwise may not have cured a patient anymore due to rising resistance trends. However, it is resistance trends with other antibiotics and a lack of clinical failures with them that have resulted in the questioning of other optimisation concepts and whether they are being applied correctly in their current format. Once the logistic issues, that currently hamper the ability to bring many of these concepts to the patient's bedside, are overcome, the true ability to use these dosing concepts will be finally recognised through the application of them in randomised, controlled clinical trials.

Summary

Although the concepts of using an antibiotic's pharmacokinetics and pharmaco-dynamics to adjust dosing and using the susceptibility of a pathogen to a specific drug have been in the literature for >40 yrs, it has not been until the last 10–15 yrs that great strides have been made using these theories. A variety of dosing concepts have been derived that when applied are thought to help ensure more optimal clinical and bacteriological outcomes in patients. While some of these have started to be applied prospectively in daily practice such as using higher doses of β-lactams against pneumococci with decreased susceptibility to penicillin, others may only represent a starting point for more research. This is especially true when attempts are made to apply these serum concentration-based concepts to drugs whose infection site concentrations are not in equilibrium with corresponding serum concentrations, as is seen with fluoroquinolones and macrolides. Along with additional research, to hone some of these dosing optimisation concepts, logistic issues may in the end limit these concepts to being applied in a population-based manner rather than as a true individualsed one.

Keywords: Dose optimisation, pharmacodynamics, pharmacokinetics.

References

1. Amsden GW, Ballow CH, Bertino JE Jr. Pharmacokinetics and pharmacodynamics of anti-infective agents. *In*: Mandell GL, Bennett JE, Dolin R eds. Principles and Practice of Infectious Diseases. 5th Edn. New York, Churchill Livingstone, 1999: pp. 253–261.
2. Eagle H. Experimental approach to the problem of treatment failure with penicillin. *Am J Med* 1952; 11: 389–399.
3. Craig WA. Pharmacokinetic/pharmacodynamic parameters: rationale for antibacterial dosing of mice and men. *Clin Infect Dis* 1998; 26: 1–12.
4. Shah PM, Junghanns W, Stille W. Dosis-Wirkungs-Beziehung der Bakterizidie bei *E. coli, K. pneumoniae*, und *Staphylococcus aureus. Dtsch Med Wochenschr* 1976; 101: 325–328.
5. Kashuba ADM, Nafziger AN, Drusano GL, Bertino JS Jr. Optimizing aminoglycoside therapy for nosocomial pneumonia caused by Gram-negative bacteria. *Antimicrob Agents Chemother* 1999; 43: 623–629.
6. Preston SL, Drusano GL, Berman AL, *et al.* Pharmacodynamics of levofloxacin: a new paradigm for early clinical trials. *JAMA* 1998; 279: 125–129.
7. Craig WA. Interrelationship between pharmacokinetics and pharmacodynamics in determining dosage regimens for broad-spectrum cephalosporins. *Diagn Microbiol Infect Dis* 1995; 22: 89–96.
8. Pallares R, LiZares J, Vadillo M, *et al.* Resistance to penicillin and cephalosporin and mortality from severe pneumococcal pneumonia in Barcelona, Spain. *N Engl J Med* 1995; 333: 474–480.
9. Friedland IR. Comparison of the response to antimicrobial therapy of penicillin-resistant and penicillin-susceptible pneumococcal disease. *Pediatr Infect Dis J* 1995; 14: 885–890.
10. Roson B, Carratala J, Tubau F, *et al.* Usefulness of beta lactam therapy for community-acquired pneumonia in the era of drug-resistant *Streptococcus pneumoniae*: a randomized study of amoxicillin-clavulanate and ceftriaxone. *Microb Drug Resist* 2001; 7: 85–96.
11. Viladrich PF, Cabellos C, Pallares R, *et al.* High doses of cefotaxime in treatment of adult meningitis due to *Streptococcus pneumoniae* with decreased susceptibilities to broad-spectrum cephalosporins. *Antimicrob Agents Chemother* 1996; 40: 218–220.
12. Schentag JJ, Nix DE, Adelman MH. Mathematical examination of dual individualization principles (I): Relationships between AUC above MIC and area under the curve for cefmenoxime, ciprofloxacin and tobramycin. *Ann Pharmacother* 1991; 25: 1050–1057.
13. Forrest A, Nix DE, Ballow CH, Goss TF, Birmingham MC, Schentag JJ. Pharmacodynamics of IV ciprofloxacin in seriously ill patients. *Antimicrob Agents Chemother* 1993; 37: 1073–1081.
14. Craig WA, Kiem S, Andes DR. Free drug 24-hr AUC/MIC is the PK/PD target that correlates with *in vivo* efficacy of macrolides, azalides, ketolides and clindamycin San Diego, 42nd Interscience Conference on Antimicrobial Agents and Chemotherapy; A1264.
15. Madaras-Kelly KJ, Ostergaard BE, Hovde LB, Rotschafer JC. Twenty-four-hour area under the concentration-time curve/MIC ratio as a generic predictor of fluoroquinolone antimicrobial effect by using three strains of *Pseudomonas aeruginosa* and an *in vitro* pharmacodynamic model. *Antimicrob Agents Chemother* 1996; 40: 627–632.
16. Lacy MK, Lu W, Xu X, *et al.* Pharmacodynamics comparisons of levofloxacin, ciprofloxacin, and

ampicillin against *Streptococcus pneumoniae* in an *in vitro* model of infection. *Antimicrob Agents Chemother* 1999; 43: 672–677.

17. Lister PD, Sanders CC. Pharmacodynamics of levofloxacin and ciprofloxacin against *Streptococcus pneumoniae*. *J Antimicrob Chemother* 1999; 43: 79–86.

18. Lister PD. Pharmacodynamics of gatifloxacin against *Streptococcus pneumoniae* in an *in vitro* pharmacokinetic model: impact of area under the curve/MIC ratios on eradication. *Antimicrob Agents Chemother* 2002; 46: 69–74.

19. Ambrose PG, Grasela DM, Grasela TH, *et al.* Pharmacodynamics of fluoroquinolones against *Streptococcus pneumoniae* in patients with community-acquired respiratory tract infections. *Antimicrob Agents Chemother* 2001; 45: 2793–2797.

20. White RL. What *in vitro* models of infection can and cannot do. *Pharmacotherapy* 2001; 21: 292S–301S.

21. Hardy DJ, Hense DM, Beyer JM, *et al.* Comparative *in vitro* activities of new 14-, 15- and 16-membered macrolides. *Antimicrob Agents Chemother* 1988; 32: 1710–1719.

22. Meyer AP, Bril-Bazuin C, Mattie H, van den Broe PJ. Uptake of azithromycin by human monocytes and enhanced intracellular antibacterial activity against *Staphylococcus aureus*. *Antimicrob Agents Chemother* 1993; 37: 2318–2322.

23. Chiu LM, Amsden GW. Intrapulmonary pharmacokinetics of antibacterial agents: implications for therapeutics. *Am J Respir Med* 2002; 1: 201–209.

24. Nix DE, Goodwin SD, Peloquin CA, Rotella DL, Schentag JJ. Antibiotic tissue penetration and its relevance: models of tissue penetration and their meaning. *Antimicrob Agents Chemother* 1991; 35: 1947–1952.

25. Ballow CH, Amsden GW, Highet VS, Forrest A. Healthy volunteer pharmacokinetics of oral azithromycin in serum, urine, polymorphonuclear leukocytes and inflammatory *vs.* non-inflammatory skin blisters. *Clin Drug Invest* 1998; 15: 159–167.

26. Kiem S, Craig WA. Why do neutrophils markedly reduce the 24-hr AUC/MIC required for efficacy of fluoroquinolones against *Streptococcus pneumoniae* (SP). San Diego, 42nd Interscience Conference on Antimicrobial Agents and Chemotherapy, 2002; A492.

27. Christianson JC, Craig WA, Kiem S, Andes DR. Impact of neutrophils on pharmacodynamic activity of clindamycin (CLINDA) and doxycycline (DOXY) against *Streptococcus pneumoniae*. San Diego, 42nd Interscience Conference on Antimicrobial Agents and Chemotherapy, 2002; A1267.

28. Quagliarello VJ, Scheld WM. Treatment of bacterial meningitis. *N Engl J Med* 1997; 336: 708–716.

29. Amsden GW, Graci DM, Cabelus LJ, Hejmanowski LG. A randomized, crossover design study of the pharmacology of extended-spectrum fluoroquinolones for pneumococcal infections. *Chest* 1999; 116: 115–119.

30. Jones RN, Pfaller MA, Doern GV, Beach M, and the SENTRY Participant Group. Antimicrobial activity of gatifloxacin, a newer 8-methoxy fluoroquinolone, tested against over 23,000 recent clinical isolates from the SENTRY antimicrobial surveillance program, 1997. San Diego, 42nd Interscience Conference on Antimicrobial Agents and Chemotherapy, 2002; E1940.

31. Blondeau JM, Laskowski R, Bjarnason J, Stewart C. Comparative *in vitro* activity of gatifloxacin, grepafloxacin, levofloxacin, moxifloxacin and trovafloxacin against 4151 Gram-negative and Gram-positive organisms. *Int J Antimicrob Agents* 2000; 14: 45–50.

32. Reinert RR, Schlaeger JJ, Lutticken R. Moxifloxacin: a comparison with other antimicrobial agents of *in vitro* activity against *Streptococcus pneumoniae*. *J Antimicrob Chemother* 1998; 42: 803–806.

33. Gotfried MH, Dattani D, Riffer E, *et al.* A controlled, double-blind, multicenter study comparing clarithromycin extended-release tablets and levofloxacin tablets in the treatment of community-acquired pneumonia. *Clin Ther* 2002; 24: 736–751.

34. Weiss LR. Open-label, randomized comparison of the efficacy and tolerability of clarithromycin, levofloxacin, and cefuroxime axetil in the treatment of adults with acute exacerbations of chronic bronchitis. *Clin Ther* 2002; 24: 1414–1425.

35. Bartlett JG, Dowell SF, Mandell LA, File TM Jr, Musher DM, Fine MJ. Practice guidelines for the management of community-acquired pneumonia in adults. *Clin Infect Dis* 2000; 31: 347–382.

36. American Thoracic Society. Guidelines for the management of adults with community-acquired pneumonia: diagnosis, assessment of severity, antimicrobial therapy, and prevention. *Am J Respir Crit Care Med* 2001; 163: 1730–1754.

37. Craig WA. Postantibiotic effects and the dosing of macrolides, azalides, and streptogramins. *In*: Zinner SH, Young LS, Acar JF, Neu HC, eds. Expanding Indications for the New Macrolides, Azalides, and Streptogramins. New York, Marcel Dekker, 1997; pp. 27–38.

38. Amsden GW, Nafziger AN, Foulds G. Pharmacokinetics in serum and leukocyte exposures of oral azithromycin, 1,500 milligrams, given over a 3- or 5-day period in healthy subjects. *Antimicrob Agents Chemother* 1999; 43: 163–165.

39. Maskell JP, Sefton AM, Williams JD. Comparative *in-vitro* activity of azithromycin and erythromycin against Gram-positive cocci, *Haemophilus influenzae* and anaerobes. *J Antimicrob Chemother* 1990; 25: Suppl. A, 19–24.

40. Amsden GW. Pneumococcal macrolide resistance – myth or reality? *J Antimicrob Chemother* 1999; 44: 1–6.

41. Baldwin DR, Wise R, Andrews JM, Ashby JP, Honeybourne D. Azithromycin concentrations at the sites of pulmonary infection. *Eur Respir J* 1990; 3: 886–890.

42. Honeybourne D, Kees F, Andrews JM, Baldwin D, Wise R. The levels of clarithromycin and its 14-hydroxy metabolite in the lung. *Eur Respir J* 1994; 7: 1275–1280.

43. Lonks JR, Garau J, Gomez L, *et al*. Failure of macrolide antibiotic treatment in patients with bacteremia due to erythromycin-resistant *Streptococcus pneumoniae*. *Clin Infect Dis* 2002; 35: 556–564.

44. Schmitz F-J, Perdikouli M, Beeck A, Verhoef J, Fluit AC. Molecular surveillance of macrolide, tetracycline and quinolone resistance mechanisms in 1191 clinical European *Streptococcus pneumoniae* isolates. *Int J Antimicrob Agents* 2001; 18: 433–436.

45. Rappaz I, Decosterd LA, Bille J, *et al*. Continuous infusion of ceftazidime with a portable pump is as effective as thrice-a-day bolus in cystic fibrosis children. *Eur J Pediatr* 2000; 159: 919–925.

46. Schentag JJ, Strenkoski-Nix LC, Nix DE, Forrest A. Pharmacodynamic interactions of antibiotics alone and in combination. *Clin Infect Dis* 1998; 27: 40–46.

47. Mouton JW, van Ogtrop ML, Andes D, Craig WA. Use of pharmacodynamic indices to predict efficacy of combination therapy *in vivo*. *Antimicrob Agents Chemother* 1999; 43: 2473–2478.

CHAPTER 2

Intrapulmonary penetration of antimicrobials and implications in the treatment of lower respiratory tract infections

M. Cazzola*, G. D'Amato*, M.G. Matera[#]

*Dept of Respiratory Medicine, Unit of Pneumology and Allergology, A. Cardarelli Hospital, and [#]Dept of Experimental Medicine, Unit of Pharmacology, Second University of Naples, Naples, Italy.

Correspondence: M. Cazzola, Via del Parco Margherita 24, 80121 Naples, Italy.

Lungs are frequent sites of infection. The place where the infection develops inevitably influences the clinical presentation. In patients with acute bronchitis (AC), acute exacerbation of chronic bronchitis (AECB), bronchiectasis, or cystic fibrosis (CF), the infection develops within the airway lumen, on the surface of mucus cells, and in the mucosa itself. In patients with bacterial pneumonia, the site of infection is in the alveolar spaces or in the pulmonary interstitium [1–3].

The efficacy of an antibiotic to treat lower respiratory tract infections (LRTIs) can depend on the levels reached by the drug and the retention times in the different pulmonary sites of infection [4–6]. For this reason, there has recently been increased interest in measuring the concentration of antimicrobial agents at these sites [7]. However, there are many host-related factors that influence the transport of antimicrobials into respiratory tissues and fluids (table 1). Moreover, the *in vivo* determination of the pulmonary concentration of an antibacterial is plagued with several methodological difficulties [9]. First and foremost an assessment should be made to ensure that the collection techniques are consistent with the current accepted practices [10], but this is not always the case. Questions can also arise regarding the ability to evaluate data that are based on different quantitative methods. For example, a microbiological technique (bioassay) monitors total inhibitory activity, which may also be due to a drug's active metabolites or other biological factors, rather than the parent drug. Alternatively, a chemical assay e.g. high performance liquid chromatography, directly measures the drug concentration regardless of the antibacterial activity at the infection site [10].

A number of models have been used with the intention of collating relevant data on the pulmonary deposition of the majority of antibiotics. This has been made possible due to the relative simplicity in obtaining respiratory tissues and fluids. During the last few years, innovative methods for the pharmacological evaluation of antimicrobial agents have been developed and the techniques have been perfected, thus allowing the attainment of more precise informations on the deposition of drugs within the lower respiratory tract.

Antibiotic penetration into sputum and bronchial secretions

For an antibiotic to pass from the bloodstream into the bronchial secretions is relatively simple, from a mechanical point of view. The antimicrobial first passes across

Eur Respir Mon, 2004, 28, 13–44. Printed in UK - all rights reserved. Copyright ERS Journals Ltd 2004; European Respiratory Monograph; ISSN 1025-448x. ISBN 1-904097-32-4.

Table 1. – Host-related factors influencing the transport of antimicrobials into respiratory tissues and fluids

Pharmacokinetic parameters
  Alteration in:
    Hepatic/renal insufficiency
    Elderly
    Underlying disease
    Intensive care hospitalization
    Cardiovascular disease
    Severe respiratory disease

Site of infection
  Intramacrophagic pathogens (atypical pneumonia)
  Parenchymal consolidation
  Endobronchial infections
  Degree of inflammation: acute inflammation, increased vascularisation and antibiotic leakage
  Mechanical injury, bleeding, fibrosis
  Role of respiratory secretions, variable in volume and composition, antibiotic clearance
  Binding and/or inactivation of antibiotics in variable degrees depending on amounts of:
    Proteins
    Nucleic acids
    Cellular membranes
    Mucopolysaccharides of mucus
  Endotracheal pH: acidic environment, intramacrophagic trapping of antibiotics, sequestrations
  Subcellular structures (leukocytic chromatin)

Accumulation and elimination of antibiotics
  Accumulation in cells, in mucus
  Reabsorption across blood-bronchus barrier
  Mechanical excretion (cough, mucociliary movement)
  Inactivation (local β-lactamase production, leukocytic enzymes)

Table adapted from BERGOGNE-BÉRÉZIN [8].

the capillary wall, hence the interstitial tissue fluid, and finally through the bronchial wall and the bronchial epithelium. It is thought that this movement occurs by simple passive diffusion across a concentration gradient according to Fick's law [11]. Passive diffusion across membranes is nonsaturable and consequently the antibiotic concentrations within the bronchial secretions reflect the serum levels. It is probable that penetration may be increased both by higher serum levels and a greater area under the curve (AUC) in a concentration/time graph.

This passive diffusion results in the accumulation of the antibiotic in interstitial fluids and bronchial secretions [12]. However, the diffusion is not solely affected by the gradient across the two sides of the blood/bronchus barrier, the membrane thickness also effects the diffusion of the antibiotic. The characteristics of biological membranes may greatly modify the crossing of an antibiotic. Under circumstances of acute infection, which may involve inflammation, vasodilation, edoema and increased permeability of biological barriers, both the protein-bound and free antibacterials may penetrate bronchial tissues more readily [1]. Alternatively, the presence of scarring tissue as a result of recurrent infections may reduce the degree of drug penetration [13].

The chemical characteristics of antibiotics may also influence passive diffusion [14]. Large molecular sized antibacterial agents have been shown to enter bronchial secretions more readily [11, 13] compared with smaller molecules, which are more likely to be trapped within the pores of a capillary wall [15] and in mucin [1]. Furthermore, only more lipophilic drugs easily cross alveolar epithelial cells, which are separated by tight junctions that presumably do not allow the passage of antibiotic molecules [16]. Also the structural characteristics of the antimicrobial, for example the presence of benzene rings within its structure (*e.g.* erythromycin), appear to enhance penetration in the secretions [1].

The propensity of the antibiotic for plasma protein binding also conditions the movement of the drug across the membrane, a high drug-protein affinity will limit its ability to cross the membrane [17]. Theoretically, only the free fraction of the drug is capable of diffusing, but the protein binding is often reversible. Alternatively, different binding sites have been described in the extravascular component (interstitial fluid), in the infection site and within cells which are nonprotein. These sites include purulent exudates, subcellular structures, cellular chromatin and other cellular components. It must be specified that the protein concentration within bronchial secretions is extremely low, and for this reason the antibiotic is present almost exclusively in the unbound form [12]. Nonetheless, in the presence of an infection, the increased leakage of proteins across the barriers may increase the accumulation of protein-bound antibiotic [14].

The possibility of an active form of transport at the bronchial level has been extensively debated, although it is still hypothetical. It is presumably a saturable mechanism dependent on the energy at disposal [17].

The penetration of different antimicrobials in bronchial secretions is shown in table 2. It is extremely low for many antibiotics. Penicillins and cephalosporins only reach marginal concentrations in bronchial secretions, in contrast with the positive clinical results obtained in controlled studies, and their sputum or bronchial secretion concentrations and blood concentration ratios vary between 0.05 and 0.25 [18–22]. However, the percentages for the extent of penetration of piperacillin and tazobactam, as defined by the bronchial secretion/serum AUC ratio, have been shown to be 35.70% and 78.42%, respectively [23]. The slight penetration is present even when a cephalosporin is administered by continuous infusion [24]. Bronchial secretion AUCs for ceftazidime almost doubled its value between 1–2 g dosing, while between 2–3 g doses only a

Table 2. – Antibiotic levels in serum and bronchial secretions

Antibiotic	Dose	Route	Serum mL·L^{-1}	Bronchial secretions mL·L^{-1}
Amoxicillin g	1	IV	6.9	0.52
Carbenicillin g	20	IV MD	130	15–49
Mezlocillin g	5	IV	140	10.0
Piperacillin g	4	IV MD	196.3	12.2±8.5
Cefaclor AF mg	750	PO MD	8.6	1.5
Cefuroxime mg	0.75	IM	10.6	1.95
Cefuroxime axetil mg	500	PO	3.4±2.4	1.0-3.5
Ceftibuten mg	400	PO	18.12±2.13	8.19±3.1
Cefotaxime g	2	IV	40	1.45
Ceftazidime g	1	IM	39.89	6.87
Imipenem g	1	IV	69	0.94
Gentamicin mg·kg^{-1}	5	MD	5.0–6.0	1.83
Amikacin mg	500	IV	11–20	6.7
Tobramycin mg·kg^{-1}	1.7		6.0–8.0	2.68
Erythromycin g	1	PO MD	1.37±0.89	0.59
Roxithromycin mg	150	PO MD	6.26±0.7	3.1±0.77
Clarithromycin mg	500	PO MD	3.96	±1.02
Azithromycin mg	500	PO	0.2–04	0.23–9.5
Dirithromycin mg	500	PO MD	0.44	2.67
Spiramycin g	2–3	PO MD	2.4	7.3
Ciprofloxacin mg	500	PO	1.64±0.42	1.3±2.33
Ofloxacin mg	200	PO MD	1.90–5.18	1.51±0.7
Lomefloxacin mg	400	PO MD	2.8±1.0	2.78±3.64
Sparfloxacin mg	400	PO	1.2	1.80±1.03
Trovafloxacin mg	200	PO MD	3.4	3.2
Doxycycline mg	100	PO	2.74	1.05
Minocycline mg	200	PO	4.6	1.7
Thiamphenicol mg	750	PO	5.8	3.4
Clindamycin mg	300	PO	2.6	1.6

IV: intravenous; MD: multiple doses; PO: *per os*; IM: intramuscular; AF: advanced formulation.

moderate and nonsignificant increase was found [25]. On the basis of these results, the existence of a saturable transport mechanism for ceftazidime from serum-to-bronchial secretions has been postulated. Apparently, there is a large variability in the penetration into sputum even for β-lactams that are similar. For example, the pharmacokinetics of ampicillin and amoxicillin following simultaneous intravenous (IV) administration are almost identical, but sputum amoxicillin concentrations are significantly higher than ampicillin [26]. It is interesting to note that by modifying the structure of an oral cephalosporin (cefaclor) it is possible to substantially increase the penetration in sputum and to prolong its presence over time [22].

Fluoroquinolones have been shown to achieve high concentrations in bronchial secretions, which are 0.8–4.0 times greater than those in the bloodstream [27–32]. These high concentrations have been attributed to an active transport across the airway epithelium. Parenteral aminoglycosides are highly polar and penetrate poorly into the endobronchial space [33]. The mean peak sputum concentration after parenteral administration is only 12–20% of the peak serum concentration [34–37]. Interestingly, concentrations in bronchial secretions of the patients treated with amikacin *b.i.d.* ranged from 3–4 mg·L^{-1}, whereas in patients treated with amikacin once daily, concentrations of bronchial secretions were more than two-fold higher, >8 mg·L^{-1} for 12 h [38]. With the use of aerosolised aminoglycosides, high concentrations of the drug can be delivered topically to the lungs and consequently, an adequate amount of aminoglycoside reaches the endobronchial site of infection but not the blood [39]. In this instance, the drug deposition and distribution into the lung is dependent on the aerosol particle size, particle velocity, and patient factors, including breathing patterns, airway anatomy, and degree of airway obstruction [40]. Tetracyclines present sputum/blood ratio values of 50–60% [41, 42], whereas macrolides show a variable penetration between 5–500% [43–45]. The latest compounds present the best penetration values; e.g. azithromycin [46] and dirithromycin [45, 47] exhibit a ratio >500% (fig. 1).

It must be noted that it is extremely difficult to elicit a definitive conclusion on the clinical significance of these pharmacokinetic data. It must be stressed that the bioactivity of antibiotics in respiratory secretions is not identical to that found *in vitro*. Laboratory

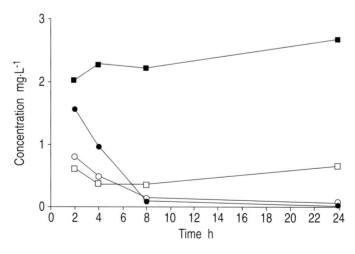

Fig. 1. – Mean concentrations of dirithromycin (DIRI) and erythromycin (ERY) in bronchial secretions. ■: DIRI bronchial secretion (BS); □: DIRI serum; ●: ERY BS; ○: ERY serum. DIRI was administered orally at a dose of 500 mg·every 24 h for a total of five doses. ERY was administered orally at a dose of 250 mg every 6 h for a total of 28 doses. The data have been adapted from MATERA *et al.* [45].

conditions are standardised and selected to approximate serum. Deviations from these conditions can markedly influence the results. Differences in composition between sputum and laboratory culture media, as well as variation in growth and metabolism of respiratory secretions must be considered when predicting *in vivo* activity in sputum [48]. Moreover, the clinical utility of penetration ratios is somewhat misleading since bacterial eradication is a function of the drug concentration at the site of infection rather than penetration ratio.

The wide variation of levels reported for each single agent may also reflect methodological difficulties. For example, some patients only present limited amounts of secretions and it is therefore necessary to add a volume of saline solution to obtain a sample, or alternatively, sputum can be induced with inhaled hypertonic saline [49], however, in this case the dilution factor cannot be accurately determined. Moreover, sputum is often diluted by saliva during sampling and this can result in false, low concentration [18]. Alternatively an antibiotic may be excreted into saliva and produce artificially high levels in sputum specimens. Moreover, the sample obtained cannot be considered homogeneous as it represents the gathering of respiratory secretion aliquots coming from different compartments of the airways and is accumulated at different times [50]. The possibility that different samples may be mixed increases when the efficiency of mucociliary clearance and cough decreases. In these circumstances there is an apparent lack of correlation between blood and sputum levels [13]. Although it is possible to avoid salivary contamination by aspirating bronchial secretions directly by a bronchoscope, the problem of endobronchial stagnation remains unfortunately insurmountable. Even the time of collection is important. Sputum collected in the morning after sleep is the expression of the accumulation of secretions during the night and this fact may contribute to the finding of high antibiotic levels. The accumulation of bronchial secretions over several hours invalidates the determination of concentrations if these are referred to the time of administration. Moreover, the accumulation of secretions allows the degradation of the drug by enzymes [51], temperature, pH, and protein modification [52].

It must be highlighted that a variety of pulmonary enzymes are capable of metabolising foreign chemicals through a combination of oxidation and conjugation reactions [53]. A large proportion of the lung's complement of cytochrome P450 enzymes, a category of enzymes that widely participates in drug metabolism, is located in the nonciliated bronchiolar (Clara) cells [53]. Furthermore, other common enzymes that relate to drug metabolism, including uridine diphosphate glucuronosyltransferase, epoxide hydrolase and glutathione S-transferase, can be found both in isolated alveolar type II cells and in Clara cells. Since no definitive information is available at present, it is difficult to say how much the presence of these enzymes affects the activity of medications [10].

As the inflammatory process dampens and clinical conditions improve, antimicrobial penetration probably decreases. This aspect is of great importance since the reduced antibiotic penetration may cause a drop in the local concentration of the drug below bactericidal levels, thereby increasing the probability of recurrence of infection [2]. Since most antibiotics, particularly β-lactams, penetrate in secretions on a reduced quantity, bacteria are probably exposed to below the minimal inhibitory concentration (MIC) of the antibiotic, at least for a part of the posologic interval. However, the exposure to sub-MIC concentrations alters the interactions between host and bacteria, reducing a microorganism's adherence to airway epithelial cells [54] and causing lesser epithelial damage [55]. The ability of bacteria to adhere to epithelial cells is a prerequisite for the colonisation of mucus surfaces and the subsequent development of infection [56]. Moreover, *in vitro* studies suggest that when sublethal concentrations of antimicrobial agents alter bacterial surfaces, microorganisms become more prone to phagocytosis by polymorphonuclear cells and macrophages and this may interfere with the bacterial factors involved in mucus colonisation [57]. It is therefore always useful to determine drug concentrations in sputum, particularly because some bacteria may persist in airway lumen and cause damage without invading mucosa.

Antibiotic penetration into bronchial mucosa

The determination of the antibacterial penetration into bronchial mucosa has been described as a more reliable indicator of intrapulmonary penetration compared to sputum concentration, because overcomes the drawbacks and the inaccuracies of the determination of antibiotics in sputum and/or bronchial secretions [58]. Unfortunately, data in this field are limited, notwithstanding the fact that the methods for determining total concentrations in samples obtained by bronchial biopsies during bronchoscopy are well standardised and are relatively simple to carry out [59]. The penetration of different antibiotics appears relatively high. This is also true for β-lactams, which usually accumulate into bronchial mucosa to 25–60% of the level attained in serum [21, 59–70] (table 3). The penetration of fluoroquinolones and macrolides is higher. In general, the levels of fluoroquinolones are 1.5–3-fold greater than those in the bloodstream [32, 71–80] (fig. 2), whereas the concentrations of macrolides are 0.9–19 times greater than those found in the blood [44, 48, 51, 81–83]. The behaviours of azithromycin and dirithromycin are interesting because these drugs persist in bronchial mucosa at high concentrations at up-to 72–96 h after the last administration, even in the presence of low or

Table 3. – Antibiotic levels in serum and bronchial mucosa

Antibiotic	Dose	Route	Serum mg·L^{-1}	Bronchial mucosa mg·kg^{-1}	% penetration
Amoxicillin mg	500	PO MD	5.9	0.5	15
Amoxicillin g	1	IV	8.4	20.8	248
Clavulanic acid mg	200	IV	2.7	306	133
Piperacillin g	4	IV MD	196.3	55.2	28
Cefuroxime axetil mg	500	PO	3.4±2.4	3.8±1.6	44–85
Cefdinir mg	600	PO	4.20	1.14	27
Ceftibuten mg	200	PO	8.77	2.25	39
Cefixime mg	400	PO	6.6	2.4	36
Ceftriaxone g	1	IV	70.9	18.1	25
Ceftazidime g	1	IV	36.04±9.21	8.14±2.23	23
Cefepime g	2	IV	40.4±28.1	24.1±17.8	59
Cefpirome g	1	IV	55.6	33.0	62
Erythromycin mg	500	PO MD	4.3	7.2	160
Roxitromycin mg	150	PO MD	6.3	5.6	90
Clarithromycin mg	500	PO MD	3.96	16.76	430
Azithromycin mg	500	PO	0.2–0.4	3.89±1.2	972–1945
Dirithromycin g	500	MD	0.61	2.71	444
Spiramycin g	2–3	PO	2.4	13–36	30-50
Telithromycin mg	800	PO MD	1.86	3.88	210
Ciprofloxacin mg	500	PO	1.64	4.4	260
Clinafloxacin mg	200	PO	1.54	2.65	172
Lomefloxacin mg	400	PO MD	2.8	6.2	221
Ofloxacin mg	200	×2 PO	1.0–5.2	10–13	250–921
Sparfloxacin mg	400	PO	1.2	2.6	217
Trovafloxacin mg	200	PO MD	1.41	1.52	110
Levofloxacin mg	500	PO	6.6	10.8	164
Moxifloxacin mg	400	PO	3.2	5.4	169
Garenoxacin mg	600	PO	10.0	7.0	70

IV: intravenous; MD: multiple dose; PO: *per os*.

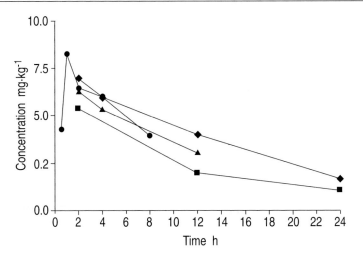

Fig. 2. – Mean concentrations in bronchial mucosa of levofloxacin (500 mg, ●), moxifloxacin (400 mg, ■), gatifloxacin (400 mg, ▲), and garenoxacin (600 mg, ◆) in patients undergoing fibre-optic bronchoscopy following a single oral dose. Adapted from ANDREWS *et al.* [76], SOMAN *et al.* [77], HONEYBOURNE *et al.* [79], and ANDREWS *et al.* [80].

nondeterminable blood concentrations [46, 47]. Ketolides also penetrate in an effective manner into bronchial mucosa [84].

It still remains unclear if the inflammatory process influences the antibiotic levels in the mucosa. This probably occurs only in a limited manner compared to sputum. However, inflammation plays an important role in determining an antibiotic's ability to cross barriers [3]. As a result of local inflammation, there is an increase in tissue vascular supply and the volume of intracellular fluids increases in relation to the total tissue mass [85]. Consequently, antibiotic tissue penetration increases [86]. Therefore, with drugs that do not cross the epithelium in a satisfying manner higher levels should be expected in the inflamed airways, whereas there should be no significant differences in the levels of drugs that easily cross membranes. If this is true, β-lactams and aminoglycosides, but not fluoroquinolones and macrolides, should present higher levels. However, for macrolides a clear correlation between the degree of inflammation and their degree of penetration into airways has been found when inflammation diminishes [43]. The effect on antibiotic penetration and the capability of different dosage regimens to modify the drug levels obtained hypothetically, played by pathologic conditions such as bronchiectasis, still remains unclear.

The principal criticism to the clinical significance of the measurement of antibiotic penetration into bronchial mucosa is that with the methods currently employed to date, it does not allow us to differentiate between intracellular and extracellular components. This information is extremely important, as the ability of an antibiotic to enter and accumulate in cells will influence the levels of drug measured. Drugs that show a high intracellular accumulation *in vitro* present higher concentrations in bronchial mucosa. Obviously, the penetration into cells of different antimicrobials differs according to their class [87] (table 4). All data show that the concentration of hydrophilic antibiotics, such as β-lactams and aminoglycosides, in extracellular pulmonary fluids reflects serum concentrations fairly faithfully, whereas lipophilic antibiotics that are taken up by cells, such as fluoroquinolones, tetracyclines, and macrolides, reach much higher concentrations in tissues [4]. However, although initial observations suggest that in contrast to the data for β-lactam agents, fluoroquinolone and macrolide tissue concentrations are higher

Table 4. – Antibiotic intracellular penetration, accumulation and release

Antibiotic	Penetration	Accumulus	Localisation	Release
Aminoglycosides	Very slow (days)	Very slow	Lysosomes	Very slow (weeks)
β-lactams	Very limited	Absent	Cytosol	Rapid
Fluoroquinolones	Rapid, similar for all compounds	4–8 fold	Phagosomes, Lysosomes	Rapid (min)
Macrolides	Slow (1–2 h) drug dependant	May reach >100 fold drug dependent	Lysosomes >90%	Slow (days)

than serum concentrations, this is not completely true [10]. The tissue concentrations are obtained by homogenisation of lung tissues, therefore there is no differentiation between intracellular and extracellular fluid in the samples. This lack of distinction can dramatically alter the resulting data; this is especially important when studying fluoroquinolones and macrolides because they penetrate both physiological compartments, whereas β-lactam agents do not. Since the drug is present in both intracellular and extracellular compartments, fluoroquinolone and macrolide tissue concentrations appear higher than serum concentrations. As β-lactam antibacterials are present only in the interstitial fluid, their actual concentrations are diluted by the contents of the intracellular compartment.

Antibiotic penetration into epithelial lining fluid

With the improvements in the technique of bronchoalveolar lavage (BAL), a mechanical procedure that avoids contamination with saliva or sputum, it has been possible to obtain samples from two further infection sites, the alveolar lining and alveolar macrophages. The epithelial lining fluid (ELF) is considered an important site of extracellular infection in pneumonia, whereas macrophages are an important site in intracellular infections [1]. The concentrations reached by antibiotics into these two distal sites are excellent predictors of their clinical efficacy in the treatment of pneumonia [4].

The alveolar epithelial membrane is a significant barrier that separates the alveolar lining from blood. Thus, the alveolar lining constitutes an important microenvironment. Clinical efficacy, particularly with pathogens that are confined to sites separated from blood by significant barriers, may be more closely related to drug concentrations at actual sites of infection [88].

Unfortunately, the technique for performing BAL can cause evaluation errors that must always be kept in mind. To perform BAL, four 50-mL aliquots of heated normal saline must be instilled into the lungs by means of a bronchoscope, and each must immediately be aspirated into a trap. It is preferable to discard the first aliquot as it corresponds primarily to lavage of the proximal airways. From the remaining three aliquots, roughly 60–70 mL are retrieved on which it is possible to perform the determination antibiotic levels [89]. Data obtained is generally not reliable, due to the dilution produced by saline introduced into airways, which makes it difficult to compare the concentration of antibiotics in aspirate lavage fluid and in blood [1]. To overcome this problem, the drug levels in blood and in BAL are compared to a reference substance, usually urea or creatinine, used as a marker of dilution [89–91]. These substances have a low molecular weight and diffuse rapidly across the alveolo-capillary membrane. It is felt that, in conditions of equilibrium, the concentration of urea in the blood is equal to that in alveolar lavage [92]. Comparing the ratio between the concentration of the antibiotic and that of the reference substance in BAL with the same ratio in blood, it is possible to calculate the relative penetration coefficient of the antibiotic into alveolar fluid. It must, however, be highlighted that the urea method does not account for the partial movement of the solute from pulmonary capillaries to the alveolar space, thus causing an underestimate of the concentration of the drug. In fact, although epithelial permeability to urea is low, redistribution of the dilution marker during lavage due to its absorption, cell binding, or metabolism may cause the erroneous estimation of the ELF volume and the corresponding drug concentrations [93]. The ratio between the concentration of the antibiotic in lavage fluid and the true concentration of the drug in the alveolar lining is nonetheless considered equal to the same ratio for the reference molecule. This represents a dilution factor.

It has been repeatedly stressed that the fluid introduced by a bronchoscope stagnates in the lungs for the time that is necessary to gather the distal alveolar lining. This interval allows the diffusion of urea from the interstitium and the blood and falsely increases its levels in the fluid obtained with BAL. This causes an overestimate of the alveolar lining volume of 100–300% after only 1 min of stagnation [94]. To overcome this limitation, the microlavage technique has been suggested. This procedure involves the introduction into the lungs of smaller volumes of saline solution by means of a minute catheter enabling the quick sampling of small quantities of fluid. However, there is the possibility of contamination with blood following mechanical trauma if personnel, lacking in expertise, perform this procedure [89].

Nevertheless, the technique of BAL has several major drawbacks. For example, many substances distribute into the ELF within minutes after entering the systemic circulation but this technique lacks the ability to monitor rapid changes in concentrations of drugs in the ELF of the lung in a single subject. Furthermore, due to the nature of the sampling process and each lavage altering the composition of the ELF, this makes frequent multiple sampling from an individual patient difficult. Therefore this technique is not generally well suited for pharmacokinetic studies. Consequently to ascertain ELF drug penetration, clinical trial designs randomise patients to different drug doses and sampling times. Analysis of these data is often limited to obtaining ratios of drug concentrations into ELF to those determined simultaneously in blood. For drugs with multi-compartmental behaviour, these ratios will change as a function of the sampling time. Such time dependency makes this measure a poor one for understanding the penetration behaviour of a drug [95]. Moreover, due to the difficulty of confining the instilled fluid to a limited area within the lung, saline distributes freely throughout the available space during lavage. As a result, the technique lacks spatial resolution and usually presents data averaged over a segment of the lung. The accuracy of the estimate can also be adversely affected by the influx of the fluid from the interstitium during lavage.

The movement of antibiotics across the blood-alveolus barrier is extremely difficult as the capillary endothelium of the pulmonary circulation is nonfenestrated and the alveolar membranes are relatively impermeable due to the presence of many tight junctions (zonulae occludens) [96]. As a consequence antimicrobials penetrate less in the alveolar lining than in the bronchial mucosa [89]. However, fluoroquinolones appear to concentrate more in alveolar lavage than in the bronchial mucosa and this behaviour makes it seem probable that this class of compound possesses additional mechanisms that allow the crossing of the membrane [90].

There are substantial differences in the concentration into ELF among the different classes of antimicrobials, and even among compounds of the same class [21, 45–47, 66, 67 75–80, 84, 98–121] (table 5). This is also true for macrolides, which are tissue-directed antibiotics [122]. Macrolides have been found to concentrate into ELF [45–47, 106, 114], with azithromycin showing a 7-fold and clarithromycin a 5.7-fold increase compared with serum levels. In particular, it has been documented that clarithromycin was concentrated in ELF (range, 72.1 ± 73.0 mg·L^{-1} at 8 h to 11.9 ± 3.6 mg·L^{-1} at 24 h),

Table 5. – Antibiotic levels in serum and epithelium lining fluid

Antibiotic	Dose	Route	Serum mg·L^{-1}	ELF mg·L^{-1}	% penetration
Amoxicillin mg	500	PO MD		2.56±1.41	
Clavulanic acid mg	250	PO MD		1.33±0.65	
Cefuroxime axetil mg	613	PO MD		1.04±0.66	
Cefpodoxime proxetil mg	220	PO	1.85±0.82	0.22±0.13	12
Ceftibuten mg	400	PO	15.2	1.6	10
Cefdinir mg	600	PO	4.20	0.49	11
Ceftazidime g	1	IM	39.89	2.71	7
Cefepime g	1	IV	40.4	3.4	8
Cefpirome g	1	IV	34.5	7.2	21
Imipenem g	1	IV	19.0±1.1	24.1±51.4	127
Meropenem g	1	IV	25.98	7.07	27
Tobramycin mg	300	IM	5.5	3	55
Erythromycin mg	250	PO MD	1.57	0.97	62
Clarithromycin mg	500	PO MD	3.96	20.46	512
Azithromycin mg	500	PO MD	0.13±0.05	1.4	1076
Dirithromycin mg	500	PO MD	0.61	2.37	388
Roxithromycin mg	300	PO MD		2.0±1.7	
Telithromycin mg	800	PO MD	1.86	14.89	800
Pefloxacin mg	800	PO	7.46±0.25	97.7±30.0	1305
Clinafloxacin mg	200	PO	1.54	2.71	176
Lomefloxacin mg	400	PO MD	3.2	6.9	216
Trovafloxacin mg	200	PO MD	1.41	4.8	340
Temafloxacin mg	600	PO MD	9.6±1.22	6.5±3.6	276
Sparfloxacin mg	400	MD	1.2±0.4	115.0±8.3	1250
Levofloxacin mg	500	PO	6.6	10.9	165
Gatifloxacin mg	400	PO	3.96	6.16	155
Moxifloxacin mg	400	PO	3.2	20,7	647
Garenoxacin mg	600	PO	10.0	14.3	143
Vancomycin mg	15	IV MD	24	4.5	19
Linezolid mg	600	PO MD	7.3±4.9	64.3±33.1	881

PO: *per os*; MD: multiple doses; IV: intravenous; IM: intamuscular.

whereas the concentrations of erythromycin in ELF were low at 4, 8, and 12 h following the last dose of the drug (range, 0–0.8±0.1 mg·L^{-1}) [113]. In another study, the azithromycin concentrations in ELF were less than half those of clarithromycin [115]. The higher apparent volume of distribution of azithromycin may explain these results. It can presumably be caused by a larger distribution of this azalide to extracellular sites than clarithromycin. Concentration in ELF of the ketolide telithromycin, a semi-synthetic derivative of the 14-membered ring macrolides, is eight times higher than in serum [84]. A recent study that has evaluated the bronchopulmonary concentrations of IV levofloxacin and azithromycin in healthy adults, showed that levofloxacin 500 and 750 mg achieved significantly higher concentrations in steady-state ELF than azithromycin 500 mg during the 24 h after drug administration. This difference was despite the values of azithromycin at 24 h sampling being higher that those of levofloxacin [121]. The hydrophilic nature of ß-lactams leads to poor penetration into the relatively impermeable alveolar space and the ELF, with levels only reaching 12–50% of serum concentration [21, 64, 66, 67, 120]. In addition aminoglycosides also penetrate poorly into ELF and high peak serum concentrations of aminoglycosides are necessary to obtain microbiologically active concentrations at the alveolar level. In fact, because of their hydrophilicity, polycationic charge and relatively large size, these antibiotics are able to diffuse only sparsely across biological membranes without active transport mechanisms [10]. In patients with pneumonia, the ratio ELF to serum concentration of tobramycin at peak serum time was 0.30 [118], whereas that of netilmicin was 0.46 [109].

Antibiotic penetration into alveolar macrophages

Although the neutrophil is the prevalent cell in bacterial infections, *in vitro* studies show that alveolar macrophage (AM) concentrates antibacterials in a manner similar to a neutrophil. Consequently the determination of antibacterial concentration in AM is a valid model for evaluating antibiotic levels in the site of infections caused by intracellular pathogens such as *Legionella pneumophila* or *Chlamydia pneumoniae* [3]. The quantity of antimicrobials passed into cells is determined using AM isolated from lavage fluid by rapid centrifugation and following equally rapid ultrasonication.

The possibility of a rapid effusion of the antibiotic from AM is a potential source of evaluation error. It has been shown that even cells that contain a high concentration of a drug rapidly lose great amounts if they are not placed in a medium containing the drug itself. This is what happens during BAL; the extracellular concentration of the antibiotics falls by at least 100 fold. *In vitro* studies have generally shown that a considerable loss of the drug takes place within 10 min from the suspension of the cellular culture in a medium lacking in antibiotic [123]. The efflux of fluoroquinolones is particularly relevant because these antimicrobials rapidly leave the cells, whereas the efflux of ß-lactams is difficult to assess considering that they penetrate very poorly into cells. Macrolides vary in their efflux capacity [90]; erythromycin exits rapidly [124], whereas the uptake of azithromycin is slow and the release rate is even slower [125].

The technique for obtaining BAL is fairly long and is conditioned by the clinical situation of each single patient. It is therefore preferable to wait for a complete equilibrium between the obtained fluid by BAL and the cellular component, even though some studies indicate that the release of antibiotics during BAL does not proceed at the same rate observed *in vitro*. There are, obviously, some discrepancies between antibiotic levels quantified in macrophages *in vitro* and those determined in BAL [83]. Alternatively, AMs must be separated in a fast manner to minimise the efflux of drug from intracellular compartments into extracellular BAL fluid. Placing the samples on ice and centrifugation of the sample as quickly as possible helps to diminish this loss [126]. The accurate quantification of the number of macrophages is also important since high degrees of variability in the cell count will lead to varying concentrations [127].

β-Lactams diffuse but do not accumulate into phagocytes, probably because of their acidic character, their activity at this site is negligible due to the low pH. However, clavulanate, but not amoxicillin, is detectable in AMs [121]. Aminoglycosides are too polar to pass across membranes and are therefore only taken up slowly by endocytosis. Lincosamides, macrolides and fluoroquinolones all accumulate in phagocytes [124]. Levels of azithromycin are up-to 23 times and clarithromycin ~70 times higher than in serum [114], whereas levofloxacin shows an 8-fold [80], gatifloxacin a 35-fold [79], and moxifloxacin a 50-fold increase [77] compared with serum levels. In 36 healthy, nonsmoking adult subjects, the concentrations in AM following IV administration of five doses of levofloxacin (500 or 750 mg) and azithromycin (500 mg) once daily were higher than concentrations in plasma [121]. However, azithromycin achieved significantly higher concentrations in AM than levofloxacin. Linezolid concentrations in AMs are less than those observed in plasma and ELF, suggesting that the drug is excluded or rapidly removed from this compartment [128]. A similar partitioning for pyrazinamide has been reported [129].

The concentration of antimicrobials in AMs is greater in inflamed airways due to macrophage activation. Moreover, smokers present higher levels since their macrophages reach a higher level of activation [130].

It is important to highlight that antibiotic disposition varies within cells (table 4). Consequently, very large differences in intracellular concentrations exist between antibiotics. This has an impact on the choice of the antibiotic treatment. Some bacteria (*e.g. Legionella sp.* and *Chlamydia sp.*) are found within subcellular compartments, such as the phagosomes. Others, such as *Staphylococcus aureus*, are mostly located within phagolysosomes.

Fluoroquinolones appear to be entirely soluble in cells,and lincosamides concentrate in both phagosomes and lysosomes. On the contrary, macrolides accumulate principally in lysosomes because the pH in these sites is extremely low and induces a high rate of protonation and aminoglycosides result in an exclusively lysosomal localisation [131, 132]. The macrolide molecule becomes more polar when it is protonated and therefore is less capable of exiting the cell [124]. It is still not known whether drugs withheld in the lysosomes are truly capable of carrying out their antimicrobial activity. A relatively new hypothesis that has started to gain acceptance is that the concentrations achieved by the macrolides within the actual phagocytic cells that will clear infecting bacteria (*i.e.* neutrophils, monocytes, macrophages) to be the drug levels that should be considered [133]. The fact that intraphagocytic concentrations of these drugs are multiple logs higher than the corresponding serum concentrations and are maintained at this level for a prolonged period, either through cellular retention (azithromycin) or dosing (erythromycin, clarithromycin), helps explain how all macrolides are active against not only susceptible bacterial isolates, but also potentially against those bacteria with "resistant" MICs [10].

Antibiotic penetration into pulmonary parenchyma

The concentrations of antibiotics in human lung pulmonary tissues have been determined diffusely in samples obtained from pulmonary resections or biopsies during thoracotomy (mostly during resection of lung carcinoma). Antibiotic levels are generally higher in lung tissues than in bronchial secretions. It is therefore possible that tissue concentrations give a better picture of the efficacy of an antibiotic treatment.

Unfortunately, antibiotic penetration in pulmonary tissues is difficult to estimate. The number of patients included in different groups and the number of consecutive samples obtainable for each subject are limited. Tissue pharmacology must be deduced by single determinations in groups of patients with an inevitable variation between individuals. Moreover, the final level of antibiotic in tissue samples is determined in a homogenate that contains unknown quantities of blood, body fluids and intracellular contents, and this explains why data from different studies evaluating the lung penetration of an antibiotic may be extremely variable from one to the other [134]. The lungs are the organs of the body with the richest blood supply and therefore their blood content is very high. As a consequence, pulmonary tissue specimens contain a considerable quantity of blood and it is well known that the presence of blood aliquots in samples can cause an increase in antibiotic levels. However, it is difficult to separate the haematic and nonhaematic components. In order to overcome this problem the concentration of the drug must be expressed after correcting for the haematic factor by means of the determination of the haemoglobin content in the tissue [135].

In studies carried out on humans, a correlation has been found between antibiotic pulmonary levels and dose, mode, and route of administration [44, 135–143] (table 6). For example, the peaks in oral cephalosporin, vancomycin, fluoroquinolone and macrolide tissue concentrations are lower than those of parenteral preparations of the same drugs [44, 138, 141]. Thus, higher concentrations of the drug in pulmonary tissue have been found after parenteral administration of 500 mg of erythromycin (6.53± 3.18 mg·kg^{-1}) compared with oral administration of 1 g of erythromycin ethylsuccinate

Table 6. – Antibiotic levels in serum and pulmonary parenchyma

Antibiotic	Dose	Route	Serum mg·L^{-1}	Pulmonary parenchyma mg·kg^{-1}	% penetration
Penicillin G mg	1–3	MU IV	25	25	10
Amoxicillin g	1	PO	5.6	2.4	43
Amoxicillin g	1	IV	6.9	4.4–5.6	60–80
Amoxicillin g	1	PO	9.9	1.3	13
Clavulanate mg	250	IV MD	3.8	0.7	19
Carbenicillin g	20	IV	130	45–75	35–58
Mezlocillin g	5	IV	140	25–35	6–9
Ticarcillin g	5	IV	469	30–45	6–10
Piperacillin g	1	IV	43.3	19	44
Imipenem g	1	IV	64	9.1	14
Cefuroxime mg	750	IV	28	9.6	35
Cefuroxime mg	750	IVx3	19	17.1	89
Cefotetan g	1	IV	104.1	39.7	38
Cefotaxime g	2	IV	40	5–14	12–30
Ceftriaxone g	2	IV	127	57.4	45
Ceftazidime g	2	IV	43	16	37
Gentamicin mg·kg^{-1}	5	MD	5	5	120
Tobramycin mg·kg^{-1}	1.7		6–8	6–9	100–150
Amikacin mg	500	IV	11–20	6–9	45–54
Erythromycin g	1	Pox2	1.4	4.2	300
Erythromycin mg	500	IV MD	3.05	6.53	210
Clarithromycin mg	500	PO MD	2.5	17.5	690
Azithromycin mg	500	PO MD	0.2–0.4	2.3–8.1	200–2000
Dirithromycin g	250	PO MD	0.08	1.6–2.4	2000–3000
Spiramycin mg	2–3	PO	2.4	19.25	802
Pefloxacin mg	400	IV	10.9	20	183
Ciprofloxacin mg	750	PO	2	4.9	275
Ciprofloxacin mg	200	IV	0.6±0.49	4.71±3.1	600
Ofloxacin mg	200	PO MD	1.90–5.18	6.7–7.3	2350
Temafloxacin mg	600	PO MD	6.05±2.19	27.97±17.02	460
Doxycycline mg	100	×3PO	2.74	5.4–23	190–840
Clindamycin mg	500	PO	3.3–10	3.2–9.3	100
Vancomycin g	1	IM	5.3	13	245
Vancomycin g	1	IV	6.7–40.6	2.8–9.6	24–41

MU: million unit; PO: *per os*; MD: multiple doses; IV: intravenous; IM: intamuscular.

(4.23±2.14 mg·kg^{-1}) [138]. Generally, the tissue concentrations of β-lactams are lower than serum levels. However, OHKUDA *et al.* [139] demonstrated that 30 min after IV injection of 1 g cefotiam, the lung tissue drug concentration was higher than the blood concentration, suggesting a higher rate of transition of the drug from the blood into the lung tissue than *vice versa*. The levels of aminoglycosides are equal to intravascular concentrations, whereas the concentrations of macrolides and fluoroquinolones are higher than peak serum levels thanks to their ability to diffuse freely and rapidly into all tissues and inside cells [8]. Recently, it has been documented that lung exposure to azithromycin is increased proportionally by doubling the dose, which results in a predictable pharmacokinetic behaviour of the drug in the lower respiratory tract [143].

In evaluating pulmonary tissue concentrations, it must always be kept in mind that their value in predicting the therapeutic efficacy is limited. They represent an average of different tissue compartments, independently from the distribution of an antibiotic into a tissue is not uniform (for example, distribution may be limited in the extracellular component if the drug is scarcely liposoluble). Tissue homogenate data can only be useful if correctly interpreted by correcting for the partitioning between the tissue components [14]. Thus, since the cellular penetration of β-lactam drugs is poor, the concentrations of the drug in the interstitial fluid of these tissues and in ELF may be higher than that revealed by the concentration in homogenate tissues [140].

Antibiotic penetration into thoracic lymph

Since the success of treatment depends upon the antibiotic levels in the site of infection, a high pneumotropism of the antibiotic is scarcely important if its penetration into the site of infection is inadequate. This occurs when lung abscesses with thick, fibrotic walls or other anatomical conditions withhold the antibiotic from reaching the infecting microorganism at therapeutically useful concentrations.

In order to identify the true pulmonary pharmacokinetic behaviour of an antibiotic, the determination of drug concentrations in the pulmonary lymph tissue has been suggested, since it reflects the extracellular and extra haemato-vascular compartments [144, 145]. Lymph is considered identical in composition to the interstitial fluid from which it stems [146]. Consequently, the antibiotic concentration in pulmonary lymph may be considered equal to the concentration surrounding lung parenchyma cells. As most infections probably develop only when microorganisms have entered epithelial cells and have possibly reached as far as the subepithelial tissues, it is likely that an antibiotic may be truly useful in the treatment of bacterial LRTIs if its consistently high concentrations are maintained in pulmonary lymph. Several experimental studies, which used a sheep model with a pulmonary fistula to collect pulmonary lymph specimens, showed that the β-lactam antibiotics and vancomycin were well distributed in lymph [144, 147, 148]. As the manipulation of the human thoracic duct is clearly unsuitable, drug concentrations in hilar lymph nodes could be determine [149].

Data in the literature on this subject is scant. CAZZOLA et al. [145] demonstrated an interesting behaviour of cefonicid following intramuscular administration of 1 g and of azithromycin, the latter maintaining high concentrations in hilar lymph nodes even at 144 h after oral treatment with 500 mg daily for 3 days [150] (fig. 3). It must be underlined that whereas lung tissue concentrations of β-lactams were lower than the corresponding hilar lymph node concentrations, higher macrolide levels were found in pulmonary tissues, probably due to the macrolides' capacity to accumulate within phagocytes.

Antibiotic penetration into interstitial space fluid

Because the majority of infections are localised within the extracellular space, the interstitial space fluid is considered an important target site for antimicrobial chemotherapy [151]. However, since ELF is obtained by bronchoscopy, and thoracic lymph by surgery, only interindividual data pooling can derive longitudinal pharmacokinetic data. Recently, a novel microdialysis-based approach for measuring drug concentrations in lung interstitial fluid has been developed [152].

The technique, which offers a number of advantages over BAL, involves the introduction of a microdialysis fiber probe into a fluid or tissue to be sampled. The fiber functions as an artificial blood capillary through which a perfusion medium (usually a physiological solution) is continuously pumped. Small molecules readily permeate the dialysis membrane driven by the concentration gradient. Substances recovered in the perforate are then analysed with suitable analytical methods either on line, or as a series of discreet samples collected over short time intervals. As a continuous sampling technique with no net fluid withdrawal, microdialysis is well suited for pharmacokinetic

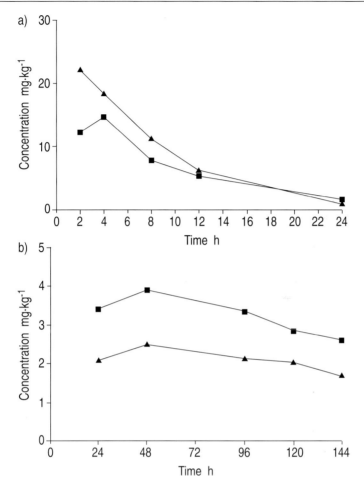

Fig. 3. – a) Penetration of cefonicid 1 g single dose intramuscular and b) azithromycin 500 mg×3 *per os* into lung tissue (■) and hylar lymphnodes (▲). Adapted from CAZZOLA *et al.* [146], and CAZZOLA *et al.* [151].

studies in the lung where a limited volume of fluid is present. Furthermore, microdialysis measures only the unbound pharmacologically active drug fraction in the interstitial space fluid [153]. The molecular cut-off weight of the membrane (20,000 daltons) is such that protein molecules, cells and protein- and cell-bound substances cannot permeate the membrane.

Microdialysis data indicates that in healthy people interstitial concentrations of ß-lactams are in the range of free serum concentrations, whereas interstitial levels of fluoroquinolones and macrolides are considerably lower than those predicted from biopsies [153]. Using this approach, it has been documented that cefpirome concentrations in lung interstitial fluid were 66% of the corresponding plasma values within the first 240 min and exceeded MICs of most relevant bacteria [152]. For several conditions, notably septicaemia and septic shock, tissue concentrations of antibiotics such as piperacillin may be subinhibitory even though effective concentrations are attained in serum [154, 155]. This may explain therapeutic failures and the emergence of drug-resistant bacteria that were exposed to subinhibitory drug concentrations in tissue. However, a recent paper has shown that maximal free concentrations of piperacillin were 176.0 ± 105.0 mg·L^{-1} in the interstitial space of pneumonic lung tissue and 326.0 ± 60.6 mg·L^{-1} in serum, respectively, following IV administration of a single dose of 4 g piperacillin and 500 mg tazobactam [156]. The intrapulmonary concentrations of piperacillin and tazobactam exceeded the MIC for most relevant bacteria for 4-6 h.

The major limitation of microdialysis is a possible error introduced when the calibration data obtained *in vitro* (the relative recovery) are extrapolated to the *in vivo* measurements [157]. Other factors such as the probe used, the perfusate flow rate, sampling time or the analysed concentration surrounding the probe or in the dialysate fluid, among others, may also influence the recovery value (fig. 4). This becomes particularly important in pharmacokinetic studies involving dynamic systems with continuous fluctuations in concentration, which may or may not be directly reflected by the perfusate concentration curve [158]. Another potential shortcoming with this technique is that the antibiotic concentrations in the interstitial fluid of normal lungs may not reflect those in the interstitial fluid of lungs in patients with pneumonia [152]. Nonetheless, closed chest microdialysis of the lung in spontaneously breathing patients has several advantages compared with the current methodological armamentarium for measuring drug concentrations in the lung these are as follows: 1) microdialysis probes can be implanted during routine surgery without major time expense; 2) continuous sampling is possible for several hours; 3) measurements can be performed under physiological and pathological conditions; and 4) bedside monitoring of target site antibiotic concentrations becomes possible as technical means for immediate analysis become available [152]. In particular, as a continuous sampling technique with no fluid introduced or withdrawn, it allows much higher temporal resolution and consequently is better suited for pharmacokinetic measurements [158]. The use of microdialysis also eliminates methodological errors associated with fluid dilution or depletion and reduces the number of patients required for the studies. As only one subject is used to construct a complete pharmacokinetic profile, minute changes in concentration can be detected. Inter-subject variation, a major concern in pharmacokinetic studies, is thus avoided.

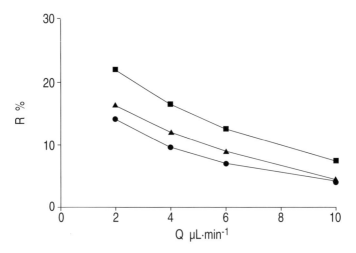

Fig. 4. – Relationship between the *in vitro* recovery (R %) determined by direct dialysis of ciprofloxacin, and dialysate flow rate (Q). ■: R%=29.56e-0.16Q; ▲: R%=21.83e-0.17Q; ●: R%=15.80e-0.14Q. Adapted from MARTÍNEZ MARTÍNEZ *et al.* [158].

Antibiotic penetration into pleural fluid

It is generally felt that pleural fluid acts as an "interstitial reservoir" in which the kinetic processes resemble those of the extravascular compartment [44]. However, only a limited number of researchers have studied the antibiotic penetration into pleural space in subjects with pleural effusion. This fact is surprising considering that pleurisy and empyema often complicate pneumonia and require adequate concentrations of antibiotic in pleural fluid, and that pleural fluid is easily obtainable.

The equilibration between an antibiotic in the serum and the pleural fluid depends on several factors. These factors include: the size of the pleural effusion (equilibration will occur less rapidly with larger pleural effusions); the thickness of the pleura (equilibration will occur less rapidly with a thicker pleura); the degree of pleural inflammation (equilibration will occur more rapidly with inflammation due to increased protein flux); and the antibiotic itself [159].

In general cephalosporins penetrate slowly into pleural space, but the concentrations reached are high and remain stable and persistent [160–165] (table 7). For example, after the administration of 1 g cefazoline in a single bolus, a level of 63.1 ± 6.7 mg·L^{-1} was reached [160], where after a bolus of 500 mg the concentration was 25.6 mg·L^{-1} with a penetration ratio of 48% [161]. Also the penetration of 1 g ceftazidime into large pleural effusion was good with concentrations from 17 ± 3–28 ± 2 mg·L^{-1} corresponding to a mean penetration ratio of 38% [162]. The concentration in pleural fluid after IV infusion of a 2-g dose of cefoperazone reached a peak of 7–25 mg·L^{-1} at 4–6 h after administration; the elimination half-life was $\sim$2–5 times longer in pleural fluid than in serum [163]. Using a drug with a high binding rate to serum proteins such as ceftriaxone the concentrations reached were lower ($\sim$2.4–3.5 mg·L^{-1} after 4–6 h) but persistent over time (1.8–2.2 mg·L^{-1} 24 h after administration) [164]. The mean ratios of pleural fluid/maximum concentrations of ceftriaxone were 9.1% in patients with transudative fluid and 13.5% in patients with exudative fluid [165]. Following oral administration of 500 mg of erythromycin *b.i.d.* pleural concentrations varied between 1.0–7.4 mg·L^{-1}; the pleura/blood ratio was

Table 7. – Antibiotic levels in serum and pleural fluid

Antibiotic	Dose and route	Route	Serum mg·L^{-1}	Pleural fluid mg·L^{-1}	Penetration %
Penicillin G g	1–3	MU IV	2–61	1–56	50–92
Ampicillin g	1	IV	3.2–30	4–11	37–125
Cerbenicillin g	5	IV	463±89	59	13
Cefazolin g	1	IV	53.5–72.5	21.3–25.6	30–48
Cefuroxime g	1.5	IV	35–40	5.5–6	15–16
Cefotaxime g	2	IV	40	4	10
Ceftazidime g	2	IV	80	17–28	21–38
Ceftriaxone g	1	IV	6–4–16	2.3–3.5	9.1–13.5
Ticarcillin g	5	IV	469	57.4	12
Piperacillin g	4	IV	196	55	28
Imipenem mg	250–500	IV	18.8–26.6	3.8–6.5	22
Doxycycline mg	200	PO	5–8	7.5-9	112–150
Streptomycin g	1	IM	26.8	20	75
Gentamicin mg·kg^{-1}	1.5	IV	5.1	2.9	57
Netilmicin mg·kg^{-1}	2	IV	5.4	3.7	69
Tobramycin mg·kg^{-1}	1.7		6–8	3.2	40–53
Amikacin mg·kg^{-1}	7.5		23.7±2.9	8.2	35
Erythromycin mg	500	PO *b.i.d.*		1.0–7.4	
Clindamycin mg	300	PO	4.0–6.0	6.9	115–172
Ciprofloxacin mg	500	PO	0.67–1.64	0.5–0.9	55–81

MU: multiple doses; IV: intravenous; PO: *per os*; IM: intamuscular; *b.i.d.*: twice daily.

approximately 70%, thus indicating a good antibiotic penetration into the extravascular space [43].

The concentration of ciprofloxacin in the pleural space was 0.9 mg·L^{-1} 6–9 h after oral administration of 500 mg, at 24 h the concentration was 0.5 mg·L^{-1}, whereas serum levels reached only 0.1 mg·L^{-1} [166]. Pleural concentrations of ciprofloxacin equalled plasma concentrations 1.5 h after 200 mg was given IV and the pleural/plasma ratio was ≥0.9 for 4 h [166]. In another study, the peak concentrations in pleural fluid 1.5 h after one and three injections of ciprofloxacin (1.5 mg·kg^{-1} of body weight) were 0.52±0.09 and 0.77±0.15 mg·L^{-1}, respectively; the corresponding 8-h concentrations were 0.19±0.05 and 0.39±0.10 mg·L^{-1}. At 1 and 8 h, the ratios of mean concentrations in pleural fluid to mean concentrations in serum were 112% and 158%, respectively, after one injection and 77% and 122% after three injections [167]. The penetration of fluoroquinolones into pleural fluid is higher than β-lactams. It has been documented that the mean ratios of concentrations in pleural fluid/maximum concentrations in serum of lomefloxacin were 66%, in patients with transudative fluid, and 69% in patients with exudative fluid [168].

With empyema, the pleural surfaces are thicker, the pleural fluid is more acidic, and more purulent material is present in the pleural space than with other conditions. It is quite possible that the diffusion of bioactive antibiotics would be hindered by the thickened pleura. Indeed, in one case of chronic tuberculous empyema with a thickened pleura (containing acidic, purulent material), the concentration of rifampin in the pleural fluid was <4% than in the serum [169]. Another report showed that aminoglycosides diffused across the normal pleura easily, but diffused into empyemic fluid much less easily [170]. Contrary to this, the penetration of oral 500 mg ciprofloxacin in empyema appeared satisfactory with a fluid/blood ratio varying between 0.4 and 1.9 [141, 168]. After 750-mg oral doses, ciprofloxacin penetrated into sterile and empyemic pleural fluid with concentrations 30–90% and 100–200% of plasma concentrations, respectively [166].

Clinical and therapeutic significance of pulmonary penetration of antibiotics

For an efficient treatment of LRTIs, physicians must try to obtain antibiotic levels equal or superior to the MIC for the pathogen in infected tissues or secretions [171]. Recent animal data indicate that the outcomes of the treatment of experimental pneumonia are influenced by the pharmacokinetic parameters of the antimicrobial in lung tissue. In the treatment of lung infection in rats, the better cure rates obtained with cefadroxil compared to cefalexin might be due to the higher drug concentration and the greater lung tissue AUC of cefadroxil [172]. In mouse experimental pneumonia, survival rates and lung clearance of the pathogen were greater when the animals were treated with temafloxacin than when they were treated with ofloxacin or ciprofloxacin [173]. This result could be related to the greater tissue concentration and longer half-life and maximum residence time over the minimal bactericidal concentration achieved in the infected lung with temafloxacin than with ciprofloxacin [174]. Similarly, lung half-lives of various macrolides have been shown to be predictive of their efficacy in treating experimental respiratory tract infection [175].

In effect, some studies have suggested that an efficient antimicrobial penetration into potential sites of pulmonary infection and its protracted permanence in active form are advantageous [7]. This is particularly true when the infection has not spread beyond the lung and there are no existing barriers to adequate lung penetration, such as lung abscess or necrotic pneumonia. The results of community-acquired pneumonia (CAP) clinical trials of the IV azithromycin are paradigmatic of this assumption. These trials have revealed that clinical outcomes were similar in bacteremic patients and in a control group treated with cefuroxime with or without erythromycin [176]. Since, with azithromycin, serum levels fall rapidly, but levels in lung parenchyma and phagocytes rise several fold, these results support the concept that pulmonary antibiotic levels may be the most significant pharmacokinetic factor in the cure of patients with CAP.

Some other studies have documented that drugs, which penetrate well and remain for long periods of time into the pulmonary site of infection, often induce therapeutic responses greater than expected on the basis of *in vitro* data. This finding seems to be independent from the class of antimicrobials used. Therefore in patients with acute exacerbations of chronic bronchitis, a 5-day treatment with dirithromycin has induced effective concentrations in different pulmonary sites of infection up-to 96 hours after the last dose. Symptom remission has progressed together with the trend of the pulmonary antibiotic concentrations independently from the length of treatment [177] (fig. 5). Interestingly, notwithstanding its poor *in vitro* activity against *Haemophilus. influenzae*, dirithromycin was effective against this microrganism *in vivo*. This discrepancy could be due to the fact that the MICs of dirithromycin in the presence of serum *in vivo* are 5-fold lower than *in vitro* in artificial media [178], but the persistence of antimicrobial activity in the tissues may as well be inhibitory for this pathogen [179]. Also the eradication of nosocomial pathogens such as *Enterobacteriaceae* or *Pseudomonas aeruginosa* correlates to the presence of relatively high pulmonary concentrations of ceftriaxone or imipenem [180].

Fluoroquinolones, which concentrate in pulmonary tissues and fluids, reach levels that are sufficient to overcome a good percentage of cases of infective processes caused by *Streptococcus pneumoniae*, which present high MICs toward these antibiotics, are another documentation of the importance of effective pulmonary disposition of antimicrobials. For example, although the serum level of ciprofloxacin (1.19 ± 0.16 mg·L^{-1}) is below the MIC$_{90}$ of *S. pneumoniae* (2.0 mg·L^{-1}), the concentrations reached in ELF are ~3 mg·L^{-1} [72]. Similarly, the mean concentration of pefloxacin is 88.2 ± 10 mg·L^{-1} in the ELF, whereas the mean serum concentration is 6.67 ± 0.47 mg·L^{-1} [181], which is below

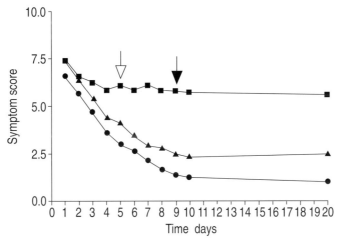

Fig. 5. – Symptom scores, in patients with acute exacerbations of chronic bronchitis (■: dyspnoea; ▲: cough; ●: sputum), after treatment with dirithromycin 500 mg·day^{-1} for 5 days. Open arrow: last dose; closed arrow: last day with effective pulmonary concentration). Effective antibacterial concentrations at different pulmonary sites of infection were achieved up to 96 h after the last dose. Symptom remission, evaluated by a decrease in arbitrary scores, progressed with trends in pulmonary antibacterial concentrations independently of the length of treatment. Adapted from CAZZOLA *et al.* [177].

the MIC_{90} of *S. pneumoniae* (8.0 mg·L^{-1}). However, failures of ciprofloxacin and pefloxacin in the treatment of pneumococcal pneumonia have been described notwithstanding the relevance of their accumulation in lower respiratory tract. BALDWIN *et al.* [72] suggested that subtherapeutic intrapulmonary concentrations might be responsible for these failures.

The studies mentioned above seem to indicate that drugs with higher intrapulmonary concentrations would have greater clinical efficacy. Nonetheless, the presence of a relationship between antibiotic levels in the site of infection and their clinical efficacy in the lung has not been clearly demonstrated due to the numerous methodological difficulties [1].

In particular, it has been suggested that experimentally determined "total tissue concentrations" are not good indicators of activity since they represent average values including unspecifically bound drug and not the actual present concentrations at the site of action [8]. For the same reason, the concept of "tissue partition coefficients" is inadequate since it implies homogenous tissue concentrations. It is the aqueous unbound concentration at the site of infection in the tissue that is most relevant for the magnitude of antibiosis [181, 182]. Therefore, if overall concentrations are measured, effect site concentrations of drugs that equilibrate exclusively with the extracellular space, such as ß-lactams, may be underestimated [183]. This, in turn, will also lead to the overestimation of effect site concentrations of drugs that accumulate intracellularly. Unfortunately, the tissue/blood ratio is equally considered not really important. The clinical utility of penetration ratios is somewhat misleading since bacterial eradication is a function of the drug concentration at the site of infection rather than penetration ratios.

Substantially, pulmonary pharmacokinetics is a very useful tool for describing how drugs behave in the human lung, but it does not promote an understanding of pharmacologic effects of a drug [169]. Instead the correlation between pulmonary disposition of the drug and its MIC values for the infectious agent is more important [11].

Various antibiotics show a link with the correlation between tissue concentrations of the drug and the MIC values for the infectious agent (known as inhibitory quotient: IQ; or as killing ratio) and the eradication of the pathogens present in the airways [180, 184, 185]. Those agents with killing ratios ≥ 2 are more likely to be associated with a favourable clinical outcome than those with lower killing ratios [186]. For example, the peak concentration in bronchial secretions to MIC ratio following a single IV administration of 1 g ceftriaxone in a patient suffering from acute exacerbation of chronic bronchitis shows that ceftriaxone is extremely active against *H. influenzae*, *Klebsiella pneumoniae*, and partially active against *S. pneumoniae*, even when its concentrations at the site of infection is considered [187]. It has also been documented that treatment is generally ineffective when the peak tissue levels are $\leq MIC$ for responsible bacteria. Therefore, in patients with exacerbations of chronic bronchitis caused by *H. influenzae*, ampicillin (which presents a MIC value of 0.12 mg/l against this pathogen) was ineffective at a dose of 200 mg because its concentration in the sputum was below the MIC value. Contrary to this, doses >400 mg were effective [188]. Patients with pneumonia or exacerbation of chronic bronchitis responded in an adequate manner to 7 days of treatment with amoxicillin, particularly when the drug sputum were >0.25 mg·L^{-1} [20]. Contrary to this, sputum concentrations <0.5 mg·L^{-1} following dosage of cefaclor of up-to 500 mg compared unfavourably with the MICs for *H. influenzae* and *Moraxella catarrhalis* and were associate with clinical failure [189].

The results of these studies seem to indicate a good correlation between pulmonary concentrations of the drug and the MIC for the pathogens, but they have only associated MIC values with the peak concentration at the site of infection. *In vivo* bacteria are not exposed to constant, but to constantly changing antibiotic concentrations, with peaks and troughs [190]. Therefore, in addition the pathogens are exposed to a gradient of antibiotic concentration according to the pharmacokinetics of the antibiotic at the pulmonary site of infection [190]. The addition of bacteriological characteristics to *in vivo* pharmacokinetic studies has triggered a "pharmacodynamic approach". Pharmaco-dynamic parameters integrate the microbiological activity and pharmacokinetics of an anti-infective drug by focusing on its biological effects, in particular growth inhibition and killing of pathogens. Therefore, they allow a better evaluation of the dosage regimen in conjunction with its clinical response [191, 192].

It is extremely difficult to define the real impact of the interrelationship between pulmonary pharmacokinetics and pharmacodynamics on clinical and microbiological outcomes. The majority of studies have only examined the interrelationship between serum pharmacokinetics and pharmacodynamics in patients with LRTIs, probably because it is easier and more ethical to sample blood than sputum, bronchial mucosa or ELF [171].

Since β-lactams exert a dose-dependent bactericidal effect on bacteria and do not possess a significant postantibiotic effect, their levels at the sites of infection should be above MIC for the entire length of treatment. A significant linear correlation exists between *t*>MIC and time to eradication of bacteria from respiratory secretions [193]. Nevertheless, the magnitude and duration by which concentrations must exceed the MIC level remain controversial. Papers that support the importance of the interrelationship between pharmacokinetics and pharmacodynamics in inducing a good clinical and bacteriological outcome are scarce [194]. Experimental research has shown that cephalosporins exert an *in vivo* bacteriostatic effect even when their concentrations are above MIC levels for only 40% of the time between administrations, whereas maximal bactericidal effect is obtained when concentrations are above MIC levels for 60–70% of time [195]. Therefore, the aim for a highly effective dosing regimen would be to provide levels above the MIC for at least 70% of the dosing interval [196].

Ceftazidime reaches significantly higher levels than the MICs of the most common respiratory pathogens in the potential sites of lung infection, even at 8–12 h after the administration of 1 g intramuscular (IM; fig. 6) [21]. For this reason, a recent study has

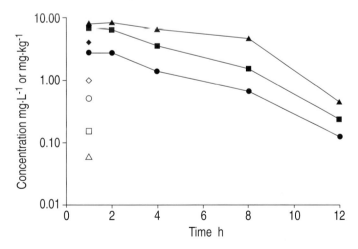

Fig. 6. – Correlation between mean pulmonary concentrations of intramuscular ceftazidime (1g) administered to patients with acute exacerbation of chronic bronchitis (■: sputum; ▲: mucosa; ●: epithelial lining fluid) and the minimal inhibitory concentration for relevant respiratory pathogens: ◆: *Staphlococcus aureus*; ◇: *Pseudomonas earuginosa*; ○: *Streptococcus pneumoniae* and *Klebsiella pneumoniae*; □: *Haemophilus influenzae*; △: *Moraxella catarrhalis*. Adapted from CAZZOLA *et al* [21].

suggested the possibility of using ceftazidime in a single daily dose of 1 g IM to treat those patients with exacerbations of chronic obstructive pulomonary disease who only present moderately impaired functional symptoms. However, this type of therapeutic approach must be used with extreme caution in subjects with marked functional damage, although a satisfactory clinical response may be obtained in some cases. The small number of patients included in this study does not allow solid conclusions to be drawn [197].

Although these data are intriguing, it is important to note that it is always best to administer high concentrations of the drug, particularly in treating patients hospitalised in intensive care units, because studies on β-lactam tissue kinetics show evidence of a decline in the antibiotic tissue levels parallel to serum concentrations [190]. It must also be highlighted that there is a close link between antibiotic dosing and antibiotic resistance. In particular, resistance follows underdosing of the AUC in relation to the MIC [198]. A major component to the selective pressure argument is dosing. For years the need to adjust antibiotic dosing as a means of lowering endemic resistance has been underappreciated, and consequences are only now been seen. As the number of really active antibiotics is declining rapidly, it is now becoming urgent to manage resistance by managing the dosing and use patterns of the remaining agents [199]. With all β-lactams, which have a slow, time-dependent antibacterial effect, the aim must be to keep the antibiotic level above the MIC for the duration of therapy. Consequently, if the drug has a long-life, single doses at long intervals can be given. However, if the half-life is short, the antibiotic should be given frequently, thus ensuring that the β-lactam is maintained at concentrations above the MIC level at all times in infected tissues.

A different study by CAZZOLA et al. [200] examined the relationship between the bacterial susceptibility to cefaclor (MIC), the achieved cefaclor advanced formulation serum and sputum concentrations, and *in vivo* eradication of the bacteria in patients with acute exacerbations of chronic bronchitis. Treatment was successful in all subjects with the per cent of time above the MIC in serum >40%, whereas the time that levels in sputum stayed above the MIC was not the pharmacodynamic parameter that correlated best with therapeutic efficacy for cefaclor [200]. This and the findings from other studies, question the role of pulmonary pharmacodynamics and seem to indicate that the correlation between clinical and microbiological outcomes and serum concentration is better than that between these outcome and pulmonary levels of the antibiotic. This is probably due to the serum concentration better reflecting the interstitial fluid concentration [201].

Conclusion

Antimicrobials show considerable variation in their ability to penetrate pulmonary tissues. Nonetheless, lung penetration is considered, in part, to be predictive of efficacy in the treatment of LRTIs. Unfortunately most studies are performed during the steady state, in uninfected individuals. This could result in bias as the pharmacokinetics of antibiotics may be altered in individuals with an infection. In order to provide the greatest insight into the utility of these agents for different pathogens causing LRTIs, it is important to examine the penetration in the presence of the pathological process for which they are being employed. The presence of LRTIs will have significant inflammation attendant to them. It is likely that this inflammation will alter penetration in a time-dependent way. The inflammation is likely to peak early in the process, with a maximal effect on tight junctions and penetration occurring in the first few days after the introduction of the drug. As the agent starts the resolution process, it is further likely that penetration will decrease. These issues need to be adequately studied to gain the full understanding of drug penetration and its effect on the pathological process of LRTIs. It is also possible that tissue penetration at steady state differs from that after a single dose. Consequently, several doses may be needed to achieve the steady state, which may also affect tissue penetration [171]. Continued research is warranted to determine the best method of assessing respiratory tract concentrations and prediction of clinical response.

Summary

The efficacy of antibiotic treatment in bacterial lower respiratory tract infections (LRTIs) is partly dependent on the levels reached by the drug and on the length of stay at the site of infection. The place where the infection develops inevitably influences the clinical presentation. Unfortunately, the *in vivo* determination of antimicrobial concentrations at these sites is plagued with several methodological difficulties. Moreover, a severe obstacle is also encountered when attempting to compare pulmonary pharmacokinetics of different antimicrobials using data present in literature as different studies conducted on a single therapeutic agent differ in terms of methods used, dosage, therapeutic interval, and route of administration. Although the presence of a correlation between antibiotic levels at the site of infection and their clinical efficacy in LRTIs has not been clearly demonstrated due to these difficulties, drugs with higher intrapulmonary concentrations would have greater clinical efficacy.

Keywords: Antibiotics, clinical relevance, pulmonary distribution.

References

1. Valcke Y, Pauwels R, van der Straeten M. Pharmacokinetics of antibiotics in the lungs. *Eur Respir J* 1990; 3: 715–722.
2. Baldwin DR, Honeybourne D, Wise R. Pulmonary disposition of antimicrobial agents *in vivo*: observations and clinical relevance. *Antimicrob Agents Chemother* 1992; 36: 1176–1180.
3. Honeybourne D, Baldwin DR. The site concentrations of antimicrobial agents in the lungs. *J Antimicrob Chemother* 1992; 30: 249–260.
4. Cazzola M. Problems and prospectives in the antibiotic treatment of lower respiratory tract infections. *Pulm Pharmacol* 1994; 7: 139–152.
5. Cazzola M, Rossi F. Pulmonary penetration of antibiotics [La penetrazione polmonare degli antibiotici]. *Gior It Chemioter* 1993; 40: 116–121.
6. Cazzola M, Diamare F, Vinciguerra A, Salzillo A, Calderaro F. Pulmonary penetration of antibiotics and its clinical impact [La penetrazione polmonare degli antibiotici e il suo impatto clinico]. *Rass Pat App Respir* 1996; 11: 134–147.
7. Honeybourne D. Antibiotic penetration in the respiratory tract and implications for the selection of antimicrobial therapy. *Curr Opin Pulm Med* 1997; 3: 170–174.
8. Bergogne-Bérézin E. New concepts in the pulmonary disposition of antibiotics. *Pulm Pharmacol* 1995; 8: 65–81.
9. Cruciani M, Gatti G, Cazzadori A, Concia E. Pharmacokinetics of antimicrobial agents in the respiratory tract. *Zentralbl Bakteriol* 1996; 284: 1–31.

10. Chiu LM, Amsden GW. Intrapulmonary pharmacokinetics of antibacterial agents. Implications for therapeutics. *Am J Respir Med* 2002; 1: 201–209.

11. Bergogne-Bérézin E, Vallée E. Pharmacokinetics of antibiotics in respiratory tissues and fluids. *In*: Pennington JE, ed. Respiratory Infections: Diagnosis and Management. 3rd Edn. New York, Raven Press, 1994; pp. 715–740.

12. Walstad RA. Concentrations of antibiotics in sputum. *Res Clin Forum* 1990; 12: 87–92.

13. Pennington JE. Penetration of antibiotics into respiratory secretions. *Rev Infect Dis* 1981; 3: 67–73.

14. Kneer J. Relevance of antibiotic tissue penetration in treating respiratory tract infections. *Respiration* 1993; 60: Suppl. 1, 32–37.

15. Smith BR, Le Frock JL. Bronchial tree penetration of antibiotics. *Chest* 1983; 83: 904–908.

16. Barza M. Principles of tissue penetration of antibiotics. *J Antimicrob Chemother* 1981; 8: Suppl. C, 7–28.

17. Dursano GL. Role of pharmacokinetics in the outcome of infections. *Antimicrob Agents Chemother* 1988; 32: 289–297.

18. Stewart SM, Fisher M, Young JE, Lutz W. Amoxycillin levels in sputum, serum and saliva. *Thorax* 1974; 29: 110–114.

19. Marlin GE, Burgess KR, Burgoyne J, Funnell GR, Guinness MDG. Penetration of piperacillin into bronchial mucosa and sputum. *Thorax* 1981; 36: 774–780.

20. Muller-Serieys C, Bergogne-Bérézin E, Rowan C, Dombret MC. Imipenem penetration into bronchial secretions. *J Antimicrob Chemother* 1987; 20: 618–619.

21. Cazzola M, Matera MG, Polverino M, Santangelo G, De Franchis I, Rossi F. Pulmonary penetration of ceftazidime. *J Chemother* 1995; 7: 5054.

22. Cazzola M, Matera MG, Cirella M, *et al.* Penetrazione del cefaclor nell'espettorato dopo somministrazione singola e multipla: confronto fra la preparazione a rilascio classico e una nuova formulazione a rilascio modificato. *GIR* 1995; 16: 37–41.

23. Jehl F, Muller-Serieys C, de Larminat V, Monteil H, Bergogne-Berezin E. Penetration of piperacillin-tazobactam into bronchial secretions after multiple doses to intensive care patients. *Antimicrob Agents Chemother* 1994; 38: 2780–2784.

24. Vinks AA, Brimicombe RW, Heijerman HG, Bakker W. Continuous infusion of ceftazidime in cystic fibrosis patients during home treatment: clinical outcome, microbiology and pharmacokinetics. *J Antimicrob Chemother* 1997; 40: 125–133.

25. Langer M, Cantoni P, Bellosta C, Boccazzi A. Penetration of ceftazidime into bronchial secretions in critically ill patients. *J Antimicrob Chemother* 1991; 28: 925–932.

26. Lovering AM, Pycock CJ, Harvey JE, Reeves DS. The pharmacokinetics and sputum penetration of ampicillin and amoxycillin following simultaneous *i.v.* administration. *J Antimicrob Chemother* 1990; 25: 385–392.

27. Bergogne-Bérézin E, Berthelot G, Even P, Sten M, Reynaud P. Penetration of ciprofloxacin into bronchial secretions. *Eur J Clin Microbiol* 1986; 5: 197–200.

28. Davies B, Maesen FPV, Geraedts W, Baur C. Penetration of ofloxacin from serum to sputum. *Drugs* 1987; 34: Suppl. 1, 26–32.

29. Bergogne-Bérézin E, Muller-Serieys C, Kafé H. Penetration of lomefloxacin into bronchial secretions following single and multiple oral administration. *Am J Med* 1992; 92: Suppl. 4A, 8S–11S.

30. Fujita A, Miya T, Tanaka R, *et al.* Levofloxacin concentrations in serum, sputum and lung tissue: evaluation of its efficacy according to breakpoint. *Jpn J Antibiot* 1999; 52: 661–666.

31. Begg EJ, Robson RA, Saunders DA, Graham GG, Buttimore RC, Neill AM, Town GI. The pharmacokinetics of oral fleroxacin and ciprofloxacin in plasma and sputum during acute and chronic dosing. *Br J Clin Pharmacol* 2000; 49: 32–38.

32. Cazzola M, Matera MG, Tufano MA, *et al.* Pulmonary disposition of lomefloxacin in patients with acute exacerbation of chronic obstructive pulmonary disease. A multiple-dose study. *J Chemother* 2001; 13: 407–412.

33. Mendelman PM, Smith AL, Levy J, Weber A, Ramsey B, Davis RL. Aminoglycoside penetration, inactivation, and efficacy in cystic fibrosis sputum. *Am Rev Respir Dis* 1985; 132: 761–765.

34. Dull WL, Alexander MR, Kasik JE. Bronchial secretion levels of amikacin. *Antimicrob Agents Chemother* 1979; 16: 767–771.
35. Klastersky J, Thys JP, Mombelli G. Comparative studies of intermittent and continuous administration of aminoglycosides in the treatment of bronchopulmonary infections due to Gram-negative bacteria. *Rev Infect Dis* 1981; 3: 74–83.
36. Alexander MR, Schoell J, Hicklin G, Kasik JE, Coleman D. Bronchial secretion concentrations of tobramycin. *Am Rev Respir Dis* 1982; 125: 208–209.
37. Braude AC, Hornstein A, Klein M, Vas S, Rebuck AS. Pulmonary disposition of tobramycin. *Am Rev Respir Dis* 1983;1 27: 563–565.
38. Santre C, Georges H, Jacquier JM, Leroy O, Beuscart C, Buguin D, Beaucaire G. Amikacin levels in bronchial secretions of 10 pneumonia patients with respiratory support treated once daily versus twice daily. *Antimicrob Agents Chemother* 1995; 39: 264–267.
39. Geller DE, Rosenfeld M, Waltz DA, Wilmott RW. Efficiency of pulmonary administration of tobramycin solution for inhalation in cystic fibrosis using an improved drug delivery system. *Chest* 2003; 123: 28–36.
40. Geller DE, Pitlick WH, Nardella PA, Tracewell WG, Ramsey BW. Pharmacokinetics and bioavailability of aerosolized tobramycin in cystic fibrosis. *Chest* 2002; 122: 219–226.
41. Gartmann J. Doxycycline concentrations in lung tissue, bronchial wall, bronchial secretions. *Chemotherapy* 1975; 21: 19–26.
42. Watanabe A, Anzai Y, Niitsuma K, Saito M, Yanase K, Nakamura M. Penetration of minocycline hydrochloride into lung tissue and sputum. *Chemotherapy* 2001; 47: 1–9.
43. Marlin GE, Davies PR, Rutland J, Berend N. Plasma and sputum erythromycin concentrations in chronic bronchitis. *Thorax* 1980; 35: 441–445.
44. Bergogne-Bérézin E. Tissue distribution of macrolide antibiotics. *In*: Bryskier AJ, Butzler J-P, Neu HC, Tulkens PM, eds. Macrolides. Chemistry, Pharmacology and Clinical Uses. Paris, Arnette Blackwell, 1993; pp. 451–484.
45. Matera MG, Tufano MA, Polverino M, Rossi F, Cazzola M. Pulmonary concentrations of dirithromycin and erythromycin during acute exacerbation of mild chronic obstructive pulmonary disease. *Eur Respir J* 1997; 10: 97–102.
46. Baldwin DR, Wise R, Andrews JM, Ashby JP, Honeybourne D. Azithromycin concentrations at the sites of pulmonary infection. *Eur Respir J* 1990; 3: 886–890.
47. Cazzola M, Matera MG, Tufano MA, *et al.* Pulmonary penetration of dirithromycin in patients suffering from acute exacerbation of chronic bronchitis. *Pulm Pharmacol* 1994; 7: 377–381.
48. Levy J. Antibiotic activity in sputum. *J Pediatr* 1986; 108: 841–846.
49. Peleman RA, Van De Velde V, Germonpre PR, Fleurinck C, Rosseel MT, Pauwels RA. Trovafloxacin concentrations in airway fluids of patients with severe community-acquired pneumonia. *Antimicrob Agents Chemother* 2000; 44: 178–180.
50. Rebuck AS, Braude AC. Assessment of drug disposition in the lung. *Drugs* 1984; 28: 544–553.
51. Lambert HP. Clinical significance of tissue penetration of antibiotics in the respiratory tract. *Scand J Infect Dis* 1978; Suppl. 14, 262–266.
52. Reynolds HY, Levine AS, Wood RE. Diminished effect of gentamicin under anaerobic or hypercapnic conditions. *Lancet* 1986; i: 447–449.
53. Cohen GM. Pulmonary metabolism of foreign compounds: its role in metabolic activation. *Environ Health Perspect* 1990; 85: 31–41.
54. Tylewska S, Hijerten S, Waldstrom T. Effects of subinhibitory concentrations of antibiotics on the adhesion of *Streptococcus pyogenes* to pharyngeal epithelial cells. *Antimicrob Agents Chemother* 1981; 20: 563–566.
55. Tsang KW, Rutman A, Kanthakumar K, *et al.* *Haemophilus influenzae* infection of human respiratory mucosa in low concentration of antibiotics. *Am Rev Respir Dis* 1993; 148: 201–207.
56. Beachey EH. Bacterial adherence: adhesion-receptor interactions mediating attachment of bacteria to mucosal surfaces. *J Infect Dis* 1981; 143: 325–345.

57. Ahlstedt S. The antibacterial effects of low concentrations of antibiotics and host defence factors: a review. *J Antimicrob Chemother* 1981; 8: Suppl. C, 59–70.

58. Marlin GE, Nicholls AJ, Funnell GR, Bradbury R. Penetration of cefaclor into bronchial mucosa. *Thorax* 1984; 39: 813–817.

59. Cox AL, Meewis JM, Horton R. Penetration into lung tissue after intravenous administration of amoxycillin/clavulanate. *J Antimicrob Chemother* 1989; 24: Suppl. B, 87–91.

60. Wise R, Baldwin DR, Honeybourne D. Penetration of antibiotics into the bronchial mucosa. *Res Clin Forums* 1990; 12: 95–100.

61. Baldwin DR, Andrews JM, Ashby JP, Wise R, Honeybourne D. Concentration of cefixime in bronchial mucosa and sputum after three oral multiple dose regimens. *Thorax* 1990; 45: 401–402.

62. Chadha D, Wise R, Baldwin DR, Andrews JM, Ashby JP, Honeybourne D. Cefepime concentrations in bronchial mucosa and serum following a single 2 gram intravenous dose. *J Antimicrob Chemother* 1990; 25: 959–963.

63. Imaizumi M, Ojika T, Watanabe H, Sakakibara M, Nishimura M, Abe T. A clinical study of transfer of cefiminox and piperacillin into pulmonary tissue. *Jpn J Antibiot* 1992; 45: 1039–1049.

64. Baldwin DR, Andrews JM, Wise R, Honeybourne D. Bronchoalveolar distribution of cefuroxime axetil and *in vitro* efficacy of observed concentrations against respiratory pathogens. *J Antimicrob Chemother* 1992; 30: 377–385.

65. Gould IM, Harvey G, Golder D, *et al.* Penetration of amoxycillin/clavulanic acid into bronchial mucosa with different dosing regimen. *Thorax* 1994; 49: 999–1001.

66. Cook PJ, Andrews JM, Woodcock J, Wise R, Honeybourne D. Concentration of amoxycillin and clavulanate in lung compartments in adults without pulmonary infection. *Thorax* 1994; 49: 1134–1138.

67. Cook PJ, Andrews JM, Wise R, Honeybourne D. Distribution of cefdinir, a third generation cephalosporin antibiotic, in serum and pulmonary compartments. *J Antimicrob Chemother* 1996; 37: 331–339.

68. Honeybourne D, Andrews JM, Ashby JP, Lodwick R, Wise R. Evaluation of the penetration of ciprofloxacin and amoxicillin into the bronchial mucosa. *Thorax* 1998; 43: 715–719.

69. Krumpe P, Lin C-C, Radwanski E, Cayen MN, Affrime MB. The penetration of ceftibuten into the respiratory tract. *Chest* 1999; 116: 369–374.

70. Byl B, Jacobs F, Roucloux I, de Franquen P, Cappello M, Thys JP. Penetration of meropenem in lung, bronchial mucosa and pleural tissues. *Antimicrob Agents Chemother* 1999; 43: 681–682.

71. Davey PG, Precious E, Winter J. Bronchial penetration of ofloxacin after single and multiple oral dosage. *J Antimicrob Chemother* 1991; 27: 335–341.

72. Baldwin DR, Wise R, Andrews JM, Gill M, Honeybourne D. Comparative bronchoalveolar concentrations of ciprofloxacin and lomefloxacin following oral administration. *Respir Med* 1993; 87: 595–601.

73. Cook PJ, Andrews JM, Wise R, Honeybourne D, Moudgil H. Concentrations of OPC-17116, a new fluoroquinolone antibacterial, in serum and lung compartments. *J Antimicrob Chemother* 1995; 35: 317–326.

74. Wise R, Honeybourne D. A review of the penetration of sparfloxacin into the lower respiratory tract and sinuses. *J Antimicrob Chemother* 1996; 37: 57–63.

75. Andrews JM, Honeybourne D, Brenwald NP, *et al.* Concentrations of trovafloxacin in bronchial mucosa, epithelial lining fluid, alveolar macrophages and serum after administration of single or multiple oral doses to patients undergoing fibre-optic bronchoscopy. *J Antimicrob Chemother* 1997; 39: 797–802.

76. Andrews JM, Honeybourne D, Jevons G, Brenwald NP, Cunningham B, Wise R. Concentrations of levofloxacin (HR 355) in the respiratory tract following a single oral dose in patients undergoing fibre-optic bronchoscopy. *J Antimicrob Chemother* 1997; 40: 573–577.

77. Soman A, Honeybourne D, Andrews J, Jevons G, Wise R. Concentrations of moxifloxacin in serum and pulmonary compartments following a single 400 mg oral dose in patients undergoing fibre-optic bronchoscopy. *J Antimicrob Chemother* 1999; 44: 835–838.

78. Honeybourne D, Andrews JM, Cunningham B, Jevons G, Wise R. The concentrations of clinafloxacin in alveolar macrophages, epithelial lining fluid, bronchial mucosa and serum after administration of single 200 mg oral doses to patients undergoing fibre-optic bronchoscopy. *J Antimicrob Chemother* 1999; 43: 153–155.

79. Honeybourne D, Banerjee D, Andrews J, Wise R. Concentrations of gatifloxacin in plasma and pulmonary compartments following a single 400 mg oral dose in patients undergoing fibre-optic bronchoscopy. *J Antimicrob Chemother* 2001; 48: 63–66.

80. Andrews J, Honeybourne D, Jevons G, *et al.* Concentrations of garenoxacin in plasma, bronchial mucosa, alveolar macrophages and epithelial lining fluid following a single oral 600 mg dose in healthy adult subjects. *J Antimicrob Chemother* 2003; 51: 727–730.

81. Lamy P, Anthoine D, Zuck P, Weber M, Baudesson D. Etude pharmacocinétique de la spiramycine en pathologie infectieuse respiratoire. *Ann Med* 1977; 16: 109–112.

82. Chastre J, Brun P, Fourtillan JB, Soler P, Basset G, Manuel C. Pulmonary disposition of roxithromycin (RU 28965), a new macrolide antibiotic. *Antimicrob Agents Chemother* 1987; 31: 1312–1316.

83. Mattie H, Hoogeterp JJ, Kaajan JPG, Hermans J. The penetration of erythromycin into human bronchial mucosa. *Br J Clin Pharmacol* 1987; 24: 179–183.

84. Khair OA, Andrews JM, Honeybourne D, Jevons G, Vacheron F, Wise R. Lung concentrations of telithromycin after oral dosing. *J Antimicrob Chemother* 2001; 47: 837–840.

85. Emmerson AM. The clinical significance of tissue concentration. *Res Clin Forums* 1990; 12: 117–121.

86. Smith BR, LeFrocq JL. Bronchial tree penetration of antibiotics. *Chest* 1983; 6: 904–908.

87. Cars O. Distribution of antibiotics into tissues and cells. *Medical Masterclasses* 1993; 1: 2–9.

88. Olsen KM, San Pedro GS, Gann LP, Gubbins PO, Halinski DM, Campbell GD Jr. Intrapulmonary pharmacokinetics of azithromycin in healthy volunteers given five oral doses. *Antimicrob Agents Chemother* 1996; 40: 2582–2585.

89. Baldwin DR, Wise R, Andrews JM, Honeybourne D. Concentrations of antimicrobials in the pulmonary alveolar epithelial lining. *Res Clin Forums* 1990; 12 (4): 103–113.

90. Rennard SI, Basset G, Lecossier D, *et al.* Estimation of volume of epithelial lining fluid recovered by lavage using urea as marker of dilution. *J Appl Physiol* 1986; 60: 532–538.

91. Braude AC, Hornstein A, Klein M, Vas S, Rebuck AS. Pulmonary disposition of tobramycin. *Am Rev Respir Dis* 1983; 127: 563–565.

92. Braude AC, Cohen RD, Penner JL, Preston MA, Rebuck AS. Pulmonary disposition of moxalactam. *Chest* 1984; 86: 881–883.

93. Chinard FP. Quantitative assessment of epithelial lining fluid in the lung. *Am J Physiol* 1992; 263: L617–L618.

94. Marcy TW, Merrill WW, Rankin JA, Reynold HY. Limitation of using urea to quantify epithelial lining fluid recovered by bronchoalveolar lavage. *Am Rev Respir Dis* 1987; 135: 1276–1280.

95. Drusano GL, Preston SL, Gotfried MH, Danziger LH, Rodvold KA. Levofloxacin penetration into epithelial lining fluid as determined by population pharmacokinetic modeling and Monte Carlo simulation. *Antimicrob Agents Chemother* 2002; 46: 586–589.

96. Staehelin LA. Structure and function of intercellular junctions. *Intern Ren Cytol* 1974; 39: 191–283.

97. Farago E, Kiss J, Gomory A, Aranyosi IJ, Juhasz I, Mihoczy L. Amikacin: *in vitro* bacteriological studies, levels in human serum, lung and heart tissue, and clinical results. *Intern J Clin Pharmacol Biopharm* 1979; 17: 421–428.

98. Unertl K, Adam D, Sunder-Plassman L, Koller H, Martin E. Serum and lung tissue concentrations of imipenem. *In*: Proceeding of Fourteenth International Congress of Chemotherapy. Kyoto. *Chemotherapy* 1985; 1216–1219.

99. Saux MC, Crockett R, Fourtillan JB, Leng B, Couraud L. Diffusion de l'amikacine dans les poumons. *Pathol Biol* 1986; 34: 113–117.

100. Benoni G, Cuzzolin L, Bertrand C, Puchetti V, Velo G. Imipenem kinetics in serum, lung tissue

and pericardial fluid in patients undergoing thoracotomy. *J Antimicrob Chemother* 1987; 20: 725–728.

101. Benoni G, Cuzzolin L, Bertrand C, Puchetti V, Velo G. Penetration of imipenem-cilastatin into the lung tissue and pericardial fluid of thoracotomized patients. *Chemoterapia* 1987; 6: 259–260.

102. Just HM, Frank U, Simon A, Kaiser D, Daschner FD. Concentrations of ceftriaxone in serum and lung tissue. *Chemotherapy* 1984; 30: 81–83.

103. Vlahov V, Dobrev P, Alexiev N, Bacracheva N, Chervenakov P. Distribution of ceftriaxone in human pulmonary and bronchial tissue. Concentrations of ceftriaxone in non-inflamed pulmonary and bronchial tissue and in blood plasma. *Clin Trials* 1987; 24: 137–142.

104. Perea EJ, Ayarra J, Garcia Iglesias MC, Garcia Luque I, Loscertales J. Penetration of cefuroxime and ceftazidime into human lungs. *Chemotherapy* 1988; 34: 1–7.

105. Panteix G, Harf R, de Montclos H, Verdier MF, Gaspar A, Leclercq M. Josamycin pulmonary penetration determined by broncho-alveolar lavage in man. *J Antimicrob Chemother* 1988; 22: 917–921.

106. Morita J, Hamaguchi N, Yoshizawa K, Niki S, Kondo K. Study on cefotaxime in respiratory surgery: transfer to lung tissue and kinetics in serum. *Jpn J Antibiot* 1989; 42: 2406–2411.

107. Reid TM, Gould IM, Golder D, *et al.* Respiratory tract penetration of ciprofloxacin. *Am J Med* 1989; 87: Suppl. 5A, 60S–61S.

108. Valcke YJ, Vogelaers DP, Colardyn FA, Pauwels RA. Penetration of netilmicin in the lower respiratory tract after once-daily dosing. *Chest* 1992; 101: 1028–1032.

109. Bergogne-Berezin E. Pharmacokinetics of antibiotics into lower respiratory tract. Limits of bringing such aninformation [Pharmacocinétique des antibiotiques dans les voies respiratoires inférieures. Limites de l'apport de cette information]. *Med Mal Infect* 1992; 22, Spécial: 103–113.

110. Martin C, Ragni J, Lokiec F, *et al.* Pharmacokinetics and tissue penetration of a single dose of ceftriaxone (1,000 milligrams intravenously) for antibiotic prophylaxis in thoracic surgery. *Antimicrob Agents Chemother* 1992; 36: 2804–2807.

111. Lamer C, De Beco V, Soler P, *et al.* Analysis of vancomycin entry into pulmonary lining fluid by bronchoalveolar lavage in critically ill patients. *Antimicrob Agents Chemother* 1993; 37: 281–286.

112. Conte JE Jr, Golden JA, Duncan S, McKenna E, Zurlinden E. Intrapulmonary pharmacokinetics of clarithromycin and of erythromycin. *Antimicrob Agents Chemother* 1995; 39: 334–338.

113. Conte JE Jr, Golden J, Duncan S, McKenna E, Lin E, Zurlinden E. Single-dose intrapulmonary pharmacokinetics of azithromycin, clarithromycin, ciprofloxacin, and cefuroxime in volunteer subjects. *Antimicrob Agents Chemother* 1996; 40: 1617–1622.

114. Patel KB, Xuan D, Tessier PR, Russomanno JH, Quintiliani R, Nightingale CH. Comparison of bronchopulmonary pharmacokinetics of clarithromycin and azithromycin. *Antimicrob Agents Chemother* 1996; 40: 2375–2379.

115. Schüler P, Zemper K, Borner K, Koeppe P, Schaberg T, Lode H. Penetration of sparfloxacin and ciprofloxacin in alveolar macrophages, epithelial lining fluid and polymorphonuclear leucocytes. *Eur Respir J* 1997; 10: 1130–1136.

116. Nix DE. Intrapulmonary concentrations of antimicrobial agents. *Infect Dis Clin North Am* 1998; 12: 631–646.

117. Imaizumi M, Niimi T, Uchida T, *et al.* Clinical study on transfer into lung tissue and postoperative prophylactic effect of new cephamycin antibiotics, particularly cefotetan and cefbuperazone]. *Jpn J Antibiot* 1998; 41: 437–459.

118. Carcas AJ, Garcia-Satue JL, Zapater P, Frias-Iniesta J. Tobramycin penetration into epithelial lining fluid of patients with pneumonia. *Clin Pharmacol Ther* 1999; 65: 245–250.

119. Allegranzi B, Cazzadori A, Di Perri G, *et al.* Concentrations of single-dose meropenem (1 g *iv*) in bronchoalveolar lavage and epithelial lining fluid. *J Antimicrob Chemother* 2000; 46: 319–322.

120. Gotfried MH, Danziger LH, Rodvold KA. Steady-state plasma and intrapulmonary concentrations of levofloxacin and ciprofloxacin in healthy adult subjects. *Chest* 2001; 119: 1114–1122.

121. Rodvold KA, Danziger LH, Gotfried MH. Steady-state plasma and bronchopulmonary

concentrations of intravenous levofloxacin and azithromycin in healthy adults. *Antimicrob Agents Chemother* 2003; 47: 2450–2457.

122. Amsden GW. Advanced-generation macrolides: tissue-directed antibiotics. *Int J Antimicrob Agents* 2001; 18: Suppl. 1, S11–S15.

123. Johnson JD, Hand WI, Francis JB, King-Thompson NL, Corwin RW. Antibiotic uptake by alveolar macrophages. *J Lab Clin Med* 1980; 95: 429–439.

124. Tulkens PM. Intracellular distribution and activity of antibiotics. *Eur J Clin Microbiol Infect Dis* 1991; 10: 100–106.

125. Gladue RP, Bright GM, Isaacson RE, Newborg MF. *In vitro* and *in vivo* uptake of azithromycin (CP-62,993) by phagocytic cells: possible mechanism of delivery and release at sites of infection. *Antimicrob Agents Chemother* 1989; 33: 277–282.

126. Steinberg TH. Cellular transport of drugs. *Clin Infect Dis* 1994; 19: 916–921.

127. Wilcox M, Kervitsky A, Watters LC, King TE Jr. Quantification of cells recovered by bronchoalveolar lavage. *Am Rev Respir Dis* 1988; 138: 74–80.

128. Conte JE Jr, Golden JA, Kipps J, Zurlinden E. Intrapulmonary pharmacokinetics of linezolid. *Antimicrob Agents Chemother* 2002; 46: 1475–1480.

129. Conte JE Jr, Golden JA, Duncan S, McKenna E, Zurlinden E. Intrapulmonary concentrations of pyrazinamide. *Antimicrob Agents Chemother* 1999; 43: 1329–1333.

130. Hand WL, Boozer RM, King-Thompson NL. Antibiotic uptake by alveolar macrophages of smokers. *Antimicrob Agents Chemother* 1985; 27: 42–45.

131. Carlier MB, Zenebergh A, Tulkens PM. Cellular uptake and subcellular distribution of roxithromycin and erythromycin in phagocytic cells. *J Antimicrob Chemother* 1987; 20: Suppl. B, 47–56.

132. De Duve C, de Barsy T, Poole B, Trouet A, Tulkens P, Van Houf F. Lysosomotropic agents. *Biochem Pharmacol* 1974; 23: 2495–2531.

133. Amsden GW. Pneumococcal macrolide resistance: myth or reality? *J Antimicrob Chemother* 1999; 44: 1–6.

134. Khor SP, Bozigian H, Mayersohn M. Potential error in the measurement of tissue to blood distribution coefficients in physiological pharmacokinetic modeling. *Drug Metab Dispos* 1991; 19: 486–490.

135. Kroening U, Liebig S, Wundschock M. Tobramycin - Spiegel in menschlichen Lungengewebe. *Infection* 1978; 6: 231–235.

136. Thadepalli H, Mandal AK, Bach VT, Oparah SS. Tissue levels of doxycycline into the human lung and pleura. *Chest* 1980; 78: 304–305.

137. Klasterky J, Thys JP. Mombelli G. Comparative studies of intermittent and continuous administration of aminoglycosides in the treatment of bronchopulmonary infections due to gram-negative bacteria. *Rev Infect Dis* 1981; 3: 74–83.

138. Brun Y, Forey F, Gamondes JP, Tebib A, Brune J, Fleurette J. Levels of erythromycin in pulmonary tissue and bronchial mucus compared to those of amoxycillin. *J Antimicrob Chemother* 1981; 8: 459–466.

139. Ohkuda K, Ichinose T, Inaba H, Sakuma T, Tanita T. Time-course of the concentration of cefotiam in human extra-vascular pulmonary tissue. *Nippon Kyobu Shikkan Gakkai Zasshi* 1991; 29: 225–230.

140. Nix DE, Goodwin SD, Peloquin CA, Rotella DL, Schentag JJ. Antibiotic tissue penetration and its relevance: impact of tissue penetration on infection response. *Antimicrob Agents Chemother* 1991; 35: 1953–1959.

141. Decré D, Bergogne-Bérézin E. Pharmacokinetics of quinolones with special reference to the respiratory tract tree. An update. *J Antimicrob Chemother* 1993; 31: 331–343.

142. Cruciani M, Gatti G, Lazzarini L, *et al.* Penetration of vancomycin into human lung tissue. *J Antimicrob Chemother* 1996; 38: 865–869.

143. Danesi R, Lupetti A, Barbara C, *et al.* Comparative distribution of azithromycin in lung tissue of patients given oral daily doses of 500 and 1000 mg. *J Antimicrob Chemother* 2003; 51: 939–945.

144. Cohen SH, Hoeprich PD, Demling R, *et al.* Entry of four cephalosporins into the ovine lung. *J Infect Dis* 1984; 149: 264–270.

145. Cazzola M, Polverino M, Guidetti E, *et al.* Penetration of cefonicid into human lung tissue and lymph nodes. *Chemotherapy* 1990; 36: 325–331.

146. Brigham KL, Snapper JR. Lung lymph composition and flow in normal and abnormal states. *In*: Fishman AP, ed. Pulmonary Diseases and Disorders. New York, McGraw-Hill, 1988; pp. 909–918.

147. Kobayashi T, Hirai K, Kawashima A, *et al.* The distribution of cefotaxime in serum, lung lymph and lung tissue of sheep. *Jpn J Antibiot* 1985; 38: 102–106.

148. May DG, Stratton CW, Denney WD, Watts FL, Bernard GR, Branch RA. Vancomycin entry into lung lymph in sheep. *Antimicrob Agents Chemother* 1987; 31: 1689–1691.

149. McGee ZA, Woods ML. Pathogenic mechanisms in bacterial respiratory tract infections. *In*: Sande MA, Hudson LD, Root RK, eds. Respiratory Infections. New York, Churchill Livingstone, 1986; pp. 1–11.

150. Cazzola M, Siniscalchi C, Vinciguerra A, Santangelo G, Matera MG, Rossi F. Evaluation of lung tissue and hilar lymph node concentrations of azithromycin. *Int J Clin Pharmacol Ther Toxicol* 1994; 32: 88–91.

151. Ryan DM. Pharmacokinetics of antibiotics in natural and experimental superficial compartments in animals and humans. *J Antimicrob Chemother* 1993; 31: Suppl. D, 1–16.

152. Herkner H, Müller MR, Kreischitz N, *et al.* Closed chest microdialysis to measure antibiotic penetration into human lung tissue. *Am J Resp Crit Care Med* 2002; 165: 273–276.

153. Muller M. Science, medicine, and the future: Microdialysis. *BMJ* 2002; 324: 588–591.

154. Joukhadar C, Derendorf H, Müller M. Microdialysis. A novel tool for clinical studies of anti-infective agents. *Eur J Clin Pharmacol* 2001; 57: 211–219.

155. Joukhadar C, Frossard M, Mayer BX, *et al.* Impaired target site penetration of ß-lactams may account for therapeutic failure in patients with septic shock. *Crit Care Med* 2001; 29: 385–391.

156. Tomaselli F, Dittrich P, Maier A, *et al.* Penetration of piperacillin and tazobactam into pneumonic human lung tissue measured by *in vivo* microdialysis. *Br J Clin Pharmacol* 2003; 55: 620–624.

157. Eisenberg EJ, Conzentino P, Eickhoff WM, Cundy KC. Pharmacokinetic measurement of drugs in lung epithelial lining fluid by microdialysis: aminoglycoside antibiotics in rat bronchi. *J Pharmacol Toxicol Methods* 1993; 29: 93–98.

158. Martínez Martínez MS, Gutiérrez Hurtado B, Colino Gandarillas CI, Martínez Lanao J, Sánchez Navarro A. *In vitro* study of experimental factors affecting the microdialysis results. *Analytica Chimica Acta* 2002; 459: 143–150.

159. Teixeira LR, Sasse SA, Villarino MA, Nguyen T, Mulligan ME, Light RW. Antibiotic levels in empyemic pleural fluid Chest 2000; 117: 1734–1739.

160. Lode H, Dzwillo G. Investigations of the diffusion of antibiotics into the human pleural space. *In*: Siegenthaler W, Luthy R, eds. Current Chemotherapy and Immunotherapy. Washington DC, American Society for Microbiology, 1978; pp. 386–388.

161. Cole DR, Pung J. Penetration of cefazolin into pleural fluid. *Antimicrob Agents Chemother* 1977; 11: 1033–1035.

162. Walstad RA, Hellum KB, Blika S, Dale LC, Dredriksen T, Myhre KI, Spencer GR. Pharmacokinetics and tissue penetration of ceftazidime: studies on lymph, aqueous humour, skin blister, cerebrospinal and pleural fluid. *J Antimicrob Chemother* 1983; 12: Suppl. A, 275–282.

163. Yamada H, Iwanaga T, Nakanishi H, Yamaguchi M, Iida K. Penetration and clearance of cefoperazone and moxalactam in pleural fluid. *Antimicrob Agents Chemother* 1985; 27: 93–95.

164. Benoni G, Arosio E, Cuzzolin L, Vaona B, Raimondi MG, Lechi A. Penetration of ceftriaxone into human pleural fluid. *Antimicrob Agents Chemother* 1986; 29: 906–908.

165. Kimura M, Matsushima T, Nakamura J, Kobashi Y. Comparative study of penetration of lomefloxacin and ceftriaxone into transudative and exudative pleural effusion. *Antimicrob Agents Chemother* 1992; 36: 2774–2777.

166. Joseph J, Vaughan LM, Basran GS. Penetration of intravenous and oral ciprofloxacin into sterile and empyemic human pleural fluid. *Ann Pharmacother* 1994; 28: 313–315.

167. Jacobs F, Marchal M, Francquen P, Kains JP, Ganji D, Thys JP. Penetration of ciprofloxacin into human pleural fluid. *Antimicrob Agents Chemother* 1990; 34: 934–936.

168. Dalhoff A. A review of quinolone tissue pharmacokinetics. *In*: Fernandes PB, ed. Quinolones. Barcelona, JR Prous Science Publ, 1989; pp. 277–312.

169. Elliott AM, Berning SE, Iseman MD, Peloquin CA. Failure of drug penetration and acquisition of drug resistance in chronic tuberculous empyema. *Tubercle Lung Dis* 1995; 76: 463–467.

170. Thys JP, Serruys-Schoutens E, Rocmans P, Herchuelz A, Vanderlinden MP, Yourassowsky E. Amikacin concentrations in uninfected postthoracotomy pleural fluid and in serum after intravenous and intrapleural injection. *Chest* 1984; 85: 502–505.

171. Cazzola M, Matera MG, Terzano C, Blasi F, Marsico SA. Delivering antimicrobials to the lungs: considerations for optimising outcomes. *Am J Respir Dis* 2002; 1: 261–272.

172. Chisholm DR, DeRegis RG, Behr DA. Therapeutic efficacy of cefadroxil and cephalexin for pneumonia in a rat test model. *Antimicrob Agents Chemother* 1986; 301: 105–109.

173. Azoulay-Dupuis E, Bedos JP, Vallee E, Hardy DJ, Swanson RN, Pocidalo JJ. Antipneumococcal activity of ciprofloxacin, ofloxacin, and temafloxacin in an experimental mouse pneumonia model at various stages of the disease. *J Infect Dis* 1991; 163: 319–324.

174. Vallée E, Azoulay-Dupuis E, Pocidalo JJ, Bergogne-Bérézin E. Pharmacokinetics of four fluoroquinolones in an animal model of infected lung. *J Antimicrob Chemother* 1991; 28: 39–44.

175. Veber B, Vallée E, Desmont JM, Pocidalo JJ, Azoulay-Dupuis E. Correlation between macrolide lung pharmacokinetics and therapeutic efficacy in a mouse model of pneumococcal pneumonia. *J Antimicrob Chemother* 1993; 32: 473–482.

176. Plouffe J, Schwartz DB, Kolokathis A, *et al.* Clinical efficacy of intravenous followed by oral azithromycin monotherapy in hospitalized patients with community-acquired pneumonia. The Azithromycin Intravenous Clinical Trials Group. *Antimicrob Agents Chemother* 2000; 44: 1796–1802.

177. Cazzola M, Caputi M, Santangelo G, Vinciguerra A, Di Perna F, Polverino M. A five-day course of dirithromycin in the treatment of acute exacerbation of severe chronic obstructive pulmonary disease. *J Chemother* 1997; 9: 279–284.

178. Neu HC. Activity of macrolides against common pathogens *in vitro*. *In*: Bryskier AJ, Butzler J-P, Neu HC, Tulkens PM, eds. Macrolides; Chemistry, Pharmacology and Clinical Uses. Arnette-Blackwell, Paris, 1993; pp. 167–182.

179. Sides GD, Cerimele BJ, Black HR, Busch U, DeSante KA. Pharmacokinetics of dirithromycin. *J Antimicrob Chemother* 1993; 31: Suppl. C, 65–75.

180. Bergogne-Bérézin E. Predicting the efficacy of antimicrobial agents in respiratory infections – is tissue concentration a valid measure? *J Antimicrob Chemother* 1995; 35: 363–371.

181. Panteix G, Harf R, Desnottes JF, *et al.* Accumulation of pefloxacin in the lower respiratory tract demonstrated by bronchoalveolar lavage. *J Antimicrob Chemother* 1994; 33: 979–985.

182. Nolting A, Costa TD, Vistelle R, Rand KH, Derendorf H. Determination of free extracellular concentrations of piperacillin by microdialysis. *J Pharm Sci* 1996; 85: 369–372.

183. Müller M, Haag O, Burgdorff T, *et al.* Characterization of peripheral-compartment kinetics of antibiotics by *in vivo* microdialysis in humans. *Antimicrob Agents Chemother* 1996; 40: 2703–2709.

184. Ellner PD, Neu HC. The inhibitory quotient. A method for interpreting minimum inhibitory concentration data. *JAMA* 1981; 246: 1575–1578.

185. Cazzola M. Pulmonary pharmacokinetics of dirithromycin allow a 5-day treatment of acute bacterial exacerbation of chronic bronchitis. *Drugs of Today* 1995; 31: 105–109.

186. Cunha BA. Antibiotic pharmacokinetic considerations in pulmonary infections. *Semin Respir Infect* 1991; 6: 168–182.

187. Fraschini F, Scaglione F, Cogo R, Casali W, Falchi M, Gattei G. Bactericidal effect of ceftriaxone versus imipenem plus cilastin in bronchial secretion. *Chemotherapy* 1988; 34: Suppl. 1, 3–15.

188. Maesen FPV, Beeuwkes H, Davies BI, Buytendijk HJ, Brombacher PJ, Wessman J. Bacampicillin

in acute exacerbations of chronic bronchitis - a dose-range study. *J Antimicrob Chemother* 1976; 2: 279–285.

189. Maesen FPV, Geraedts WH, Davies BI. Cefaclor in the treatment of chronic bronchitis. *J Antimicrob Chemother* 1990; 26: 456–457.

190. Cazzola M, Matera MG, Noschese P. Parenteral antibiotic therapy in the treatment of lower respiratory tract infections. Strategies to minimize the development of antibiotic resistance. *Pulm Pharmacol Ther* 2000; 13: 249–256.

191. Delacher S, Derendorf H, Hollenstein U, *et al.* A combined *in vivo* pharmacokinetic–*in vitro* pharmacodynamic approach to simulate target site pharmacodynamics of antibiotics in humans. *J Antimicrob Chemother* 2000; 46: 733–739.

192. Cazzola M, Matera MG. Interrelationship between pharmacokinetics and pharmacodynamics in choosing the appropriate antibiotic and the dosage regimen for treating acute exacerbations of chronic bronchitis. *Respir Med* 1998; 92: 895–901.

193. Odenholt-Tornqvist I, Lowdin E, Car O. Pharmacodynamic effects of subinhibitory concentrations of ß-lactam antibiotics *in vitro. Antimicrob Agents Chemother* 1991; 35: 1834–1839.

194. Cazzola M, Matera MG, Donner CF. Pharmacokinetics and pharmacodynamics of newer oral cephalosporins: implication for treatment of community-acquired lower respiratory tract infections. *Clin Drug Invest* 1998; 16: 335–346.

195. Vogelman B, Gudmundsson S, Leggett J, Turnidge J, Ebert S, Craig WA. Correlation of antimicrobial pharmacokinetic parameters with therapeutic efficacy in an animal model. *J Infect Dis* 1988; 158: 831–847.

196. Craig WA. Interrelationship between pharmacokinetics and pharmacodynamics in determining dosage regimens for broad-spectrum cephalosporins. *Diagn Microbiol Infect Dis* 1995; 22: 89–96.

197. Cazzola M, Noschese P, Vinciguerra A, Di Perna F, Califano C, Berra A. Le correlazioni esistenti tra farmacocinetica polmonare e farmacodinamica permettono di ipotizzare l'utilizzo del ceftazidime alla dose di 1 g una sola volta al giorno nel trattamento delle riacutizzazioni batteriche della broncopneumopatia cronica ostruttiva con danno funzionale moderato. *Minerva Med* 1998; 89: 15–22.

198. Thomas JK, Forrest A, Bhavnani SM, *et al.* Pharmacodynamic evaluation of factors associated with the development of bacterial resistance in acutely ill patients during therapy. *Antimicrob Agents Chemother* 1998; 42: 521–527.

199. Highet VS, Forrest A, Ballow CH, Schentag JJ. Antibiotic dosing issues in lower respiratory tract infection: population-derived area under inhibitory curve is predictive of efficacy. *J Antimicrob Chemother* 1999; 43: 55–63.

200. Cazzola M, Di Perna F, Boveri B, Di Marco F, Diamare F, Centanni S. Interrelationship between the pharmacokinetics and pharmacodynamics of cefaclor advanced formulation in patients with acute exacerbation of chronic bronchitis. *J Chemother* 2000; 12: 216–222.

201. Vallée E, Azoulay-Dupuis E, Bauchet J, Pocidalo JJ. Kinetic disposition of temafloxacin and ciprofloxacin in a murine model of pneumococcal pneumonia. Relevance for drug efficacy. *J Pharmacol Exp Ther* 1992; 262: 1203–1208.

CHAPTER 3

Interaction of antibacterial agents with host respiratory defences

M.T. Labro

Correspondence: M.T. Labro, NSERM U479, CHU X. Bichat, 16 rue Henri Huchard, Paris, 75018, France.

Respiratory tract diseases are a major cause of morbidity and mortality worldwide [1]. Indeed, the respiratory tract is one of the main routes in which pathogens can gain access to the body. The lung maintains a highly sophisticated defence system, enabling it to combat permanent aggressions. This defence system consists of structural, mechanical, secretory and cellular mechanisms. The pathogenetic mechanisms of microorganisms and the clinical status of the host may explain the panorama of the main respiratory pathogens involved in respiratory infections. In addition, a dysregulation of the defence system itself can generate many respiratory diseases, with/without superinfections.

This chapter will discuss the host's respiratory immune system, the main effects of antibacterial agents on immunomodulatory characteristics, and the antibiotics which have given promises for the treatment of respiratory and other noninfectious diseases.

The respiratory immune system

Respiratory Defences

The respiratory defence system and its various components have been dealt with in many papers and will be only reviewed briefly (table 1) [2–4]. The first line of defence comes from barriers such as mucus and cilia, followed by a battery of mediators (lactoferrin, lysozyme, immunoglobulins, antimicrobial proteins, collectins and defensins) and phagocytic cells that constitute the innate response. Activation of these components can lead directly to lysis of pathogens, or to destruction through opsonisation or the recruitment of inflammatory cells. Alveolar macrophages are the most common cells in the lower respiratory tract and have several important roles in both the innate and acquired immune response to bacterial infections. Various pathogens have evolved strategies to persist and multiply within macrophages. Alveolar macrophages are also important in the acquired immune response as they present antigens to T cells and produce a large number of regulatory cytokines and mediators. Even in the absence of inflammation, polymorphonuclear neutrophils (PMN) are concentrated in the pulmonary capillaries compared to the systemic blood. Inflammatory stimuli such as bacteria or mediators increase the number of PMN within the capillaries. PMN recruitment into the lung upon bacterial/inflammatory challenge is dependent upon various families of adhesion molecules including selectins and the β2-integrins. Adaptive immune responses are required to defend the lung against pathogens that survive in normal macrophages and extracellular organisms that evade phagocytosis. Lymphocytes determine the specificity of the immune response. Activated T-lymphocytes provide

Eur Respir Mon, 2004, 28, 45–63. Printed in UK - all rights reserved. Copyright ERS Journals Ltd 2004; European Respiratory Monograph; ISSN 1025-448x. ISBN 1-904097-32-4.

Table 1. – Respiratory defence mechanisms

Factors	Role
Airway Defences	
Anatomical barriers	
Airway reflexes	Clearance of entrapped material
Muco-ciliary clearance	
Immunological defences	Bacterial killing
Innate	
Lactoferrin	Opsonin, complement binding, virus
Antimicrobial peptides and proteins	neutralisation, agglutination,
Neutrophils	
Epithelia	
Adaptive	
Ig (secretory IgA, IgG)	
LT (adenoids, tonsils, bronchus-associated LT 80% B cells),	Local immunity
Ag-presenting cells,	Antigen capture and processing.
Alveolar unit	
Alveolar lining fluid: surfactant	Opsonisation
Collectins SPA, SPD	ROS activation (SPA *in vitro*)
Phospholipids	Killing;
Enzymes	Antiprotease action
IgG complement	Defence, mediator release
α1 antitrypsin	Specific immune response, inflammation
Cells: macrophages (85%)	
Neutrophils (2%)	
Lymphocytes (10%; T>B cells)	

Ig: immunoglobulin; LT: lymphoid tissue: Ag: antigen; SPA: surfactant protein A; SPD: surfactant protein D.

cytokines which activate macrophages and lyse infected antigen-presenting cells. Antibodies produced by plasma cells facilitate microbial clearance through opsonisation, complement fixation and antibody-dependent cytotoxicity. Different populations of T lymphocytes may dramatically alter the balance between clearance of the pathogen and induction of tissue damage depending on the cytokines they secrete.

Inflammation

The respiratory tract is a fragile tissue so that the price of excessive or inappropriate inflammatory responses may itself be very high. Reactive oxygen and nitrogen species are generated by several inflammatory and structural cells of the airways. These oxidant species may have important effects on different lung cells as regulators of signal transduction, activators of key transcription factors, and modulators of gene expression and apoptosis. An increased oxidative stress accompanied by reduced endogenous antioxidant defences may have a role in the pathogenesis of a number of inflammatory pulmonary diseases including asthma and cystic fibrosis. An imbalance between oxidants and antioxidants has also been considered in the pathogenesis of smoking-induced lung diseases, such as chronic obstructive pulmonary disease (COPD), particularly emphysema. Tumour necrosis factor (TNF), and interleukin (IL)-8 strongly prime the PMN oxidative burst in response to bacterial peptides in whole blood; these cytokines may play a critical role in bacterial killing *in vivo* and in the surrounding tissue injury, secondary to pathological inflammatory reactions. For instance, TNF and IL-8 plasma levels have been correlated with the production of reactive oxygen species (ROS) by stimulated PMN and with the lung injury score in patients with Adult Respiratory Distress Syndrome.

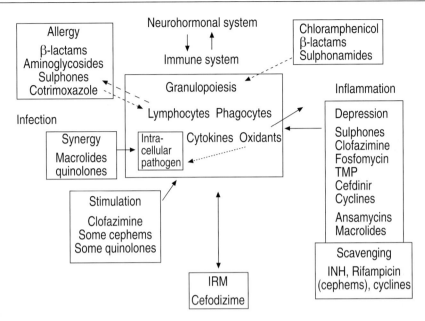

Fig. 1. – Schematic presentation of the classification of immunoregulatory properties.

Antibacterial agents as immunomodulators

General aspects

The immunomodulatory properties of antimicrobial agents and their clinical impact, have been a focus of worldwide interest in recent years [5–8]. A rough classification of the immunoregulatory properties of antibacterial agents has been proposed [5] and slightly modified [7]. A schematic presentation is given in figure 1.

There are many possibilities in the host-(microbe)-antibiotic interplay. These general aspects have been reviewed by LABRO [7]. The focus here is on two aspects in relation to the host's respiratory defences, firstly the cellular accumulation which underlies intracellular bioactivity, and secondly the modulation of cellular functions, which can interfere with antibacterial defences and/or the inflammatory response.

Cellular accumulation and intracellular bioactivity

Extensive studies have been made on the cellular penetration, location and bioactivity of antibacterial agents [5, 7, 9–11]. The cell subsets which have been preferentially analysed in this context are the phagocytes, in particular PMN owing to their large numbers and easy recovery from venous blood. The main parameter used to compare drugs is the ratio of accumulation, *i.e.* the ratio between the cellular (cell-associated) and extracellular concentrations (C/E). A simplified presentation of the accumulation of most antibacterial agents within human phagocytes is given in table 2.

An important question raised by these experiments is the impact of cellular accumulation on intracellular bioactivity. Intracellular uptake, although a necessary condition for bioactivity, is not the sole factor involved [5, 9–11]. Antibiotic accumu-lation is also the basis of tissue-directed pharmacokinetics, and the direct modulation of

Table 2. – Schematic classification of phagocytic uptake of antibacterial agents

Drugs	PMN C/E	Mo/MP	Characteristics
Poor Accumulation			
β-Lactams	<1		Passive difusion
Meropenem	2–10	3–12	
Imipenem	3–0.3	3.7–0.8	Transient accumulation
Aminoglycosides	<1	2–4	Slow accumulation pinocytosis
Daptomycin	0.6		
Moderate accumulation (*e.g.* passive diffusion, lipophilicity)			
Cyclines	1–3	2–4	Cytoplasm, nucleus
Fosfomycin	~2		
Isoniazid	~1	~1	Cytosol
Ethambutol	1–5	0.1–9.5	
Chloramphenicol	3–10	2–4	
Sulfamethoxazole	1.7		
Metronidazole	1	0.5	
Lincomycin	1.6–3	0.6–2	
Trimethoprim	6–21	3	
Brodimoprim	74		
Quinolones (most)	3–10	4–10	Cytosol, rapid efflux
Grepafloxacin	66		
Pefloxacin	4–10		Active transport systems
Ciprofloxacin	4–10		Two active transport systems
Lomefloxacin, ofloxacin, norfloxacin, possibly others			Two active transport system?
Fusidic acid	2–4		
Rifampicin	2.4–9.2		
Rifabutin			
Rifapentin	88	6	
Strong accumulation (*e.g.* active mechanisms)			
Macrolides	>10–>100		Active transport (uptake/efflux)
Clindamycin	~10	8–24	Possible nucleoside transport system
Coumermycin	11–17[#]		
Teicoplanin	52 (13)[¶]	41	Membrane associated
Streptogramins			
RP 54476	34 (120 min)[¶]		
RP 57669	50 (120 min)[¶]		

C/E: cellular/extracellular concentration ratio; Mo: monocyte; MP: macrophage; PMN: polymorphonuclear neutrophils; [#]: measured by bioactivity; [¶]: measured in J 774 cells.

phagocyte functions or metabolism by high drug concentrations. Tissue-directed pharmacokinetics has mainly been studied with macrolides and may explain the low serum level of these agents relative to their high tissue concentrations. This concept is based on the rapid and massive accumulation by blood PMN, which are rapidly attracted to the infected site and supposes that the intracellular drug is slowly released in its bioactive form along the migration route up to its final destination. Some elegant *in vitro* experiments have lent weight to this concept but no consensus has yet been reached. Another point of importance relative to the intracellular accumulation of antibiotics, is the understanding of the mechanisms which underlie the entry and efflux of drugs. Highlights on cellular uptake mechanisms have been provided [5] Macrolides, particularly erythromycin A derivatives, have been extensively studied in this context [10–12]. An active transport system has been suggested and the putative carrier seems to be common to all macrolides, irrespective of their chemical structure. Various data also favour the existence of an active efflux system in PMN. There are some arguments suggesting a link between the P-glycoprotein (P-gP) family involved in the active efflux of various hydrophobic compounds and the macrolide carrier. Theoretically, the analysis of drug uptake by host cells *ex vivo, i.e.* after drug administration to volunteers, patients or infected/noninfected animals, is a more clinically relevant approach than *in vitro* studies. However, the possibility of drug efflux during cell recovery can lead to understatement of the results. Despite these difficulties, the majority of studies have confirmed the cellular concentration of macrolides, particularly those with moderate efflux, and their persistent accumulation in lung tissues and alveolar macrophages [12, 13].

Immunomodulatory effects of antibacterial agents in vitro

The modulation of immune activity in vitro may involve a direct modulation of cell functions or an interference with immune by-products, for instance oxidants or enzymes.

Direct interference with immune by-products. Artefactual conditions such as scavenging of oxidant species may lead to false appreciations of the actual effect of an antibiotic on phagocyte activity [7, 14]. Appropriate controls using cell-free oxidant generating systems can help to characterise the target of antibiotic action. Rifampicin quenches superoxide anions and cyclines scavenge hypochlorous acid (HOCl) as do clofazimine and various aminothiazolyl cephalosporins. Penicillin G and ampicillin inhibit the chemiluminescence of PMN and cell-free systems by scavenging HOCl and hydrogen peroxide (H_2O_2), whereas chloramphenicol increases it. Dapsone and isoniazid directly interfere with myeloperoxidase (MPO) and impair the production of HOCl by the MPO-H_2O_2-halide system. Cefdinir, a hydroxy-imino-aminothiazolyl cephalosporin, impairs MPO activity in the external medium but not in the phagolysosome, likely because it does not enter neutrophils. The impact of these effects on bactericidal function and the tissue destructive potential of neutrophils has been questioned. Various *in vitro* experiments suggest, for instance, that some β-lactams may have a cytoprotective role or can prevent antiprotease inactivation by activated neutrophils. Other direct interferences with immune factors concern the modulation of enzyme activities, *e.g.* metallo-proteinases, collagenase, gelatinase, which are crucial in inflammation. Rifamycins, cyclines and macrolides show a marked inhibition of various enzyme activities, which may at least partly, correlate to the antiinflammatory activity of these molecules.

Modulation of immune cell activities. The modulation (stimulation/inhibition) of immune cell activities is the most widely investigated and controversial area. Owing to their critical role in host defence and pathological inflammation, as well as in the generation of the adaptive immune response, phagocytes represent a privileged target to the immunomodulatory potential of antibacterial agents. The main effects of the different families of antibacterial agents (and where possible, the molecular mechanism) will be given below. For simplification, only references not cited in LABRO [7] will be given.

Aminoglycosides. There are controversial data on the inhibitory effect of amino-glycosides at therapeutic concentrations on PMN chemotaxis (oriented migration), oxidative metabolism and yeast killing. Various mechanisms have been advanced: they include binding to negatively charged membrane phospholipids leading to membrane disturbances, specific binding to inositol biphosphate resulting in the inhibition of phospholipase C, and inhibition of protein kinase C.

Ansamycins. Two functional activities seem to be modified by ansamycins: chemotaxis and oxidant production. Rifampicin competes for receptors on neutrophils with small peptide chemoattractants, *e.g.* N-formyl-methionyl-leucyl-phenylalanine, but not with serum-derived chemoattractants. These effects occur at concentrations attained during rifampicin therapy and are not due to rifampicin toxicity. Rifamycin SV, rifampicin and rifapentine inhibit *in vitro* neutrophil chemotaxis in the range of their therapeutic levels. The effect of rifamycin SV, rifamycin B, rifampicin and 30 semisynthetic derivatives on human neutrophil functions such as locomotion, superoxide production and degranulation stimulated by specific agonists has been investigated by SPISANI *et al.* [15, 16]. The derivatives displayed inhibitory activities covering the whole range of activities tested. Among the newly synthesised compounds, the most active were the derivatives carrying an acidic substituent at C3. Rifampicin decreases phyto-haemaglutinin (PHA) and concanavalin A (ConA)-induced proliferation, and inhibits also leukocyte-induced angiogenesis *in vitro*. A suppression of interferon (IFN)-γ production by mouse T lymphocytes cultivated 4 days with *Listeria monocytogenes* has been observed with rifampicin. Recently, two new ansamycin derivatives which induce a heat shock response *in vitro* were shown to increase messenger ribonucleic acid (mRNA) levels of the inhibitory IκBα protein, suggesting that inhibition of nuclear factor κB (NFκB) activation could contribute to their suppressive effects [17]. One of these compounds, geldamycin, inhibits both IL-2 and IFN-γ production induced by anti-CD3 and anti-CD28 or phorbol myristate acetate (PMA) and anti-CD28. Lastly, PAHLEVAN *et al.* [18] have demonstrated that rifamycin B, rifapentine, rifamycin SV, rifabutin and rifampicin inhibited both TNF-α and PMA-induced NF-κB activation in Jurkat T cells.

β-lactam antibiotics. Many data are available on the *in vitro* immunomodulatory effects of β-lactam antibiotics but no class or subgroup effects have been demonstrated, however, particular aspects linked to chemical features have been identified. With the exception of cefodizime, which seems to be endowed with immune response modifier (IRM) activity, β-lactam induced modulation of immune responses does not appear to be of major clinical relevance. Scarce and often controversial data have been reported on the effect of β-lactams on cytokine release. The amoxycillin-clavulanic acid combination, which increases the phagocytic and microbicidal activity of PMN, also elicist the production of IL-1β and IL-8 by lipopolysaccharide (LPS)- and Klebsiella-stimulated PMN. The IRM antibiotic cefodizime [19] stimulates the proliferative response of lymphocytes, increases the phagocytotic and bactericidal activity of PMN, and down-modulates the production of pro-inflammatory cytokines by stimulated monocytes. Contrary to all β-lactams, cefodizime significantly increases colony formation by granulocyte-monocyte progenitors.

Benzylpyrimidines. Trimethoprim (TMP) alone or in combination with sulphamethoxazole, has an inhibitory effect on PMN functions. Brodimoprim, in which the methoxy group in position four of the benzyl ring of the TMP molecule is replaced by a bromine atom, displays greater lipophilicity and cellular uptake than TMP, and no inhibitory effect on PMN function.

Cyclines. The first report of a depressive effect of cyclines on phagocytosis dates back to the early 1950s. Since then, these drugs have been widely studied in this context, with most reports confirming an inhibitory action on various phagocyte functions at therapeutic concentrations. Few studies have investigated the effect of cyclines on cytokine production, paradoxically minocycline and to a lesser extent tetracycline, increases IL-1β secretion by LPS-stimulated human monocytes. Various mechanisms (chelation of Ca^{2+}, binding of intracellular Mg^{2+}, photodamage of PMN, and artefactual scavenging of HOCl) have been proposed to explain the inhibitory action of cyclines. Structure-activity relationships indicate a parallel increase in lipid solubility and inhibitory properties.

Fosfomycin. Fosfomycin has demonstrated imunomodulatory activity on B and T lymphocyte functions, and also inhibits histamine release from basophils; it decreases the production of various inflammatory cytokines by phagocytes and interferes with neutrophil functions [20]. Fosfomycin decreases the rate of synthesis of TNF-α and IL-1, but increases that of IL-6.

Fusidic acid. Fusidic acid inhibits PMN functions *in vitro*, without markedly altering those of monocytes. Its possible value as an immunosuppressive agent has been promoted in human immunodeficiency virus infection, although direct antiviral activity has also been forwarded.

Gyrase B inhibitors. At therapeutic concentrations coumermycin impairs chemotaxis, superoxide anion production and intracellular killing of PMN. Novobiocin effectively suppresses the production of various cytokines (IL1, IL-6 and IL-10) by LPS-stimulated monocytes.

Isoniazid. The antimycobacterial activity of isoniazid has been attributed to its oxidative metabolism by mycobacterial peroxidases. This chemical reactivity explains its inhibition of the MPO-H_2O_2-halide system and also its potential toxicity after oxidisation by activated leukocytes.

Lincosamides. Clindamycin has long appeared as a forerunner in antimicrobial chemotherapy and presented as a possible immunomodulator in infection in the early 1980s. Since then, controversial data (enhancement, decrease or no effect) on phagocyte functions have been reported with various techniques, depending on drug concentrations.

Macrolides. An extended classification of macrolides from the classical definition of Woodward presents a vast continuum of macrocyclic lactonic structures in which some molecules are mainly antibacterial (true macrolides) whereas others possess mainly immunosuppressant activity (FK 506, rapamycin) or antifungal activity with host cell inhibitory properties (bafilomycins, concanamycins). Over the past few years, there has been continuous research into the development of new macrolide antibiotics by chemical modifications of the existing natural derivatives. All these compounds display a homogeneous antimicrobial spectrum and the capability to concentrate within host cells. This property has been the major reason behind the search for new compounds targeting intracellular pathogens. Renewed interest in this family has come from the demonstrated therapeutic efficacy of various erythromycin A derivatives in noninfectious inflammatory diseases. Updates in this area have been provided recently [7, 21–24]. Down-modulation of pro-inflammatory cytokine and oxidant production by phagocytes seems to be the two key events supporting the anti-inflammatory activity of some macrolides. Individual susceptibility to the immunomodulating activity of macrolides has been shown for both cytokine production and oxidant production. Structure activity studies have shown that only erythromycin A derivatives, including the azalide azithromycin, impair the phagocyte oxidative burst in a time- and concentration-dependent manner and directly stimulate exocytosis by human neutrophils. The chemical entity responsible for these effects was shown to be the L cladinose at position three of the lactone ring, but this does not rule out the possibility that other structures may also interfere with phagocytic transductional targets [25, 26]. Roxithromycin also inhibits the release of reactive oxygen species from eosinophils, which are believed to injure epithelial cells at inflamed sites, resulting in airway hyperresponsiveness [27].

The clinical relevance of the antioxidant properties of macrolides is difficult to establish. High concentrations of the drugs, which impair the PMN oxidative burst, do not alter the bactericidal activity [28]. The antioxidant properties of macrolides could be beneficial in airway inflammation by protecting the ciliated epithelium against damage inflicted by bioactive phospholipid sensitised phagocytes. Macrolides interfere with cytokine production *in vitro*, generally decreasing pro-inflammatory cytokine production by stimulated phagocytes while increasing that of the anti-inflammatory cytokine IL-10 [21–23, 29]. Modulation of pro-inflammatory cytokine production has also been observed in eosinophils, mastocytes, lymphocytes and in nonphagocytic cells including nasal epithelial cells from polyps of patients with chronic sinusitis, human bronchial epithelial cells and a lung fibroblast cell line. In general, the suppression of cytokine release is accompanied by a parallel decrease in mRNA expression. Transcription of the genes for the pro-inflammatory cytokines is regulated by NFκB). Clarithromycin suppresses NFκB activation induced by TNF-α in human monocytic U-937 cells, a T cell line (Jurkat), and a pulmonary epithelial cell line (A549), and by staphylococcal enterotoxin A in peripheral blood mononuclear cells. This inhibition is not linked to the expression preservation of the IκBα protein [30]. In the human bronchial epithelial cell line BET-1A, clarithromycin inhibits TNF-α induced IL-8 gene expression, mainly *via* the AP-1 binding site [31]. In T cells, erythromycin downregulates IL-8 gene expression by inhibiting transcriptional activation of NF-κB, whereas the macrolide-like immunosuppressive agent FK506 inhibits both NF-κB and NF-AT [32]. Clarithromycin suppresses IL-8 production by bacterial extracts-stimulated monocytes and THP-1 and modifies the expression of other genes through AP-1 and NF-κB [33]. The effects of erythromycin, clarithromycin and josamycin on gene expression profiles have been studied in long-term cultures of small airway epithelial cells [34]. Among ~20,000 genes examined only nine revealed changes in cells treated with erythromycin (including filamin Aα and HSP70/HSP90-organising protein (HOP), both being repressed by erythromycin). Filamin interacts with TNF receptor-associated factor 2 which is required for signal transduction from TNFR and can also mediate activation of NF-κB. HOP could be the target of macrolides in psoriasis, since psoriatic keratinocytes express higher levels of this protein than normal cells. In addition, clarithromycin and erythromycin, but not josamycin, altered the expression of four genes whose functions are unknown, but could represent molecular targets for development of new anti-inflammatory drugs.

In human umbilical vein endothelial cells infected with *Chlamydia pneumoniae* or stimulated with TNF-α, azithromycin and roxithromycin but not clarithromycin, cause significant decreases in neutrophil and monocyte transendothelial migration (TEM), compared with antibiotic-free controls [35]. Azithromycin decreases IL-8 and monocyte chemotactic protein-1, whereas roxithromycin only decreases IL-8. These latter effects may, partly at least effect monocyte and neutrophil TEM inhibition by azithromycin and roxithromycin. Other macrolide-induced modifications of mammalian cell functions or metabolism have been described (modulation of adhesion molecules, accelerated apoptosis of neutrophils, inhibition of HL-60 cell growth, decreased glycoconjugate secretion by cultured human airway cells, and decrease in nitric oxide synthase and cyclooxygenase expression in rat macrophages). Although clarithromycin does not display direct cytotoxicity for tumour cells, it inhibits expression of the genes coding for tumour necrosis factor (TNF)-α, and matrix metalloproteinase-9 by tumour cells. A direct inhibitory effect on tumour cell growth has been shown with roxithromycin and a 17-membered-ring azalide. The proliferation of nasal polyp fibroblast lines is also inhibited by roxithromycin *in vitro*. The resistance of cancer cells to anticancer drugs is mediated by membrane-associated proteins belonging to the adenosine triphosphate binding cassette (ABC) transporter proteins, that include P-glycoproteins (P-gp) and multidrug resistance-associated protein (MRP). Macrolides interfere with the functioning of P-gp or MRP, and reverse the multiple drug resistance phenotype. The diversity of effects of macrolides on host cells raises the possible existence of a common (possible multiple) cellular target of macrolide action. It is tempting to link these effects to those of the immunosuppressanst FK506 or rapamycin and, by analogy to the mechanism of action of these drugs, to look for a putative macrolide-specific immunophilin governing the cellular action of these drugs.

Peptides. In general, peptide antibiotics do not significantly alter immune functions at therapeutic concentrations. The ability of polymyxin B to bind the lipid A portion of LPS is unfortunately associated with toxicity, which contraindicates its general use in septic shock.

4-Quinolones. No class effect has been shown with quinolones, however, significant synergy with oxidative species for intracellular bactericidal activity has been reported with some molecules. High concentrations of ofloxacin and fleroxacin potentiate the chemiluminescence response of PMN, whereas other quinolones (sparfloxacin, lomefloxacin, grepafloxacin, AM-1155, *etc.*) significantly decrease it. Norfloxacin increases oxidant production by mouse macrophages and enhances the mobilisation of reduced nicotinamide adenine dinucleotide phosphate (NADPH) oxidase subunits [36]. The effects of 4-quinolones on mediator (cytokine) production by monocytes are widely documented. At high concentrations pefloxacin and ciprofloxacin decrease IL-1 production by LPS-stimulated human monocytes, and ciprofloxacin and ofloxacin decrease TNF-α production, this is possibly due to the cyclic adenosine monophosphate accumulation. A suppressive effect of therapeutically achievable concentrations of trovafloxacin on the synthesis of IL-1-α and β, IL-6, IL-10, granulocyte-monocyte colony-stimulating factor and TNF-α by LPS-stimulated human monocytes has been observed. A similar effect has been reported with moxifloxacin although the authors noted a strong interindividual variability [37]. Grepafloxacin inhibits the production of IL-1α and β, and the expression of IL-1α and β, IL-6 and IL-8 mRNA, suggesting an effect at the gene transcription level [38]. In addition, various authors have observed that 4-quinolones alter T and B lymphocyte functions and delay or suppress the proliferative response of human mononuclear cells.

Riminophenazines. Clofazimine increases superoxide anion production and degranulation by stimulated neutrophils, and TNF-α potentiates this enhancement. The pro-oxidative effect of clofazimine analogs is dependent on the nature of the alkylimino group at position 2 on the phenazine nucleus and, to a lesser extent, on halogenation. The underlying mechanism seems to involve a stimulation of phospholipase A2 activity with subsequent accumulation of arachidonic acid and lysophospholipids which act as second messengers to activate the oxidase.

Sulphones and sulphonamides. Dapsone inhibits neutrophil function such as chemotaxis and oxidant production. Dapsone impairs the production of prostaglandin E2 (PGE_2) by neutrophils, a possible explanation for dapsone-induced potentiation of cell-mediated immunity. In general, sulfonamides exert an inhibitory effect on phagocyte functions, and many agents in this class have been switched from infections to inflammatory diseases. Inhibition of the intracellular Ca^{2+} increase after stimulation has been reported with sulfasalazine and sulphapyridine.

In vivo *and* ex vivo *immunomodulatory effects of antibacterial agents*

Ansamycins. Rifampicin has been controversially described as an immunosuppressant. In a model of *Streptococcus pneumoniae*-induced meningitis in the rabbit, the leukocytes (neutrophils and monocytes) from rifampicin treated rabbits produced less reactive oxygen species than those from ceftriaxone treated animals. Whereas rifampicin releases less pro-inflammatory derivatives from bacteria than β-lactams, a direct effect on leukocytes present in the cerebrospinal fluid cannot be excluded. In B6AF1 mice, long-term treatment with rifampicin slightly stimulates production of antisheep red blood cell antibodies and suppresses cellular response. Little investigation has been undertaken in the *ex vivo* modulation of cytokine production by ansamycins. In a model of experimental chronic osteomyelitis due to *Staphylococcus. aureus* the antibacterial activity of the combination azithromycin and rifampicin was successful as determined by dramatic reduction in bone bacterial counts, but the levels of TNF-α (activity and mRNA) remained elevated throughout the observation period. In C57BL/6 mice actively immunised to develop experimental autoimmune encephalomyelitis, a single injection of geldanamycin at 3 days after immunisation reduced disease onset >50% suggesting that ansamycins can exert potent anti-inflammatory effects on brain glial cells and provide therapeutic benefit in neuroinflammatory diseases [17].

β-Lactams. A direct effect of ceftazidime on cytokine production has been suggested in a model of septic and nonseptic rats [39]. IL-6 concentrations were significantly elevated after ceftazidime administration to both septic (independently of LPS levels) and nonseptic rats, and TNF-α was also increased in nonseptic rats. Other authors have also suggested that the myelosuppressive effect of this drug is mediated by TNF release. However, in a randomised trial comparing imipenem and ceftazidime for the treatment of urosepsis, no differences in plasma endotoxin, IL-6 or TNF levels, or urinary endotoxin, IL-6 or IL-8 levels were found between the two treatment groups [40]. Among cephalosporins, cefodizime represents a peculiar case, whose immunomodulatory potential has been suggested by many *in vivo* and *ex vivo* experiments.

Fosfomycin. The immunomodulatory activity of fosfomycin has been demonstrated in two animal models. Fosfomycin and its enantiomer, which lacks antimicrobial activity, significantly increases the survival rate in a model of gut-derived *Pseudomonas. aeruginosa* sepsis and reduces serum levels of TNF-α, IL-1 and IL-6. In mice injected with LPS, fosfomycin significantly lowers the peak serum levels of TNF-α and IL-1β. The therapeutic benefit of fosfomycin has recently been investigated in a murine model of Sjögren's syndrome.

Fusidic acid. Fusidic acid protects mice from LPS and staphylococcal enterotoxin B induced lethality and suppresses the release of TNF-α and IFN-γ. Prophylactic administration of fusidin significatly increases survival in neonatal mice challenged with *Salmonella enteritidis* LPS and decreases peak values of TNF-α. The potential immunomodulatory effect of fusidic acid has also been demonstrated in a model of ConA-induced liver lesions.

Lincosamides. Renewed interest in clindamycin has been generated by its potential prophylactic effect in LPS-induced septic shock by inhibiting pro-inflammatory cytokine release [41].

Macrolides. Various aseptic animal models have emphasised the anti-inflammatory role of macrolides: in guinea pigs, clarithromycin suppresses the systemic and local inflammatory response after surgical trauma, and roxithromycin>erythromycin= clarithromycin>>azithromycin decreases the exudate volume, leukocyte accumulation and exudate PGE2 and TNF levels in rats with carrageenin induced pleurisy. Erythromycin (not josamycin) suppresses acute neutrophil influx into the lung and the intradermal Arthus reaction and intracellular adhesion molecule (ICAM)-1 adhesion molecule expression in the lesion of experimental extrinsic allergic alveolitis in mice after *Trichosporon mucoides* challenge [42]. In an experimental model of bleomycin-induced acute lung injury in mice [43] erythromycin, clarithromycin, and roxithromycin clearly inhibit the induction of vascular cell adhesion molecule-1 mRNA, and attenuate that of ICAM-1 and TNF-α mRNA; subsequently they inhibit leucocyte, especially PMN migration into the airspace during the early phase of lung injury and finally inhibit lung fibrosis. In calves experimentally infected with *Pasteurella haemolytica*, tilmicosin promotes neutrophil apoptosis and prevents further amplification of inflammatory injury in the infected lungs [44]. Control of bacterial growth may provide additional protection from deleterious inflammatory reactions, as shown in a mouse model of *S. pneumoniae* experimental pneumonia [45]. Erythromycin A-derived macrolides decrease the production of inflammatory cytokines *ex vivo* [46]. In an open-label pilot study 500 mg of clarithromycin, given *b.i.d.* to seven patients with mild-to-moderate asthma, acted synergistically with dexamethasone in suppressing lymphocyte activation. Nasal polyp fibroblast lines generated from patients treated with roxithromycin (300 mg·day^{-1} for 1 month) exhibit a lower proliferation rate *in vitro* as compared to lines from the same patients before roxithromycin treatment. Macrolides can decrease nitric oxide levels in nasal fluid, serum and spontaneous, or antigen-stimulated mononuclear cells from patients with allergic rhinitis, sinusitis, and asthma. Clarithromycin and roxithromycin may affect the functions of PMN in chronic sinusitis by modulating the expression of L-selectin and Mac-1 molecules, thereby attenuating PMN adhesion [47].

Quinolones. The potential *in vivo* suppressive effects of some quinolones has been noted in animal models. In mice injected with a lethal dose of LPS, trovafloxacin, ciprofloxacin and tosufloxacin significantly increase survival and reduce serum levels of IL-6 [48]. To date, the use of quinolones in inflammatory diseases has not proved beneficial. By contrast, new interest is stating to emerge the potential "immunostimulating" properties of some fluoroquinolones. *In vivo* treatment with ciprofloxacin enhances the repopulation of haematopoietic organs in sublethally irradiated mice and in lethally irradiated bone marrow transplanted mice. Accelerated recovery of neutrophils following prophylactic ciprofloxacin treatment of bone marrow transplant patients has also been observed.

Therapeutic use of immunomodulatory antibacterial agents

Immunodepression

The immunomodulatory activity of cefodizime has been investigated worldwide *in vitro*, *ex vivo* and *in vivo*, in humans and animals (both healthy and immunocompromised) [20]. Experimental models using immunocompromised animals have confirmed the improved efficacy of cefodizime compared to other cephalosporins. In addition, cefodizime modulated the inflammatory pulmonary response to heat-killed *Klebsaella pneumoniae* or *S. pneumoniae*. In humans, contrasting results have been obtained in healthy subjects and immunocompromised patients, immune parameters in healthy individuals given cefodizime are modestly affected or not modified, whereas in the case of depressed phagocytic functions, cefodizime administration restores the deficient parameter. Despite the abundance of published data, the development of cefodizime as an immunomodulatory antibiotic has been unsuccessful. No reports are available on the consequences of prophylactic administration of cefodizime in patients at risk of infections.

Inflammatory diseases

Because microorganisms can initiate an exaggerated inflammatory reaction and as pathogens which persist in cryptic reservoirs can be the underlying cause of chronic inflammation, the hypothesis that antibacterials can down regulate inflammation by suppressing its bacterial origin has held widespread support. A recent review has summarised the data concerning the anti-inflammatory potential of antibiotics [8]. Among the antibacterial agents of recognised value in this context are clofazimine, dapsone, sulfonamides, cyclines, ansamycins and macrolides. A summary of the latter three families is given in table 3.

Cyclines. Acne is a therapeutic target of cyclines. Inhibition of the proliferation of *Propionibacterium acnes* and interference with the inflammatory reaction seem to be involved. The efficacy of minocycline in rheumatoid arthritis (RA) has been reported in two open trials and in three double-blind controlled studies. A small trial performed in early diffuse scleroderma generated promise. Cyclines are also effective in various skin diseases including immunobullous disorders. Various models have assessed the benefit of cyclines in ischemia-reperfusion damages. Recently minocycline was shown to have neuroprotective effects in animal models of stroke/ischemic injury and Huntington's disease, and to prevent nigrostriatal dopaminergic neurodegeneration in the mouse model of Parkinson's disease. The inhibitory effect of these drugs on the activity of degradative enzymes such as matrix metalloproteinases (MMP) has been suggested to play a role in the improvement in periodontal disease. Tetracyclines by virtue of their MMP-inhibiting effect have been proposed as a novel therapeutic strategy in abdominal aortic aneurysms. However, MMPs play a pivotal role in protecting against pulmonary remodeling, and rats under chronic hypoxia treated with doxcline have higher pulmonary artery pressure and right heart ventricular more severe than controls. Further interesting hypotheses include the potential antitumor activity of doxycycline. The anti-inflammatory action of tetracycline has been proposed to be of benefit to prevent endotoxic shock by a blockade of LPS-induced TNF-α and IL-1 β secretion.

Ansamycins. The antimicrobial activity of ansamycins has been proposed to play a role in the treatment of various inflammatory diseases. Controversial results have been reported on the potential benefit of rifampicin in RA, but rifamycin displays antiarthritis activity in ankylosing spondylitis and juvenile pauci-or polyarticular RA. Treatment with rifabutin and clarithromycin or azithromycin may result in a substantial clinical improvement in Crohn's disease and justify the conduct of a randomised controlled trial. Paradoxical pro-inflammatory side-effects of various ansamycins have been described. Adverse effecst are more frequent with higher doses and in combination with the use of macrolide antibiotics.

Macrolides. The question of whether macrolides can attenuate inflammation was first raised some 20 yrs ago, when erythromycin and troleandomycin were shown to favourably affect the clinical status of patients with severe asthma. The recent interest in the anti-inflammatory potential of macrolides has been renewed with the Japanese experience of treating patients with diffuse panbronchiolitis (DPB) with erythromycin A or derivatives. In addition to the direct anti-inflammatory activity of some macrolides, it has also been suggested that these drugs could act indirectly by eliminating persistent pathogens, a possible source of chronic inflammation in atherosclerosis, asthma and arthritis. Since the initial publication of two small trials of roxithromycin and azithromycin in the prevention of acute ischemic events in patients with coranory artery disease (CAD), there has been phenomenal interest in the role of macrolides to

Table 3. – Summary of the therapeutic applications of immunomodulatory antibacterial agents

Antibacterial agents	Diseases	Mechanisms

Ansamycins
  C/E
    2–14 rifampicin
    61–88 rifapentine
	Rheumatoid arthritis[#]
	Ankylosing spondylitis
	Juvenile pauci/poly RA
	  (rifamycin SV)
	Crohn's disease
	  (rifabutin+macrolides)
	Atherosclerosis?
	  (CGP 43371 an ansamycin)
	Paradox
	  rifabutin+macrolides
	Uveitis[#] polyarthralgia/arthritis.
		Antibacterial activity
		  Mycobacteria plus possisbly others
		Hypolipidemic compounds
		Immunomodulatory effects
		  Phagocyte functions (oxidants, Chemotaxis)
		  Scavenging O_2^-
		  Metalloproteases
		    rifamycin
		  Cellular immunity
		    CD1b expression.
		  Angiogenesis[#]
		    P-gP expression[#]
		    Ligand for FMLP- R
		
		  Possible effect on NF-κB[#]
		  Possible effect on tyrosine kinase inhibition[#]

Cyclines
 	
  Cellular uptake
    C/E=2–4
	Acne
	RA
	  Minocycline
	Reactive arthritis
	Scleroderma
	  Minocycline
	Skin diseases
	Ischemia/reperfusion injury
	Abdominal aortic aneurysm
	Endotoxic shock
	Cancer
	  mouse model: Parkinson's
	    disease[#]
		Antibacterial activity
		  Chlamydia pneumonia
		  Mycoplasma sp.
		  Propionibacterium sp.
		  Possibly others
		
		Immunomodulatory effects
		  ↓ Phagocyte functions
		    Oxidants, cytokines, TNF, IL-1-[#]
		  ↓ Metalloproteinases
		  ↓ Angiogenesis
		  Scavenging
		    HOCl
		  ↓ NO synthase
		    PKC inhibition, Ca^{2+} chelation
		  ↑ P-gP expression[#]

Macrolides
 	
Only erythromycin A derivatives
  display anti-inflammatory
  activity)
C/E≥10–≥300
Active mechanism, relation
  with P-gP[#]
	Asthma[#]
	DPB
	
	CF?
	Bronchiectasis
	Sinusitis
	Polyposis
	Psoriasis
	
	Crohn's disease
	Acute inflammatory syndrome
	Arthritis?
	  (various animal models)
	Atherosclerosis[#]
	Cancer[#]
	  Lung cancer
		Antibacterial activity
		  C. pneumoniae, mycoplasma, H pylori,
		    P. aeruginosa[#]
		Bacterial virulence
		Steroid-sparing effect
		Immunomodulatory effects
		  phagocyte functions
		  ↓ oxidants, CT[#]
		
		Cytokines ↓ TNF, IL-1-, -8, -6; ↑ IL-10
		
		↓ LTB4
		↓ NO
		↑ Apoptosis
		↓ Angiogenesis
		↓ Bronchial responsiveness
		↓ Mucus production
		↓ Proliferation (fibroblasts)
		Cancer cells
		  ↓ proliferation?
		  ↓ production:TGF-β, TNF-α
		Metalloproteases
		Reverse MDR
		Modulation of the PLD-PPH pathway (PMN)
		  ↓ Ca^{2+}influx]
		Modulation of genes

57

Table 3. Continued

Antibacterial agents	Diseases	Mechanisms
		Induction of protein expression P-gP, others ↓ NF-κB in T cells, AP-1 in bronchial cells ↓ ↑ Gene expression.

C/E: Cellular/extracellular concentration; RA: rheumatoid arthritis; P-gP: P-glycoproteins; FMLP-R: N-formyl-methionyl-leucyl-phenylalanine receptor; NF-κB: nuclear factor- κB; TNF: tumour necrosis factor; IL: interleuken; HOCl: hypochlorous acid; NO: nitrous oxide; PKC: protein kinase C; DPB: diffuse panbronchiolitis; CF: cystic fibrosis; CT: chemotaxis; LTB4: leukotriene B4; TGF: tumour growth factor; MDR: multiple drug resistence; PLD-PPH: phospholipase D-phosphatidate-phosphohydrolase; PMN: polymorphonuclear neutrophils; AP-1: activator protein-1; ↑: increase; ↓: decrease.

prevent acute events in CAD [49]. Various large trials are ongoing, which involve mainly azithromycin. Other anti-inflammatory therapeutic effects of macrolides have been shown: clarithromycin modulates the acute inflammatory response associated with mastectomy resulting in better clinical outcome and oral erythromycin was used successfully to treat blepharokeratitis in five children. Macrolides have also been recently proposed to improve the clinical outcome of psoriasis. Recently an open label study has shown an impressive response to clarithromycin in a group of patients with active Crohn's disease.

Therapeutic uses of macrolides. Some examples of the therapeutic use of macrolides are given below:
Diffuse panbronchiolitis and cystic fibrosis. The revival of macrolides as anti-inflammatory agents was triggered by their phenomenal activity in DPB, in which they dramatically improve the prognosis. DPB is characterised by chronic inflammation of the bronchioles, which progresses insidiously and results in respiratory failure caused by repeated episodes of respiratory infections due mainly to *P. aeruginosa*. The prognosis of this disease has been radically transformed by the empirical use of long-term low-dose erythromycin. Only erythromycin A and its derivatives (including azithromycin) are effective. Various inflammatory parameters such as neutrophil infiltration and IL-8, leukotreine B4 and elastase levels in bronchoalveolar lavage fluid fall parallel to the disease improvement during erythromycin A therapy. Recently the relationships between radiological findings and pulmonary functions were evaluated in 24 patients before and 3 months after low-dose erythromycin therapy [50]. Positive correlations were observed between the improvement in centrilobular nodules, peripheral bronchial wall thickness and peripheral bronchiectasis, and the increase in percentage vital capacity.

Cystic fibrosis (CF) is the most common autosomal recessive disorder in Caucasians. The disease results from defects in a gene which encodes the cystic fibrosis transmembrane conductance regulator involved in the transport of electrolytes across cell membranes. Many clinical manifestations are related to defects in the epithelial transport of electrolytes and of fluid. However, it is in the lung that the most dramatic and life-threatening manifestations occur. The airways in the CF lung exhibit an extremely active inflammatory response which is greatly enhanced by the presence of bacteria but does occur early in life, perhaps as an intrinsic feature of CF epithelial cells. Inflammation leads to progressive bronchiectasis. There are remarkable similarities between CF and DPB in clinical and bacteriological aspects, although DPB only occurs in adults and does not appear to have a genetic basis. Due to the success of macrolides to treat patients with DPB, interest in these antibiotics to treat CF patients has increased. So far only limited trials have been conducted in CF [51–53].

Bronchiectasis. Bronchiectsis is a pathological feature of DPB and CF. The potential benefit of macrolides in non-CF bronchiectasis has also been assessed [54, 55]. A.low-dose erythromycin given for 8 weeks to 21 adult patients resulted in a significant increase in pulmonary parameters compared to a placebo-treated group and in a significant reduction in 24-hr sputum production [54]. However, roxithromycin given for 12 weeks to children did not modify lung function, although there was a significant reduction in airway responsiveness and an improvement in sputum properties in the treated group [55].

Asthma. The interest of macrolides in treating asthma was raised ~40 yrs ago with the use of troleandomycin. There are many trials demonstrating a reduction in steroid use in adult, steroid-dependent asthmatics and in children. However, other studies suggest that macrolides confer additional anti-inflammatory properties [56].

Other respiratory inflammatory diseases may benefit from macrolide therapy. Middle lobe syndrome is a distinct clinical entity characterised by right middle lobe atelectasis; latent lesional inflammation can be detected even when acute symptoms have disappeared. It was found two cases were resolved completely after the administration of a low dose of roxithromycin [57]. Although no placebo-controlled studies have been published, there are a number of clinical reports stating that long-term, low-dose macrolides are effective in treating chronic sinusitis incurable by surgery or glucocorticoids. The exact mechanism of action is not known, but it probably involves downregulation of the local host immune response as well as a downgrading of the virulence of the colonizing bacteria.

Lung cancer. Most studies dealing with the potential benefit of macrolides in cancer have involved Japanese patients with lung cancer. Long-term treatment with clarithromycin (400 mg·day^{-1} if the patient could tolerate it) was beneficial for patients with unresectable nonsmall cell lung cancer and appeared to increase the median survival of patients with advanced disease (535 *versus* 277 days) [58]. Various animal studies have been performed to analyse the benefit of macrolides in cancer.

Conclusions

The interest in the immunomodulatory potential of antibacterial agents is spreading worldwide. Outside their antibacterial activity, antibacterials can display immunomodulating properties that can have therapeutic importance. The clinical benefit of the immunostimulating/restoring effects of antibacterial agents is considered of minimal importance, compared to their direct antibacterial activity in the context of infectious diseases. In contrast to this new expectations are arising in antibacterials with immunodepressive/anti-inflammatory potential. The most important families of antibiotics of recognised value are cyclines, ansamycins and macrolides.

The potential danger of using antibacterial drugs outside their current indications (for example in inflammatory diseases), with a theoretically lengthy administration schedule is the induction of microbial resistance. This phenomenon has not yet been described after 10 yrs of the administration of macrolide to DPB patients in Japan. However the risk cannot be ignored. In a recent study, 18 episodes of acute exacerbations in chronic lower respiratory tract infections caused by *S. pneumoniae* during long-term macrolide therapy were investigated [59]. Intermediate resistance or resistance rates were 100% to erythromycin, 67% to clindamycin or minocycline and 11% to ampicillin, with coresistance to erythromycin, clindamycin and minocycline in one half of the episodes. All episodes were cured successfully with β-lactams or fluoroquinolones. The author concludes that attention should be paid to the trend of antibiotic susceptibility in *S. pneumoniae*. The search for antibiotic derivatives devoid of antibacterial activity but retaining immunomodulatory potential is of major interest. This has been proposed for instance with tetracycline and sulfamide derivatives. The use of the fosfomycin enantiomer may also be considered in the near future.

Summary

The respiratory tract is constantly confronted with a multitude of noxious agents that abound in the environment, including a variety of microbial pathogens. To cope with permanent aggressions, the lung maintains a highly sophisticated defence system. However, excessive or inappropriate inflammatory responses may have a role in the pathogenesis of a number of pulmonary diseases including asthma, diffuse panbronchiolitis, cystic fibrosis and chronic obstructive pulmonary disease, particularly emphysema. Outside their antibacterial activity, it is obvious that antibacterials can display immunomodulating properties that can have therapeutic importance. The modulation of immune functions is receiving major attention, particularly in the field of inflammatory diseases. Two nonmutually exclusive hypotheses are forwarded to explain the anti-inflammatory activity of various antibiotics. Firstly that inflammation is triggered by a latent/chronic infection due to a pathogen susceptible to the antibiotic, which generally, resides within host cells and secondly that antibiotics modulate one (various) components of the inflammatory response. Because phagocytes by uncontrolled use of the same mechanisms as those used to destroy pathogens (*i.e.* oxidative species, enzymes and mediators) can have detrimental effects on the host itself, they have a fundamental role in the pathogenesis of exaggerated inflammatory responses and are critical targets for the immunomodulatory effects of antibacterial agents.

The most important family of antibacterial agents of recognised value in this context are cyclines, ansamycins and macrolides.

Keywords: Antibacterial agents, inflammation, phagocytes, respiratory defences.

References

1. Murray CJL, Lopez AD. Mortality by cause for eight regions of the world. Global burden of disease study. *Lancet* 1997; 349: 1269–1276.
2. Reynolds HY. Normal and defective respiratory host defenses. *In*: Pennington JE ed. 3rd Edn Respiratory infections. Diagnosis and Management. New York, Raven Press, 1994; pp. 1–34.
3. Boyton RJ, Openshaw PJ. Pulmonary defences to acute respiratory infection. *Br Med Bull* 2002; 61: 1–12.
4. Labro MT. Immunopathology of respiratory infections. *Clin Microb Infect* 1998; 4: Suppl. 2, 1–7.
5. Labro MT. Immunomodulation by antibacterial agents. Is it clinically relevant? *Drugs* 1993; 45: 319–328.
6. Labro MT. Effect of antimicrobial agents on polymorphonuclear neutrophil functions. *In*: D. Raoult, ed. Antimicrobial Agents and Intracellular Pathogens. Boca Raton, CRC Press, 1993; pp. 87–135.

7.   Labro MT. Interference of antibacterial agents with phagocyte functions: immunomodulation or "immuno-fairy tales"? *Clin Microbiol Rev* 2000; 13: 615–650.

8.   Labro MT. Antibiotics as antiinflammatory agents. *Curr Op Inves Drugs* 2002; 3: 61–68.

9.   Silverstein SC, Kabbash C. Penetration, retention, intracellular localization, and antimicrobial activity of antibiotics within phagocytes. *Curr Op Hematol* 1994; 1: 85–91.

10. Labro MT. Intraphagocytic penetration of macrolide antibiotics. *In*: Bryskier AJ, Butzler JP, Neu HC, Tulkens PM, eds. Macrolides: Chemistry, Pharmacology and Clinical Uses. Paris, Arnette-Blackwell, 1993; pp. 379–381.

11. Labro MT. Effecs of macrolides on leukocytes and inflammation. *In*: S.H. Zinner, L.S. Young, J.F. Acar, H.C. Neu, eds. Expanding Indications for the New Macrolides, azalides and streptogramins. New York, Dekker, 101–116.

12. Labro MT. Cellular accumulation of macrolide antibiotics. Intracellular bioactivity. *In*: Schönfeld W, Kirst H, eds. Macrolide Antibiotics. Basel, Birkhäuser verlag AG. 2002; pp. 37–52.

13. Khair OA, Andrews JM, Honeybourne D, Jevons G, Vacheron F, Wise R. Lung concentrations of telithromycin after oral dosing. *J Antimicrob Chemother* 2001; 47: 837–840.

14. Labro MT, El Benna J. Interaction of antibiotics with the phagocyte oxidative burst. *In*: Faist E, Meakins JL, Schildberg FW, eds. Host Defense Dysfunction in Trauma, Shock and Sepsis. Berlin, Springer-Verlag, 1993; pp. 953–964.

15. Spisani S, Traniello S, Martuccio C, Rizzuti O, Cellai L. Rifamycins inhibit human neutrophil functions: new derivatives with potential antiinflammatory activity. *Inflammation* 1997; 21: 391–400.

16. Spisani S, Traniello S, Onori AM, Rizzuti O, Martuccio C, Cellai L. 3-(Carboxyalkylthio) rifamycin S and SV derivatives inhibit human neutrophil functions. *Inflammation* 1998; 22: 459–469.

17. Murphy P, Sharp A, Shin J, *et al.* Suppressive effects of ansamycins on inducible nitric oxide synthase expression and the development of experimental autoimmune encephalomyelitis. *J Neurosci Res* 2002; 67: 461–470.

18. Pahlevan AA, Wright DJ, Bradley L, Smith C, Foxwell BM. Potential of rifamides to inhibit TNF-induced NF-kappaB activation. *J Antimicrob Chemother* 2002; 49: 531–534.

19. Labro MT. Cefodizime as a biological response modifier: a review of its in-vivo, ex-vivo and in-vitro immunomodulatory properties. *J Antimicrob Chemother* 1990; 26: Suppl. C, 37–47.

20. Krause R, Patruta S, Daxböck F, Fladerer P, Wenisch C. The effect of fosfomycin on neutrophil function. *J Antimicrob Chemother* 2001; 47: 141–146.

21. Labro MT. Antiinflammatory activity of macrolides: a new therapeutic potential? *J Antimicrob Chemother* 1998; 41: Suppl. B, 37–46.

22. Labro MT. Immunological effects of macrolides. *Curr Op Infect Dis* 1998; 11: 681–688.

23. Labro MT. Antibiotics as anti-inflammatory drugs. *Curr Op Investig Drugs* 2002; 3: 61–68.

24. Jaffé A, Bush A. Anti-inflammatory effects of marolides in lung disease. *Pediatr Pulmonol* 2001; 31: 464–473.

25. Vazifeh D, Bryskier A, Labro MT. Effect of proinflammatory cytokines on the interplay between roxithromycin, HMR 3647, or HMR 3004 and human polymorphonuclear neutrophils. *Antimicrob Agents Chemother* 2000; 44: 511–521.

26. Abdelghaffar H, Kirst H, Soukri A, Babin-Chevaye C, Labro MT. Structure-activity relationships among 9-N-alkyl derivatives of erythromycylamine and their effect on the oxidative burst of human neutrophils *in vitro*. *J Chemother* 2002; 14: 132–139.

27. Cui CH, Honda K, Saito N, *et al.* Effect of roxithromycin on eotaxin-primed reactive oxygen species from eosinophils. *Int Arch Allergy Immunol* 2001; 125: Suppl. 138–41.

28. Vazifeh D, Abdelghaffar H, Labro MT. Effect of telithromycin (HMR 3647) on poly-morphonuclear neutrophil killing of *Staphylococcus aureus* in comparison with roxithromycin. *Antimicrob Agents Chemother* 2002; 46: 1364–1374.

29. Schultz MJ, Speelman P, van der Poll T. Erythromycin inhibits *Pseudomonas aeruginosa*-induced

tumor necrosis factor alpha production in human whole blood. *J Antimicrob Chemother* 2001; 48: 275–278.

30. Ichiyama T, Nishikawa M, Yoshitomi T, Hasegawa S, Matsubara T, Hayashi T, Furukawa S. Clarithromycin inhibits NF-kappaB activation in human peripheral blood mononuclear cells and pulmonary epithelial cells. *Antimicrob Agents Chemother* 2001; 45: 44–47.

31. Abe S, Nakamura H, Inoue S, *et al.* Interleukin-8 gene repression by clarithromycin is mediated by the activator protein-1 binding site in human bronchial cells. *Am J Respir Cell Mol Biol* 2000; 22: 51–60.

32. Aoki Y, Kao PN. Erythromycin inhibits transcriptional activation of NF-κB, but not NFAT, through calcineurin-independent signaling in T cells. *Antimicrob Agents Chemother* 1999; 43: 2678–2684.

33. Kikuchi T, Hagiwara K, Honda Y, *et al.* Clarithromycin suppresses lipopolysaccharide-induced interleukin-8 production by human monocytes through AP-1 and NF-kappa B transcription factors. *J Antimicrob Chemother* 2002; 49: 745–755.

34. Yamanaka Y, Tamari M, Nakahata T, Nakamura Y. Gene expression profiles of human small airway epithelial cells treated with low doses of 14- and 16-membered macrolides. *Biochem Biophys Res Comm* 2001; 287: 198–203.

35. Uriarte SM, Molestina RE, Miller RD, *et al.* Effect of macrolide antibiotics on human endothelial cells activated by *Chlamydia pneumoniae* infection and tumor necrosis factor-alpha. *J Infect Dis* 2002; 185: 1631–1636.

36. El Bekay R, Alvarez M, Carballo M, *et al.* Activation of phagocytic cell NADPH oxidase by norfloxacin: a potential mechanism to explain its bactericidal action. *J Leukoc Biol* 2002; 71: 255–261.

37. Araujo FG, Slifer TL, Remington JS. Effect of moxifloxacin on secretion of cytokines by human monocytes stimulated with lipolysaccharide. *Clin Microbiol Infect* 2002; 8: 26–30.

38. Ono Y, Ohmoto Y, Ono K, Sakata Y, Murata K. Effect of grepafloxacin on cytokine production *in vitro*. *J Antimicrob Chemother* 2000; 46: 91–94.

39. Alkharfy K, Kellum JA, Frye RF, Matzke GR. Effect of ceftazidime on systemic cytokine concentration in rats. *Antimicrob Agents Chemother* 2000; 44: 3217–3219.

40. Luchi M, Morrison DC, Opal S, *et al.* A comparative trial of imipenem versus ceftazidime in the release of endotoxin and cytokine generation in patients with gram-negative sepsis. *J Endotoxin Res* 2000; 6: 25–31.

41. Hirata N, Hiramatsu K, Kishi K, Yamasaki T, Ichimaya T, Nasu M. Pretreatment of mice with clindamycin improves survival of endotoxic shock by modulating the release of inflammatory cytokines. *Antimicrob Agents Chemother* 2001; 45: 2638–2642.

42. Miyajima M, Suga M, Nakagawa K, Ito K, Ando M. Effect of erythromycin on experimental extrinsic allergic alveolitis. *Clin Exp Allergy* 1999; 29: 253–261.

43. Li Y, Azuma A, Usuki J, Matsuda K, Aoyama A, Kudoh S. Attenuated mRNA induction of molecules associated with neutrophil migration by 14-membered ring macrolides inhibits bleomycin induced acute lung injury in mice. *J Nippon Med Sch* 2002; 69: 252–61.

44. Chin AC, Morck DW, Merrill JK, *et al.* 1998 Anti-inflammatory benefits of tilmicosin in calves with *Pasteurella haemolytica*-infected lungs. *Am J Vet Res* 1998; 59: 765–771.

45. Duong M, Simard M, Bergeron Y, Bergeron MG. Kinetic study of the inflammatory response in *Streptococcus pneumoniae* experimental pneumonia treated with the ketolide HMR 3004. *Antimicrob Agents Chemother* 2001; 45: 252–262.

46. Schultz MJ, Speelman P, Hack CE, Buurman WA, van Deventer SJH, van der Poll T. Intravenous infusion of erythromycin inhibits CXC chemokine production but augments neutrophil degranulation in whole blood stimulated with *Streptococcus pneumoniae*. *J Antimicrob Chemother* 2000; 46: 235–240.

47. Enomoto F, Andou I, Nagaoka I, Ichikawa G. Effect of new macrolides on the expression of adhesion molecules on neutrophils in chronic sinusitis. *Auris Nasus Larynx* 2002; 29: 267–269.

48. Khan AA, Slifer TR, Araujo FG, Suzuki Y, Remington JS. Protection against lipolysaccharide-induced death by fluoroquinolones. *Antimicrob Agents Chemother* 2000; 44: 3169–3173.

49. Grayston JT. Antibiotic treatment trials for secondary prevention of coronary artery disease events. *Circulation* 1999; 99: 1538–1539.

50. Yamada G, Igarashi T, Itoh E, Tanaka H, Sekine K, Abe S. Centrilobular nodules correlate with air trapping in diffuse panbronchiolitis during erythromycin therapy. *Chest* 2001; 1120: 198–202.

51. Jaffe A, Francis J, Rosenthal M, Bush A. Long-term azithromycin may improve lung function in children with cystic fibrosis. *Lancet* 1998; 351: 420.

52. Anstead ML, Kuhn RJ, Hartford LH, Craigmyle L, Halsey S, Kanga JF. Effect of chronic azithromycin on lung functions in cystic fibrosis. *Pediatr Pulmonol* 1999; 28: Suppl. 19, 283.

53. Ordonez CL, Stulbarg M, Grundland H, Liu JT, Boushey HA. Effects of clarithromycin on airway obstruction and inflammatory markers in induced sputum in cystic fibrosis: a pilot study. *Pediatr Pulmonol* 2001; 32: 29–37.

54. Tsang KW, Ho PI, Chan KN, *et al.* A pilot study of low-dose erythromycin in bronchiectasis. *Eur Respir J* 1999; 13: 361–364.

55. Koh YY, Lee MH, Sun YH, Sung KW, Chae JH. Effect of roxithromycin on airway responsiveness in children with bronchiectasis: a double-blind, placebo-controlled study. *Eur Respir J* 1997; 10: 994–999.

56. Cazzola M, Salzillo A, Diamant F. Potential role of macrolides in the treatment of asthma. *Monaldi Arch Chest Dis* 2000; 55: 231–236.

57. Kawamura M, Arai Y, Tani M. Improvement in right lung atelectasis (middle lobe syndrome) following administration of low-dose roxithromycin. *Respiration* 2001; 68: 210–214.

58. Mikasa K, Sawaki M, Kita E, *et al.* Significant survival benefit to patients with advanced non-small-cell lung cancer from treatment with clarithromycin. *Chemother* 1997; 43: 288–296.

59. Maeda K, Mikasa K, Konishi M, *et al.* Acute exacerbations due to *Streptococcus pneumoniae* in chronic lower respiratory infections during long-term macrolide therapy. *Kansenshogaku Zasshi* 2001; 75: 846–850.

β-Lactams and the lung

S. Gatermann*, T.T. Bauer#

*Dept of Medical Microbiology, University Hospital-Bergmannsheil, and #Dept of Internal Medicine III, Pneumology, Allergology and Sleep Medicine, Ruhr-University, Bochum, Germany.

Correspondence: T.T. Bauer, University Hospital-Bergmannesheil, Medical Clinic III, D-44789, Bochum, Germany.

Pulmonary infections are one of the leading causes of death to-date. An early randomised and placebo controlled trial with aminobenzene-sulphonamidopyridine in hospitalised patients with community-acquired pneumonia (CAP), showed a marked reduction in mortality [1]. However, beneficial effects for majority of patients with pulmonary infections, was only found after the introduction of penicillin. Penicillin belongs to the group of β-lactam antibiotics which nowadays comprise of an exceptionally large group of antibacterial compounds that share the β-lactam nucleus as a common structure for their antimicrobial activity. The β-lactam antibiotics act by binding to transpeptidases involved in cell wall synthesis. The antibiotic is cleaved during this process and binds irreversibly to the active centre of the transpeptidase, thereby inactivating the enzyme. Cell death is most likely to occur due to the unbalanced activity of the cell wall building enzymes, leading to an unstable cell wall which makes the bacterium prone to osmotic lysis [2]. Apart from the common β-lactam ring, a large number of different substitutients and structural features exist that define the different β-lactam classes and both their antibiotic spectrum and pharmacological properties. There are four different classes of β-lactams which have gained clinical importance these are penicillins, cephalosporins, carbapenems and to a lesser extent monobactams. The chemical structures of theses classes are summarised in figure 1.

Penicillins

Penicillins can be divided into several classes based on their main antibacterial activities [3, 4]. Natural penicillins like penicillin G are most active against non β-lactamase producing Gram-positive bacteria, anaerobes, Neisseria and *Treponema pallidum*. If natural penicillins are active against bacterial isolates, these agents are generally more active than semisynthetic penicillins. Therefore, the drugs of choice for a susceptible organism are the natural penicillins.

Penicillinase-resistant penicillins

Penicillinase-resistant penicillins are the drugs of choice for infections caused by β-lactamase producing staphylococci [3, 4]. For non β-lactamase producing strains these drugs are less active than their natural counterparts. They are not active against methicillin-resistant *Staphylococcus aureus* (MRSA).

Eur Respir Mon, 2004, 28, 64–77. Printed in UK - all rights reserved. Copyright ERS Journals Ltd 2004; European Respiratory Monograph; ISSN 1025-448x. ISBN 1-904097-32-4.

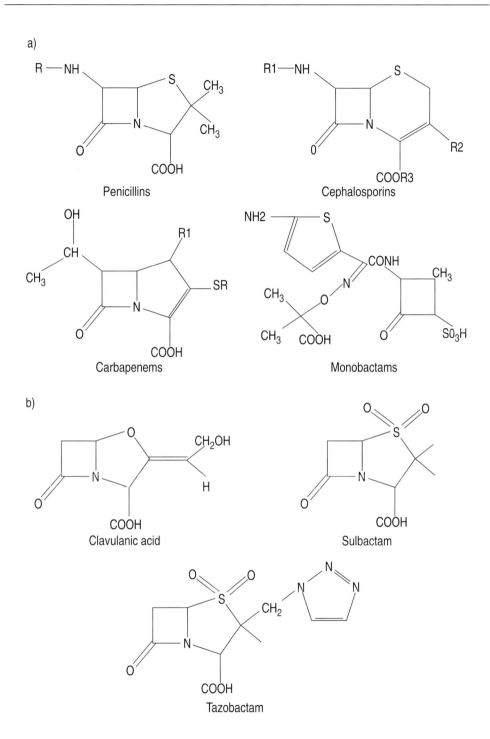

Fig. 1. – General structural formula of a) β-lactams and b) β-lactamase inhibitors. R1, R2, R3: substituents that determine antimicrobial spectra and bioavailability.

Aminopenicillins

Ampicillin and amoxicillin have spectra similar to that of natural penicillins [3, 4] but are also active against a number of Gram-negative bacteria like Enterobacteriaceae and *Haemophilus sp*. These penicillins are also the drugs of choice for the treatment of infections with Listeria or enterococci. Ampicillin is poorly absorbed after oral administration whereas amoxicillin is absorbed almost completely.

Ureidopenicillins

Ureidopenicillins extend the activity of ampicillin and include some ampicillin-resistant Enterobacteriaceae and strains of *P. aeruginosa* [3, 4]. Susceptibility, however, varies from hospital-to-hospital and even from ward-to-ward. In addition, ureidopenicillins may seem active against some ampicillin-resistant Enterobacteriaceae but may give rise to therapy failures when used in patients infected with these strains [5]. Mezlocillin is an ureidopenicillin with a spectrum similar to that of ampicillin. Its activity against many Enterobacteriaceae is higher than that of ampicillin although its *in vivo* activity is difficult to predict. Mezlocillin is not active against *P. aeruginosa* but its activity against Enterobacteriaceae supersedes that of ampicillin. Piperacillin is an ureidopenicillin that has an activity against Enterobacteriaceae that is comparable to that of mezlocillin, however, it is more active against *P. aeruginosa*. Piperacillin activity against enterococci, especially *Enterococcus faecium*, is lower than mezlocillin. Azlocillin is similar to acylaminopenicillin in that it has good activity against *P. aeruginosa* but reduced activity against Enterobacteriaceae when compared with mezlocillin and piperacillin.

Penicillin, penicillinase inhibitor combinations

The presently available β-lactamase inhibitors are β-lactams that do not have anti-bacterial activity (with the exception of *Acinetobacter sp.*) [6, 7]. These inhibitors bind to the β-lactamase and are cleaved by the enzyme, thereby they remain covalently attached to the active centre of the β-lactamase. Consequently, these molecules have been called suicide inhibitors. The β-lactamases produced by staphylococci, *Haemophilus spp., Neisseria spp., Moraxella catarrhalis, Escherichia coli* and *Klebsiella* are inhibited by these drugs. However other Enterobacteriaceae *e.g. Enterobacter sp.* or *Citrobacter freundii* produce β-lactamases that are not susceptible to the inhibitory action of β-lactamase inhibitors. Amoxicillin/clavulanic acid and ampicillin/sulbactam combinations are all active against β-lactamase producing *Staphylococci spp., Haemophilus influenzae, M. catarrhalis*, many *Klebsiella spp. and* many ampicillin resistent *E. coli*, in addition to microorganisms that are susceptible to ampicillin or amoxicillin. As the β-lactamase inhibitors do not inhibit chromosomally encoded AmpC β-lactamase, *Enterobacter spp., Citrobacter freundii, Morganella, Serratia* and *Providencia* are resistant. Piperacillin/tazobactam combines the spectra of amoxicillin/clavulanic acid and piperacillin and is also active against some strains of *Morganella morganii* and *Providencia sp*. In some countries an inhibitor *e.g.* sulbactam is available for free combination with other β-lactam anti-biotics. The spectra available for the combination usually include the active combination partner and the bacteria that produce staphylococcal or TEM and SHV β-lactamases.

Cephalosporins

The cephalosporins are arbitrarily grouped into "generations" (table 1) although this classification has been challenged by some authorities [8]. The first generation of

Table 1. – Overview of β-lactam properties

β-Lactam group	Substances	Important properties
Penicillins		
Natural penicillins	Penicillin G	IV application only. Active against non-β-lactamase-producing Gram-positive bacteria, Neisseria, *Treponema pallidum*.
	Penicillin V	Same spectrum as penicillin G, but orally available, not useful against syphilis.
Penicillinase-resistant penicillins	Oxacillin	Agent solely against β-lactamase-producing staphylococci.
	Flucloxacillin	Same as oxacillin.
Aminopenicillins	Ampicillin	IV, Spectrum similar to penicillin, but also active against some Enterobacteriaceae and non-β-lactamase producing *Haemophilus*; active against enterococci and Listeria.
	Amoxicillin	Same as ampicillin, but well absorbed after oral administration.
Ureidopenicillins	Mezlocillin	Similar to ampicillin but somehow more active against some Enterobacteriaceae; more active against enterococci than ampicillin.
	Piperacillin	Similar to mezlocillin but higher intrinsic activity to Enterobacteriaceae; also active against *Pseudomonas aeruginosa*, less active against enterococci, especially *Enterococcus faecium*.
	Azlocillin	Increased anti-pseudomonas activity relative to piperacillin or mezlocillin but less active against Enterobacteriaceae.
Penicillin/β-lactamase-inhibitor combinations	Ampicillin/ sulbactam	Spectrum includes organisms susceptible to ampicillin and some. Enterobacteriaceae resistant to ampicillin, Neisseria, *Moraxella catarrhalis*, Haemophilus, penicillinase-producing staphylococci.
	Amoxicillin/ clavulanic acid	Same as ampicillin/sulbactam but may have more adverse effects (hepatotoxicity).
	Piperacillin/ tazobactam	Includes organisms susceptible to piperacillin plus many. Enterobacteriaceae and penicillinase-producing staphylococci, *M. catarrhalis*, Haemophilus.
Cephalosporins		Cephalosporins are not active against enterococci and Listeria, only few are active against obligate anaerobes.
First generation cephalosporins	Cefazolin	Good activity against streptococci and staphylococci (except MRSA); some activity against *Escherichia coli*, but lower activity against other Enterobacteriaceae.
Second generation cephalosporins	Cefuroxim	Similar to cefazolin but more active against other *Enterobacteriaceae*.
	Cefotiam	Similar to cefuroxim.
	Cefoxitin	Good activity against Enterobacteriaceae and obligate anaerobes; not active against staphylococci and streptococci.
	Cefotetan	Same spectrum as cefoxitin.
Third generation cephalosporins	Cefotaxim	Increased activity against Enterobacteriaceae, highly active against streptococci, especially *Streptococcus pneumoniae*, including penicillin-resistant strains, Haemophilus, Neisseria, somehow reduced activity against staphylococci.
	Ceftriaxon	Main difference to cefotaxim is the exceptionally long half life allowing longer application intervals.
Cephalosporins with antipseudomonas activity	Ceftazidim	Especially active against Enterobacteriaceae, also active against *Pseudomonas aeruginosa*; reduced activity against staphylococci and streptococci.
	Cefepime	Spectrum includes Enterobacteriaceae and Gram-positive bacteria; also active against Pseudomonas but less so than ceftazidim.
	Cefpirome	Same as cefepime.
Carbapenems		
	Imipenem	Gram-positive and gram-negative bacteria. Including *Enterococcus faecalis*, but not *Enterococcus faecium*, Listeria and many strains of *Pseudomonas aeruginosa*. Active against many obligate anaerobic bacteria. *Stenotrophomonas maltophilia* is resistant as is *Burkholderia cepacia*.
	Meropenem	Similar to imipenem, but less active against gram-positive bacteria.

Table 1. Continued

β-Lactam group	Substances	Important properties
	Ertapenem	Spectrum similar to that of imipenem but somehow less active against Gram-positive microorganisms. Superior to imipenem in Enterobacteriaceae, enterococci are resistant, as are many pseudomonads.
Monobactams		
	Aztreonam	Only active against facultatively anaerobic Gram-negative bacteria and *Pseudomonas sp.* Gram-positive bacteria and anaerobic bacteria are always resistant.

IV: intavenous; MRSA: methicillin-resistant *Staphylococcus aureus.*

cephalosporins cefalotin and cefazolin show good activity against Gram-positive cocci but have only limited use against Gram-negative bacteria including *H. influenzae*. Second generation cephalosporins retain their good activity against Gram-positive cocci but are also active against some Enterobacteriaceae and *H. influenzae*. Cephalosporins of the third generation can be separated into two subgroups. The first subgroup has activity against a wide range of Enterobacteriaceae *e.g.* cefotaxim, and retain some activity against Gram-positive cocci especially pneumococci. The second subgroup *i.e.* ceftazidime has activity against Gram-negative bacteria especially Enterobacteriaceae and Pseudomonas but are only of limited use against Gram-positive cocci. Several new compounds, especially cefpirome and cefepime have been proposed to form a fourth generation of cephalosporins since these compounds have activity against Gram-positive cocci and Gram-negative bacteria including Pseudomonas. Most cephalosporins have only limited activity against anaerobic bacteria especially *Bacteorides fragilis*. Only the cefamycines *e.g.* cefoxitin show activity against these anaerobic bacteria. However, the position of the methoxy-group within these antibiotics results in the decreased activity these drugs have against Gram-positive cocci. No cephalosporin has activity against enterococci or Listeria.

First generation cephalosporins

The first generation cephalosporins, cefalotin and cefazolin show good activity against Gram-positive cocci but are of limited use for infection with Gram-negative bacteria including *H. influenzae*. The clinical use is nowadays mostly limited to prophylaxis during surgery.

Second generation cephalosporins

Cefuroxim and cefotiam show activities to Gram-positive cocci that are comparable to those of the first generation cephalosporins. Both agents are also active against a number of Enterobacteriaceae and *H. influenzae* as well as *M. catarrhalis*. In contrast, cefamandol has good activity against *S. aureus* but is an unreliable agent against β-lactamase producing *H. influenzae*. Cefamycines, *e.g.* cefoxitin and cefotetan, show increased activity against anaerobic bacteria and some Enterobacteriaceae. However, these agents have limited activity against Gram-positive cocci.

Third generation cephalosporins

Third generation cephalosporins cefotaxim, ceftizoxim and ceftriaxon possess superior activity against *Streptococcus pneumoniae*, *S. pyogenes*, *H. influenzae* and Neisseria. The agents are also active against *E. coli, Proteus mirabilis, Klebsiella sp.* and many other Enterobacteriaceae [9]. Their activity against *Pseudomonas sp., Stenotrophomonas maltophilia* and other nonfermentative Gram-negative rods is not clinically useful. The main difference between these various substances is the pharmakokinetic properties of ceftriaxon. The drug is mostly (90%) protein bound and has a half life of 8 h allowing a single dose per day and is excreted biliary and renally. Cefodizim has a similar spectrum of activity as cefotaxim but has limited activity against staphylococci.

Cephalosporins with antipseudomonal activity

Ceftazidim has excellent activity against many Gram-negative bacteria including *P. aeruginosa* but its activity against staphylococci and *B. fragilis* is low [10]. The more recent cephalosporins *e.g.* cefepime and cefpirome have broad antimicrobial activity including Gram-positive cocci, Haemophilus, Neisseria and many Enterobacteriaceae [8, 11]. They also have some activity against Pseudomonas since ~50% of strains are susceptible to these drugs.

Oral cephalosporins

Although orally available cephalosporins may be grouped with some effort into the categories mentioned above, it is more appropriate to group them in accordance with their clinical activity rather than their *in vitro* activity. This approach is more helpful in clinical/diagnostic terms as many of the oral cephalosporins are only partially absorbed and oral dosages are often much lower than the parenteral counter parts. Consequently, serum and tissue levels tend to be much lower with the oral cephalosporins in comparison with parenteral administration.

Cefalexin, cefadroxil and cefaclor have antimicrobial spectra similar to that of cefazolin, a first generation cephalosporin [12]. These antibiotics are active against Gram-positive bacteria but have low activity against Enterobacteriaceae. All have some activity against *H. influenzae* and *M. catarrhalis* although the β-lactamases of these species tend to destroy the agents. Loracarbef is a carbacefem antibiotic that has activity against staphylococci and streptococci including *S. pneumoniae* but has increased activity against *H. influenzae* and *M. catarrhalis*, particularly those strains that produce β-lactamase [13]. Cefixim is a derivative of cefotaxim and has an increased spectrum of activity especially against Gram-negative bacteria. It is active against *H. influenzae, S. pyogenes, Klebsiella spp., P. mirabilis, M. catarrhalis* and *S. pneumoniae*. It has low activity against staphylococci. Cefpodoxim proxetil and cefuroxim axetil are both only partially absorbed. Both are active against Gram-positive cocci, *H. influenzae*, staphylococci, *M. catarrhalis* and some *Enterobacteriaceae spp.* Ceftibuten has an *in vitro* activity similar to cefixim. It is active against *S. pyogenes, H. influenzae* and *M. catarrhalis* but not against staphylococci. However, it has low activity against pneumococci, but is highly active against many Enterobacteriaceae.

Carbapenems

Carbapenems are structurally related to the penicillins (fig. 1) and are extremely stable to most β-lactamases with the exception of metallo-β-lactamases [7, 14]. Currently there are three carbapenems available these are: imipenem, meropenem and ertapenem.

Imipenem

Imipenem differs from other β-lactam antibiotics because it is degraded by the renal dehydropeptidase I enzyme. Imipenem is therefore presently administered in combination with cilastatin, which is an inhibitor of dehydropeptidase, to prevent imipenem from being degraded. Imipenem is active against staphylococci, streptococci including *S. pneumoniae*, *Listeria sp.* and *Bacillus sp.* [15]. Most strains of *Enterococcus faecalis* are inhibited by imipenem although its action is only bacteriostatic not bactericidal however, *E. faecium* is resistant to imipenem. The drug is very active against Enterobacteriaceae and resistant strains have only rarely been described. Imipenem is also active against many strains of *P. aeruginosa* and Acinetobacter. However, *S. maltophilia* is resistant due to its production of a metallo-β-lactamase as is *Burkholderia cepacia*. Imipenem is active against many anaerobic bacteria, although resistant strains of Bacterioides have been described.

Meropenem

Meropenem is stable to dehydropeptidase I and can therefore be administered without cilastatin. The activity of meropenem towards Gram-negative bacteria supersedes that of imipenem although it is less active against Gram-positive bacteria [15]. Similarly to imipenem, meropenem is not active against *S. maltophilia* and *E. faecium*.

Ertapenem

Ertapenem is also stable to the dehydropeptidase enzyme. It has superior activity towards Enterobacteriaceae but is less active than Imipenem and Meropenem against Gram-positive bacteria and Pseudomonas [16]. Enterococci, including *E. faecalis*, are resistant to ertapenem. In contrast to imipenem and meropenem, ertapenem can be administered with a single, daily dose.

Monobactams

Monobactams have a unique structure and are monocyclic β-lactam antibiotics [14]. Aztreonam is currently the only monobactam available. The drug is active only against facultatively anaerobic Gram-negative bacteria like the Enterobacteriaceae and *Pseudomonas sp.* Gram-positive microorganisms and anaerobic bacteria are resistant. In Gram-negative bacteria the activity of this antibiotic is dependent on the β-lactamase that is produced by an individual bacterial strain. Strains of *Enterobacter cloacae* and *Citrobacter freundii* hyperproducing the chromosomal AmpC-β-lactamase are resistant, whereas strains of *M. morganii* and *Providencia stuartii* producing depressed AmpC-β-lactamases may be susceptible. *Haemophilus sp.*, *Neisseria sp.* and *Acinetobacter sp.* are usually susceptible, whereas *S. maltophilia* is resistant.

Adverse reactions

The main adverse effects from the administration of β-lactams are hypersensitivity reactions. Immediate anaphylactic immunoglobulin E (IgE)-mediated reactions and urticaria are rare, whereas skin rash is more common [17, 18]. It is important that the history of hypersensitivity reactions with a β-lactam antibiotic is carefully assessed as imprecise history could result in the patient not being administered with the most appropriate therapy for their infection. Several strategy management procedures have been described These comprise of detailed medical histories, skin testing and even desensitisation regimens [17–19]. Cross reactivity between penicillins and cephalosporins is probably less common than is usually assumed, however this is a matter of controversy. Cross reactions to carbapenems have been shown in 50% of penicillin skin-test-positive patients. Cross reactions to aztreonam are very weak if existing at all. Other adverse effects like neutropaenia, renal toxicity and seizures have been described to occur in penicillins but are usually rare events. Apart from hypersensitivity reactions cephalosporins can alter hemostasis mechanisms by acting as a vitamin K antagonist. This effect has especially been described for compounds carrying the methyl-thiotetrazol-group at position three. The same substituent is responsible for desulfiram-like reactions with these cephalosporins. With the administration of an antibiotic with clavulanic acid, hepatotoxicity may be more frequent than with other β-lactamase inhibitors [20].

Resistance

Bacteria that do not possess a cell wall, e.g. Mycoplasma sp., are always resistant to β-lactam antibiotics. Likewise, intracellular bacteria e.g. Chlamydia sp. or Legionella sp. are clinically resistant because the antibiotics never atain an intracellular concentration within the patients' cells that could inhibit the organism. There are three different mechanisms for acquired resistance towards β-lactam antibiotics in otherwise susceptible microorganisms [2, 4] these are as follows: 1) The production of an enzyme/s that can degrade the β-lactam antibiotic (β-lactamases). β-lactamases are enzymes that can cleave the β-lactam antibiotic and release it without being inactivated by it. 2) The alteration of the target enzymes which the β-lactam antibiotics combine with, either by point mutations or by the acquisition of alternative enzymes that are resistant to β-lactam activity. 3) The impeded diffusion of the antibiotic towards its target, this mechanism is restricted to Gram-negative bacteria and is especially frequent in P. aeruginosa.

β-lactamases

Until now >300 different β-lactamases have been described [7]. The enzymes differ in their capacity to cleave various β-lactams and some may be inhibited by β-lactamase inhibitors while others are inhibitor resistant. It is of great importance to recognise the more common enzymes as some bacteria harboring these β-lactamases may appear susceptible on routine testing but are known to respond poorly to the substances in vivo [2, 5, 21]. β-lactamases are usually grouped according to their activity towards various β-lactam classes, their susceptibility towards inhibition by β-lactamase inhibitors and according to their molecular properties. The identification of the enzymes enables the valuable prediction of in vivo activity of β-lactam antibiotics.

Target alteration

The affinity of the cell wall synthesising enzymes (also called penicillin-binding proteins) may be altered by point mutations. This mechanism is responsible for the development of penicillin-resistant pneumococci. In this species certain strains have acquired a number of mutations in genes for different penicillin-binding proteins that render these enzymes less susceptible to the action of penicillin and other β-lactams. In contrast the methicillin resistant *S. aureus* have acquired an additional penicillin binding protein called "MecA" that clearly does not originate in *S. aureus*. This enzyme also has a low affinity for β-lactams.

Impeded diffusion

In Gram-negative bacteria proteins of the outer membrane, called porins, govern the exchange of substances between the environment and the periplasmatic space and *vice versa*. Porins of many Gram-negative bacteria hinder access of penicillin G into the periplasmatic space. However, other more charged compounds can pass through the porins and exert the intended activity. It has been demonstrated that in some species *e.g.* *P. aeruginosa*, certain β-lactams (*e.g.* carbapenems) are transported across the outer membrane *via* a specific porin. Mutations that abolish production of this protein therefore cause *P. aeruginosa* to be resistant towards the antibiotic. In many other Gram-negative bacteria and with many other compounds, the subsequent consequences due to mutation are less clear but may lead the bacterial strain towards a less susceptible state [22].

Clinical use of β-lactams in pulmonary infections

All β-lactams are drugs of choice in pulmonary infections due to their favourable antimicrobial activity. However, the selection of the most appropriate β-lactam antibiotic for the patient must be governed by the answer to two questions: 1) what is the most probable bacteria that is causing the infection; and 2) what are the anticipated susceptibility properties of these infecting organisms. All the major properties of the β-lactams are summarised in table 1, this knowledge is crucial for the clinical success when administering these antibiotics. If infection with *Mycoplasma sp.*, *Chlamydia sp.* or *Legionella sp.* is suspected, β-lactams should not be used or must be used in combination with an antibiotic active against these bacteria, *e.g.*, a macrolide or a quinolone. There are three major classes of infection that can be treated with such agents: 1) acute exacerbations of chronic obstructive pulmonary disease (AE-COPD); 2) CAP; 3) nosocomial pneumonia.

There has been an ongoing debate on whether antibiotics are appropriate for the treatment of AE-COPD, as bacterial infection is a common, but probably not the only aetiology for this disorder [23–26]. The study by ANTHONISEN *et al.* [27] and co-workers is still a cornerstone for this debate. Their work demonstrated how patients with a Type I exacerbation (increase sputum volume, purulent sputum, and dyspneoa) appeared to benefit from the administration of antibiotic in comparison with those patients who only had less than two of the symptoms. More recent studies have also indicated that the severity of symptoms could be a guide for therapy with antibiotics[28, 29]. SOLER *et al.* [30] confirmed that >50% of patients with severe exacerbations and required mechanical ventilation had community-acquired endogenous pathogens in combination with Gram-negative Enterobacteriaceae, *P. aeruginosa* and/or a *Stenotrophomonas spp.* present in the tracheobronchial tree. Most of these pathogens were present in quantities acceptable for the diagnosis of pneumonia [30]. However, the additional evaluation of paired serologies revealed that ~20% of patients had also atypical bacterial pathogens (including *Chlamydia pneumoniae* in 12%), an observation confirmed by BLASE *et al.* [31]. However in severe exacerbations there is strong evidence that bacterial infection plays a crucial role in the majority of occasions. Since the evidence regarding the use of antibiotics is sparse and the placebo controlled trial yielded controversial results, it is not surprising that studies comparing β-lactams with other antibiotic are sparse [32–36]. CHODOSH *et al.* [37] compared the second-generation cephalosporin cefuroxim axetil with ciprofloxacin, in its ability to cure. The group not only examined the improvement or eradication rates for bacterial pathogens but they also examined the potential differences in the infection-free intervals after the antimicrobial treatment. Ciprofloxacin resulted equipotent as regards clinical resolution but had statistically significant higher eradication rates (96% *versus* 82%). However, this advantage did not translate into a longer infection-free interval. A similar design was performed with levofloxacin as a comparator, it also established equality of treatments [38].

In CAP *S. pneumoniae*, *H. influenzae*, and *S. aureus* are pathogens that can be potentially treated with β-lactams. In some situations Gram-negative bacteria *e.g.* Enterobacteriaceae may be suspected as the spectrum for which the β-lactam should be adapted [39]. As ~10–20% of *Haemophilus sp.*, 80–90% of *S. aureus* and all *Klebsiella sp.* produce a β-lactamase that would cleave susceptible penicillins, a β-lactam/lactamase inhibitor combination like ampicillin/sulbactam or a second generation cephalosporin like cefuroxim may be appropriate in this situation. In the presence of a previous hospitalisation, corticosteroid medication and/or structural lung disease infection with *P. aeruginosa* cannot be ruled out and piperacillin or ceftazidim may be appropriate. As both antibiotics are not active against β-lactamase-producing bacteria that may also be involved in the infection, it is probably advisable to combine piperacillin with a β-lactamase inhibitor and broaden the spectrum of ceftazidim through combination therapy [40]. Carbapenems may also be an appropriate treatment for CAP in settings where high resistance to other antibiotics is expected, however, costs are considerable and therapy should be well targeted [41–43].

Causative microorganisms of nosocomial pneumonia vary according to the individual patient-risk profile. Risk profiles derive from the knowledge of the severity of the nosocomial pneumonia, type and number of risk factors, and the time of onset of nosocomial pneumonia [44]. Gram-negative bacilli, Enterobacteriaceae, *H. influenzae* and methicillin sensitive *S. aureus* are frequent causative agents in early-onset nosocomial pneumonia. However, TROUILET *et al.* [45] showed that in cases with prolonged mechanical ventilation and antibiotic pretreatment, *P. aeruginosa* and other potentially drug resistant microorganisms (MRSA, *Acinetobacter basmati*, and *S. maltophilia*) play an important role. Just like AE-COPD and CAP are nosocomial pneumonia subject to empirical treatment with parenteral broad spectrum antibiotics, the use of monotherapy especially with β-lactams is only warranted in selected cases [44]. FINK *et al.* [46] compared imipenem monotherapy with ciprofloxacin monotherapy in 78% of 405 cases and rated both regimens effective provided that *P. aeruginosa* was not present. Therapy with ciprofloxacin was associated with a better clinical efficacy and a better rate of eradication in the presence of Enterobacteriaceae. This study was repeated by TORRES *et al.* [47] who found an equality of treatments between the carbapenem Imipenem and ciprofloxacin, however when *P. aeruginosa* was present a higher level of resistence was found in patients undergoing monotherapy treatment with Imipenem. COLARDYN AND FAULKNER [48] compared two carbapenems for the treatment of nosocomial bacterial infections. The clinical response rates were comparable for imipenem/cilastatin (75%) and meropenem (75%) in the subanalysis of nosocomial pneumonia [48].

COMETTA *et al.* [49] evaluated the efficacy of imipenem to the combination of imipenem plus netilmycin in patients with severe nosocomial pneumonia or sepsis. In that particular study, the clinical success rate with imipenem monotherapy (80%) appeared to be similar to that of the tested combination (86%). In another randomised trial, combination therapy with ceftazidime plus tobramycin was compared to meropenem alone [50]. A satisfactory clinical response occurred significantly more often with monotherapy (89%) when compared with the combination therapy (72%). However, the ceftazidime dosage given in this study was lower than recommended. Finally, RUBINSTEIN *et al.* [51] comparing ceftazidime monotherapy with the combination of ceftriaxon and tobramycin, showed a better clinical response rate in the monotherapy group of pneumonia (73% *versus* 65%), as well [51]. Moreover, none of the patients receiving ceftazidime in this study evidenced nephrotoxicity, compared to nine patients in the combination arm. Equality of treatments was also established for the comparison of ceftazidime versus piperacillin/tazobactam combined with amikacin for the treatment of nosocomial pneumonia [52] and ventilator-associated pneumonia [53].

Conclusions

β-lactams remain a cornerstone of the therapy of pulmonary infections due to the broad spectrum antimicrobial activity. They comprise three major groups with penicillins, cephalosporins and carbapenems. All betalactams may be useful in AE-COPD if certain criteria are met or in severe cases. However, atypical organisms like *Chlamydia sp.* play a role in AE-COPD and are not covered by β-lactams. Antibiotic use is compulsory in CAP and β-lactams are appropriate. In severe cases *Legionella pneumophilia* may be involved and a combination therapy is needed. In cases with *Mycoplasma sp.* and/or other atypical agents, β-lactams may be inappropriate for therapy. Nosocomial pneumonia is often complicated by infections with Gram-negative bacteria that are not susceptible to most β-lactams. In patients with risk factors for suspected or proven infection with such microorganisms third generation cephalosporins, acylureidopenicillins with β-lactamase inhibitors and/or carbapenems may be required.

Summary

Antibiotic and especially β-lactams are frequently used in the treatment of pulmonary infections, ranging from exacerbation of chronic obstructive pulmonary disease to severe cases of nosocomial pneumonia. The comprise of three major groups, penicillins, cephalosporins and carbapenems agents with broad spectrum antimicrobial activity. This article is comprised of the major features associated with the three groups of β-lactams and points out special capabilities of the most frequently used drugs. Indications of β-lactam use in infective lung disease is rehearsed and selected clinical trials in this field are referenced.

Keywords: Antibiotics, chronic obstructive pulmonary disorder, infection, mechanisms, pneumonia, resistance.

References

1.   Evans GM, Gaisford WF. Treatment of pneumonia with 2(*p*-aminobenzenesulphonamido) pyridine. *Lancet* 1938; 14–19.
2.   Livermore DM, Williams JD. β-Lactams: Mode of action and mechanisms of bacterial resistance. *In*: Lorian V, ed. Antibiotics. *In*: Laboratory Medicine. Philadelphia, Williams and Wilkins, 1996

3. Wright AJ. The penicillins. *Mayo Clin Proc.* 1999; 74: 290–307.
4. Sutherland R. *β–lactams: penicillins.* In: *O'Grady F*, Lambert H, Finch R. eds. Antibiotic and Chemotherapy. London, Churchill Livingstone, 1997; pp. 256–305.
5. Livermore DM. beta-Lactamases in laboratory and clinical resistance. *Clin Microbiol Rev* 1995; 8: 557–584.
6. Lister PD. Beta-lactamase inhibitor combinations with extended-spectrum penicillins: factors influencing antibacterial activity against Enterobacteriaceae and *Pseudomonas aeruginosa. Pharmacotherapy* 2000; 20: 213S–218S.
7. Bush K. Other β-lactams. *In*: O'Grady F, Lambert H, Finch R, eds. Antibiotic and Chemotherapy. London, Churchill Livingstone, 1997; pp. 306–327.
8. Marshall WF, Blair JE. The cephalosporins. *Mayo Clin Proc* 1999; 74: 187–195.
9. Karlowsky JA, Jones ME, Mayfield DC, Thornsberry C, Sahm DF. Ceftriaxone activity against Gram-positive and Gram-negative pathogens isolated in US clinical microbiology laboratories from 1996 to 2000: results from The Surveillance Network (TSN) Database-USA. *Int J Antimicrob Agents* 2002; 19: 413–426.
10. Rains CP, Bryson HM, Peters DH. Ceftazidime. An update of its antibacterial activity, pharmacokinetic properties and therapeutic efficacy. *Drugs* 1995; 49: 577–617.
11. Wilson WR. The role of fourth-generation cephalosporins in the treatment of serious infectious diseases in hospitalized patients. *Diagn Microbiol Infect Dis* 1998; 31: 473–477.
12. Greenwood D. Beta-lactams cephalosporins. *In*: Finch RG, Greenwood G, Norrby SR, Whitley RJ, eds. Antibiotics and Chemotherapy, 8th Edn. London, Churchill Livingstone, 2003; pp. 325–347.
13. Schatz BS, Karavokiros KT, Taeubel MA, Itokazu GS. Comparison of cefprozil, cefpodoxime proxetil, loracarbef, cefixime, and ceftibuten. *Ann Pharmacother* 1996; 30: 258–268.
14. Hellinger WC, Brewer NS. Carbapenems and monobactams: imipenem, meropenem, and aztreonam. *Mayo Clin Proc.* 1999; 74: 420–434.
15. Pfaller MA, Jones RN. A review of the *in vitro* activity of meropenem and comparative antimicrobial agents tested against 30,254 aerobic and anaerobic pathogens isolated world wide. *Diagn Microbiol Infect Dis* 1997; 28: 157–163.
16. Odenholt I. Ertapenem: a new carbapenem. *Expert Opin Investig Drugs* 2001; 10: 1157–1166.
17. Salkind AR, Cuddy PG, Foxworth JW. The rational clinical examination. Is this patient allergic to penicillin? An evidence-based analysis of the likelihood of penicillin allergy. *JAMA* 2001; 285: 2498–2505.
18. Kelkar PS, Li JT. Cephalosporin allergy. *N Engl J Med* 2001; 345: 804–809.
19. Goodman EJ, Morgan MJ, Johnson PA, Nichols BA, Denk N, Gold BB. Cephalosporins can be given to penicillin-allergic patients who do not exhibit an anaphylactic response. *J Clin Anesth* 2001; 13: 561–564.
20. Zaidi SA. Hepatitis associated with amoxicillin/clavulanic acid and/or ciprofloxacin. *Am J Med Sci* 2003; 325: 31–33.
21. Livermore DM, Winstanley TG, Shannon KP. Interpretative reading: recognizing the unusual and inferring resistance mechanisms from resistance phenotypes. *J Antimicrob Chemother* 2001; 48: Suppl. 1, 87–102.
22. Frere JM. Beta-lactamases and bacterial resistance to antibiotics. *Mol Microbiol* 1995; 16: 385–395.
23. Hirschmann JV. Do bacteria cause exacerbations of COPD? *Chest* 2000; 118: 193–203.
24. Murphy TF, Sethi S, Niederman MS. The role of bacteria in exacerbations of COPD. A constructive view. *Chest* 2000; 118: 204–209.
25. Wilson R. Bacteria, antibiotics and COPD. *Eur Respir J* 2001; 17: 995–1007.
26. Sohy C, Pilette C, Niederman MS, Sibille Y. Acute exacerbation of chronic obstructive pulmonary disease and antibiotics: what studies are still needed? *Eur Respir J* 2002; 19: 966–975.
27. Anthonisen NR, Manfreda J, Warren CPW, *et al.* Antibiotic therapy in exacerbations of chronic obstructive pulmonary disease. *Ann Intern Med* 1987; 106: 196–204.

28. Eller J, Ede A, Schaberg T, Niederman MS, Mauch H, Lode H. Infective exacerbations of chronic bronchitis: relation betwen bacteriologic etiology and lung function. *Chest* 1998; 113: 1542–1548.

29. Ewig S, Soler N, Gonzalez J, Celis R, El-Ebiary M, Torres A. Evaluation of antimicrobial treatment in mechanically ventilated patients with severe chronic obstructive pulmonary disease exacerbations. *Crit Care Med* 2000; 28: 692–697.

30. Soler N, Torres A, Ewig S, *et al.* Bronchial microbial patterns in severe exacerbations of chronic obstructive pulmonary disease (COPD) requiring mechanical ventilation. *Am J Respir Crit Care Med* 1998; 157: 1498–1505.

31. Blasi F, Damato S, Cosentini R, *et al.* Chlamydia InterAction with COPD (CIAC) Study Group. Chlamydia pneumoniae and chronic bronchitis: association with severity and bacterial clearance following treatment. *Thorax* 2002; 57: 672–676.

32. Allegra L, Konietzko N, Leophonte P, *et al.* Comparative safety and efficacy of sparfloxacin in the treatment of acute exacerbations of chronic obstructive pulmonary disease: a double-blind, randomised, parallel, multicentre study. *J Antimicrob Chemother* 1996; 37: Suppl. A, 93–104.

33. Weiss LR. Open-label, randomized comparison of the efficacy and tolerability of clarithromycin, levofloxacin, and cefuroxime axetil in the treatment of adults with acute bacterial exacerbations of chronic bronchitis. *Clin Ther* 2002; 24: 1414–1425.

34. Haczynski J, Chyczewska E, Grzelewska-Rzymowska I, *et al.* Comparative study of cefaclor AF *versus* cefuroxime axetil in acute exacerbations of chronic bronchitis. *Med Sci Monit* 2002; 8: PI1–7.

35. Hamacher J, Vogel F, Lichey J, *et al.* Treatment of acute bacterial exacerbations of chronic obstructive pulmonary disease in hospitalised patients–a comparison of meropenem and imipenem/cilastatin. COPD Study Group. *J Antimicrob Chemother* 1995; 36: Suppl. A, 121–133.

36. Phillips H, Van Hook CJ, Butler T, Todd WM. A comparison of cefpodoxime proxetil and cefaclor in the treatment of acute exacerbation of COPD in adults. *Chest* 1993; 104: 1387–1392.

37. Chodosh S, McCarty J, Farkas S, *et al.* Randomized, double-blind study of ciprofloxacin and cefuroxime axetil for treatment of acute bacterial exacerbations of chronic bronchitis. The Bronchitis Study Group. *Clin Infect Dis* 1998; 27: 722–729.

38. Shah PM, Maesen FP, Dolmann A, Vetter N, Fiss E, Wesch R. Levofloxacin versus cefuroxime axetil in the treatment of acute exacerbation of chronic bronchitis: results of a randomized, double-blind study. *J Antimicrob Chemother* 1999; 43: 529–539.

39. Arancibia F, Bauer TT, Ewig S, *et al.* Community-acquired Pneumonia caused by Gram-negative bacteria: Incidence and risk and prognosis. *Arch Intern Med* 2002; 162: 1849–1858.

40. Speich R, Imhof E, Vogt M, Grossenbacher M, Zimmerli W. Efficacy, safety, and tolerance of piperacillin/tazobactam compared to co-amoxiclav plus an aminoglycoside in the treatment of severe pneumonia. *Eur J Clin Microbiol Infect Dis* 1998; 17: 313–317.

41. Ortiz-Ruiz G, Caballero-Lopez J, Friedland IR, Woods GL, Carides A, Protocol 018 Ertapenem Community-Acquired Pneumonia Study Group. A study evaluating the efficacy, safety, and tolerability of ertapenem versus ceftriaxone for the treatment of community-acquired pneumonia in adults. *Clin Infect Dis* 2002; 34: 1076–1083.

42. Ho A, Leung R, Lai CK, Chan TH, Chan CH. Hospitalized patients with community-acquired pneumonia in Hong Kong: a randomized study comparing imipenem/cilastatin and ceftazidime. *Respiration* 1997; 64: 224–228.

43. Lin JC, Yeh KM, Peng MY, Chang FY. Efficacy of cefepime *versus* ceftazidime in the treatment of adult pneumonia. *J Microbiol Immunol Infect* 2001; 34: 131–137.

44. American Thoracic Society. Hospital-acquired pneumonia in adults: Diagnosis, assessment, initial therapy, and prevention: A consensus statement. *Am J Respir Crit Care Med* 1996; 153: 1711–1725.

45. Trouillet JL, Chastre J, Vuagnat A, *et al.* Ventilator-associated pneumonia caused by potentially drug-resistant bacteria. *Am J Respir Crit Care Med* 1998; 157: 531–539.

46. Fink MP, Snydman DR, Niederman MS, *et al.* Treatment of severe pneumonia in hospitalized patients: Results of a multicenter, randomized, double blind trial comparing intravenous ciprofloxacin with imipenem/cilastatin. *J Antimicrob Chemother* 1994; 38: 547–557.

47.   Torres A, Bauer TT, Leon C, *et al.* Treatment of severe nosocomial pneumonia requiring mechanical ventilation: A prospective randomized comparison of intravenous ciprofloxacin with imipenem/cilastatin. *Thorax* 2000; 55: 1033–1039.

48.   Colardyn F, Faulkner KL, Meropenem Serious Infection Study Group. Intravenous meropenem versus imipenem/cilastatin in the treatment of serious bacterial infections in hospitalized patients. *J Antimicrob Chemother* 1996; 38: 523–537.

49.   Cometta A, Baumgartner JD, Lew D. Prospective randomized comparison of imipenem monotherapy with imipenem plus netilmycin for treatment of severe infections in nonneutropenic patients. *Antimicrob Agents Chemother* 1994; 38: 1309–1313.

50.   Sieger B, Jon Berman S, Geckler RW, Farkas SA, Meropenem Lower Respiratory Infection Group. Empiric treatment of hospital-acquired lower respiratory tract infections with meropenem or ceftazidime with tobramycin. *Crit Care Med* 1997; 25: 1663–1670.

51.   Rubinstein E, Lode H, Grassi C, Antibiotic Study Group. Ceftazidime monotherapy vs. Ceftriaxone/Tobramycin for serious hospital-acquired Gram-negative infections. *Clin Infect Dis* 1995; 20: 1217–1228.

52.   Alvarez-Lerma F, Insausti-Ordenana J, Jorda-Marcos R, *et al.* Efficacy and tolerability of piperacillin/tazobactam versus ceftazidime in association with amikacin for treating nosocomial pneumonia in intensive care patients: a prospective randomized multicenter trial. *Intensive Care Med* 2001; 27: 493–502.

53.   Brun-Buisson C, Sollet JP, Schweich H, Briere S, Petit C. Treatment of ventilator-associated pneumonia with piperazillin-tazobactam/amikacin versus ceftazidime/amikacin: a multicenter, randomized controlled trial. *Clin Infect Dis* 1998; 26: 346–354.

CHAPTER 5

Macrolides and lower respiratory tract infections

J. Dorca, S. Padrones, F. Manresa

Pneumology Dept, Bellvitge University Hospital, Dept of Medicine, University of Barcelona, L'Hospitalet de Llobregat, Barcelona, Spain.

Correspondence: J. Dorca, Pneumology Dept, Bellvitge University Hospital, Feixa llarga s/n, 08907 L'Hospitalet de Llobregat, Barcelona, Spain.

Since their introduction over half a century ago, the macrolides have been used as valid alternatives in the treatment of respiratory tract infections, particularly those caused by Gram-positive bacteria and atypical agents. In the case of *Streptococcus pneumoniae*, the leading respiratory pathogen, erythromycin has been a valuable alternative to penicillin G and other β-lactams. More recently, other macrolide compounds have been developed in order to improve the pharmacokinetic and the antimicrobial activity available. Newer molecules such as clarithromycin and azithromycin display notable advantages over erythromycin and other older compounds in terms of clinical efficacy and side effects.

Structure

The first macrolide compound, the erythromycin, was obtained from a strain of *Streptomyces erythreus* Its basic chemical structure is based on a 14-member macrocyclic lactone ring, which was the origin for the class name the macrolides. Since then different molecules have been derived in order to improve the phamacokinetic and pharmaco-dynanic properties of the original antibiotic [1]. In some cases, the original 14-member macrocyclic lactone ring has been substituted by 15 or 16-member ones. The macrolide antibiotics are currently classified according to the characteristics of this basic structure as shown in table 1.

Mechanism of action

All the macrolide compounds display a similar mechanism of action by inhibiting the ribonucleic acid (RNA)-dependent protein synthesis at the step of chain elongation in the susceptible organism. The macrolide molecule reversibly binds to the 50S ribosomal

Table 1. – Clasification of macrolides according to the number of atoms in the macrolactonic ring

14 atoms	15 atoms	16 atoms
Clarithromycin	Azithromycin	Midecamycin
Dirithromycin		Josamycin
Erithromycin		Miokamycin (diacetyl-midecamycin)
Roxithromycin		

Eur Respir Mon, 2004, 28, 78–93. Printed in UK - all rights reserved. Copyright ERS Journals Ltd 2004; European Respiratory Monograph; ISSN 1025-448x. ISBN 1-904097-32-4.

subunit resulting in blockage of the transpeptidation and/or translocation reaction. In addition, the macrolides can also promote the dissociation of peptidyl transcriptional RNA from the ribosomes and in some bacterial species, they also inhibit the formation of the 50S ribosomal subunit. This mechanism of action is similar to that of other chemically unrelated antibiotics such as the lincosamide and the streptogramins b [2].

The macrolides display a broad-spectrum of antimicrobial activity [3], including multiple respiratory pathogens such as Gram-positive and Gram-negative bacteria, actinomycetes, mycobacteria, and the atypical bacteria *Mycoplasma pneumoniae*, *Chlamydia sp.* and *Coxiella burnetii*.

Mechanisms of resistance

To date only three main mechanisms of bacterial resistance to the macrolides have been identified these are as follows: 1) alteration of the ribosomal binding site; 2) alteration of the antibiotic transport; and 3) modification antibiotic molecular structure.

Alteration of the ribosomal binding side is the more relevant type of resistance involving modifications of the ribosomal proteins or the ribosomal RNA (rRNA). Alteration of the 23S rRNA of the 50S ribosomal subunit by methylation of the adenine induces high-level resistance to erythromycin ($MIC \geq 64$ mL·L^{-1}) and many other macrolides. In addition, structurally different antibiotics showing similar mechanism of action such as clindamycin and streptogramins type b, are often described under the combined term of the macrolide-lincosamide-streptogramin b (MLSb) group [4, 5]. The *erm* gene encodes this pattern of resistance, known as the MLSb phenotype. The MLSb phenotype resistance may be constitutive, but exposing bacterial species to subinhibitory concentrations of the antibiotic can also induce it. Only the 14- and 15-membered macrolides and not the 16-membered ones, or clindamycin, can induce this kind of resistance. Considering the major respiratory pathogens, *S. pneumoniae*, other streptococci, *Staphylococcus aureus*, *M. pneumoniae* and *Legionella pneumophila* exhibit the MLSb phenotype resistance.

A second mechanism of resistance is based on the alteration in the uptake or accumulation of the antibiotic, which involved an active efflux mechanism [6]. In the case of *S. pneumoniae* and *Streptococcus pyogenes*, an efflux pump mechanism encoded by the *mef*E gene generates resistance to 14- and 15-membered macrolides, but not to the 16-membered ones, clindamycin and streptogramins. This phenotype M mechanism is associated with low-level erythromycin resistance (minimal inhibitory concentrations (MIC) 1–16 mg·L^{-1}). In contrast, the MLSb phenotype resistance is associated with high-level erythromycin resistance.

Finally, enzymatic inactivation of 14- and 15-membered macrolides by esterases and other enzymes has been described in strains of Enterobacteriaceae, but this mechanism is not found among major respiratory pathogens.

Pharmacokinetics

Erythromycin, the first macrolide, had several pharmacokinetic limitations such as poor oral bioavailability caused by acid instability and erratic absorption; short serum half-life; gastrointestinal side effects; a high rate of phlebitis when administered by intravenous (IV) route and some clinically relevant drug interactions. The new macrolide compounds have been developed to improve the pharmacokinetic properties *i.e.* increase activity against certain pathogens and to minimise their side effects [7]. However, these new macrolides display quite different properties with wide variations in the elimination of the half-life, tissue concentrations, and intracellular penetration. Among the new 14-membered agents, roxitromycin achieves high serum concentrations, the highest of the macrolides, and consequent high sustained tissue levels. Dirithromycin has an extremely long half-life elimination. After absorption, it undergoes a nonenzymatic hydrolysis process that converts it to erythromycylamine, an active substance. Although serum concentrations are low in comparison with that of other macrolides, it reaches high tissue concentrations with a very low rate of elimination, making a once a day dosage possible. The naturally occurring 16-membered macrolides *e.g.* josamycin and midecamycin and some of its synthetic derivates such as rokitamycin and miokamycin may offer minor pharmacokynetic advantages. By contrast, two modern macrolide compounds: clarithromycin and azithromycin, display relevant properties.

Clarithromycin, a 14-membered compound, has an excellent bioavailability thanks to a rapid and near complete absorption [8]. Its half-live ranges between 4–7 h hence permiting a twice a day schedule. It has an excellent tissue penetration and the intracellular concentrations are also very high. A clarithromycin 14-hydroxy metabolite also has antimicrobial activity, in addition to that of the original structure.

Azithromycin, is the only 15-membered macrolide and is classified in a different subgroup of macrolides known as azalides [9]. This molecule includes a nitrogen atom added to the 15-membered ring. Azithromycin has an excellent absorption and has an extremely prolonged serum and tissue half life, up to 4 days. In addition it has a very high affinity for the tissues, leading to concentrations 100 times higher than those of blood, it also has an excellent intracellular penetration. Owing to these notable pharmacokinetic properties it can be administered in a once a day regimen and for a short period of time, over just 3–5 days, obtaining high tissue levels that can last for a long time. Nevertheless the low serum concentrations of azithromycin may be a problem in patients with bacteremia associated with community-acquired pneumonia (CAP).

Apart from dirithromycin, the 14-membered macrolides have an affinity for cytochrome P450 (CYP). Consequently, these antibiotics may have interactions with other drugs displaying CYP affinity, *e.g.* carbamazepine, cyclosporin, theophylline, antihistamines, digoxin, warfarin and benzodiazepines. This is not the case with azithromycin and 16-membered compounds, which do not share this trend.

Macrolide excretion is through the bile. Dosage adjustments are required in patients with hepatic dysfunction except roxithromycin. Clarithromycin is the only macrolide with significant renal excretion, therefore dosage reduction may be necessary in patients displaying renal failure.

Pharmacodynamics

The macrolides interact with specific targets that are located on bacterial ribosomes. The relationship between drug concentration and antibacterial effect describes the pharmacodynamic characteristics of a drug. There are two patterns of antibacterial activity these are as concentration-dependent and time-dependent. However, the macrolide serum concentrations are not a good predictor of macrolide activity and consequently it is difficult to classify the macrolides as concentration-dependent or time-dependent antibiotics [10].

The macrolides display a postantibiotic effect (PAE), they have a persistent antibacterial activity time after the exposure to the antibiotic. This is important when the antibiotic concentration falls below the MIC level. Agents with prolonged PAE can be administered in fewer numbers of doses. The macrolide PAE appears to be important against Gram-positive cocci.

The macrolide antibacterial activity may be bacteriostatic or bactericidal depending upon the drug concentration in the infected tissue, the specific bacterial species, its concentration and the phase of growth.

Antimicrobial activity

The *in vitro* susceptibility of the major respiratory pathogens to the more common macrolides *i.e.* erythromycin, clarithromycin and azithromycin [11–17] are summarised in table 2.

Streptococcus pneumoniae

Classically, macrolides have been considered the alternative to penicillin G for the treatment of pneumococcal infections. For decades they have been used widely in the community for the treatment of upper and lower respiratory infections, both in adult and paediatric populations, primarily because of their excellent activity and safety. Unfortunately pneumococcal antibiotic resistance has developed in certain geographical locations, implying a threat to the classical antibiotic strategies for respiratory infections [18–19].

To-date, through different mechanisms, pneumococci have developed resistance to six different categories of antibiotics these are: β-lactams, macrolides, clindamycin, chloranphenicol, tetracyclines, cotrimoxazole and quinolones. From a clinical prospective resistance to β-lactams and especially to penicillin, deserves particular attention, as this group of antibiotics were the cornerstone for the treatment of pneumococcal infections. After β-lactams resistance, pneumococcal macrolide resistance is the most clinically relevant. It is important to note that pneumococcal macrolide resistance is more prevalent among β-lactam resistant strains. During the last decade macrolide resistance has progressively increased throughout Europe reaching 40% in France and 30% in Italy, Spain and Hungary [20]. To a lesser degree, it is also present in the US.

Pneumococci display two basic mechanisms of resistance to macrolides. One involves target-site modification by a methylase that is encoded by a specific gene. These strains

Table 2. – *In vitro* minimum inhibitory concentration of 90% of bacteria activity of macrolides against major respiratory pathogens [9, 8, 11, 15–21]

	Erithromycin mg·L^{-1}	Clarithromycin mg·L^{-1}	Azithromycin mg·L^{-1}
Gram-positive cocci			
Streptococcus pneumoniae PS	0.06	0.06	0.12
S. pneumoniae PI	16	8	8
S. pneumoniae PR	>32	32	32
Streptococcus pyogenes	0.12	0.12	0.12
Staphylococcus aureus MS	2	1	2
S. aureus MR	>128	>128	>128
Gram-negative bacilli			
Moraxella catharralis	0.25	0.25	0.12
Haemophilus influenzae	8	4	2
Intracellular bacteria			
Chlamydia pneumoniae	0.12	0.03	0.25
Mycoplasma pneumoniae	≤0.01	0.012	≤0.01
Legionella pneumophila	2	0.25	2

PS: penicillin sensitive; PI: penicillin intermediate; PR: penicillin resistant; MS: methicillin sensitive; MR: methicillin resistant.

express the MLSb phenotype, which implies cross-resistance to macrolides, clindamycin and streptogramins b [4, 5]. This mechanism implies a high-level resistance that affects all members of the macrolide group. A second mechanism of resistance, encoded by a different gene, involves an active efflux pump that removes the antibiotic from the cell. This is known as phenotype M and causes low-level resistance affecting 14- and 15-membered macrolides, but not 16-membered ones [6].

The prevalence of these two mechanisms of resistance seems to vary among the different geographical locations. Recently, a multicentric study carried out in the USA [21] concluded that the phenotype M mechanism of resistance, implying low-level resistance, was predominant in the USA representing 60% of all macrolide-resistant pneumococci. However, it is important to note that phenotype MLSb, expressing high-level resistance, was found in one third of the total number of cases. This situation seems to be different within European countries. According to recently published multicentric data in Spain [22], nearly all the macrolide-resistant pneumococci harbour the phenotype MLSb, implying high-level resistance. Similar results have recently been found in Italy. This raises the question regarding the usefulness of macrolides for the treatment of pneumococcal infections in these areas.

Currently there is considerable controversy regarding the use of macrolides to treat pneumococcal infections. This is reflected in the literature. Some authors [23] support the view that pneumococcal macrolide resistance is more of a myth than a reality. These authors propose the following arguments to support their arguement: 1) different technical problems affecting susceptibility data provided by clinical laboratories decreases their reliability and magnifies the resistance; 2) at least in the USA, most of the resistant strains display low level resistance; 3) because of its specific pharmaco-kinetics and better compliciance, azitromycin may be more active than other macrolide compounds in this setting; and 4) many reports show favourable results which have been obtained by different clinical trials and the scarcity of reports about macrolide clinical failure does not validate the theory. Others however [24] considers macrolide resistance a real threat, for the following reasons: 1) *in vitro* susceptibility studies in clinical laboratories are reliable; 2) phenotype MLSb high-level resistance is near absolute in some European locations; 3) antibiotic concentrations obtained in the site of infection are in fact well below the reported MICs; and 4) most of the clinical trials are incorrectly designed and therefore macrolide efficacy in macrolide-resistant pneumoccocal infections has still to be proven in practice.

Recent episodes of macrolide treatment failure in pneumocooccal pneumonia have presently been described [25].

Haemophilus influenzae *and other Gram-negative pathogens*

The activity of erythromycin against *Haemophilus influenzae* is low. With the exception of clarithomycin and azitromycin, other macrolide compounds are no better. Compared with clarithromycin, azitromycin has increased *in vitro* activity against *H. influenzae*. Although *in vitro* activity of clarythromycin against *H. influenzae* appears to be roughly equal to that of erythromycin, routine susceptibility testing underestimates the potential of this macrolide. It has been shown recently that clarithromycin susceptibility studies against *H. influenzae* based on broth microdilution technique using Haemophilus test medium (HTM) underestimates clarithromycin activity in comparison with tests using Mueller-Hinton broth with lysed horse blood (LHB) or disk diffusion tests on HTM. In additon, clarithromycin has an *in vivo* synergy with its microbiologically active metabolite 14-hydroxy-clarithromycin and a postantibiotic effect that in practice increase its activity [26].

All macrolides display good activity against *M. catarrhalis*. Some studies indicate that azithromycin is somewhat more active than clarithromycin against this organism (27).

Atypicals

All macrolides exhibit excellent activity against intracellular bacteria causing lower respiratory tract infections (LRTIs) *e.g. M. pneumoniae, Clamydia pneumoniae* and *Clostridium. burnetii*. The macrolides also have excellent intracellular penetration into macrophages and polymorphonuclear cells, a very important fact. Intracelullar concentrations achieved vary among the macrolides, with azithromycin and dirithromycin exhibiting the highest intracellular concentrations.

Legionella pneumophila

Clarithromycin and azithromycin have a slightly better activity than erythromycin against *L. pneumophila*. In addition, their intracellular penetration is higher. In animal models, azithromycin was found to be more effective than claritromycin and erythromycin [28–30]. However, because in some of these series the animals received only a 2-day treatment it has been suggested that given the longer intracellular half-life of azitromycin this superiority could be fictitious.

Other respiratory pathogens

Macrolides have a minor activity against *Mycobacterium tuberculosis*. Nevertheless, clarithromycin and azithromycin display a good activity against *Mycobacterium avium* complex as well as other atypical mycobacteria such as *Mycobacterium kansasii, Mycobacterium chelonae* and *Mycobacterium fortuitum*.

Role of macrolides in lowere respiratory tract infections

Acute bronchitis

Acute bronchitis (AB) is a very common infection of the tracheobronchial tree affecting both the adult and paediatric population in the community. The major pathogens involved are respiratory viruses, atypical bacteria such as *M. pneumoniae* and *C. pneumoniae*. The role of pyogenic bacteria such as *S. pneumoniae, H. influenzae* or *M. catarrhalis* as cause of primary bronchial infection or superinfection appears to be much less relevant. As AB is a benign and self-limited infection within the healthy population antibiotics are not routinely needed. However, in old patients or in those already suffering chronic debilitating diseases antibiotics can be prescribed. Considering the causative spectrum described earlier, the macrolides may be the treatment of choice rather than β-lactams, owing to the possibility of an atypical agent.

Acute exacerbation of chronic bronchitis

Infection is generally considered to be one of the leading causes of acute exacerbation of chronic obstructive pulmonary disease (COPD), however in practice several potential precipitating factors need to be taken into account in this setting. Increased purulent expectoration is the best indicator of bacterial bronchial infection, much more reliable than other symptoms *e.g.* fever, dispnoea, or a nonproductive cough.

There is a general agreement in the literature about the limited number of bacterial species implicated in the acute exacerbation of chronic bronchitis (AECB) episodes, these include: *H. influenzae*, the pneumococcus and *Moraxella catarrhalis*. Other pyogenic bacteria *e.g.* streptococci, Gram-negative bacilli and staphylococci are occasionally identified. *Pseudomonas aeruginosa* has to be taken into consideration only among the more severe COPD patients. The relative importance of *Mycoplasma* and viruses seems to be smaller than it was previously thought. More recently studies have suggested that *C. pneumoniae* could be an infrequent endemic cause of COPD exacerbation.

Among all aforementioned pathogens, *H. influenzae* is by far the most relevant causative organism being implicated in nearly two thirds of all episodes. Several studies have demonstrated that nontypable *H. influenzae* strains colonise the lower tracheo-bronchial tree in a large percentage of stable COPD patients. According to the vicious circle hypothesis, this bacterial colonisation plays an important role because some bacteria, *H. influenzae* in particular, cause an alteration in the host respiratory tract defenses, perpetuating their presence in the lower airway. In addition, certain circumstances *e.g.* viral infection, exposition to irritants, *etc*, may eventually facilitate bacterial overgrow leading to periodic episodes of bacterial infection. It has been suggested that bacterial eradication after antibiotic treatment may play a crucial role in prolonging the length of intercritical episodes thereby decreasing the number of exacerbations and hospital admissions.

From a practical point of view, the empirical antibiotic treatment in AECB must at least be active against the three major pathogens: *H. influenzae*, pneumococcus and *M. catarrhalis*. Theoretically macrolides fulfill this goal, as well as many other alternatives such as aminopenicillins alone or in combination with β-lactamase inhibitors, cephalosporins, quinolones, cotrimoxazole, tetracyclines which are currently recommended in the literature.

Different authors who compared their results against different alternatives such as amoxicillin/clavulanate, quinolones and other macrolides have analysed the efficacy of macrolides in AECB. The combined analysis of these [31–38], (summarised in table 3) is difficult for several reasons. Most are industry-sponsored studies designed to demonstrate equivalence but not superiority, they often display methodological flaws (inhomogeneous populations, inadequate comparators and/or low dosages), and quite often, the microbiological follow-up is poor. In addition, owing to geographical differences in bacterial antibiotic resistance amongst *H. influenzae* and *S. pneumoniae* strains, it is very difficult to draw a general conclusion. Nevertheless, there is some evidence indicating that macrolides may not be so active in this setting compated to certain comparators *e.g.* amoxillin/clavulanate [32] or the quinolones [34].

The usefulness of the macrolides where *H. influenzae* and *S. pneumoniae* are the major pathogens may present some concerns. Considering *H. influenzae* the activity of all other macrolides, except azithromycin and clarithomycin, appears to be poor. It is important to note there are other alternatives for instance the quinolones and amoxicillin/clavulanate, which are more active against *H. influenzae* obtaining higher rates of eradication in respiratory secretions that could lead to a prolonged intercritical period. Alternatively high-level pneumococcal macrolide resistance, which is currently high in different European countries, supposes a risk of failure in the case of pneumococcal bronchial infections.

In conclusion, although azithromycin and clarithromycin may be useful in the treatment of AECB in milder forms of COPD, amoxicillin/clavulanate or quinolones should be preferred for the treatment of bronchial infections in patients with "complicated COPD". That is those with the poorest lung function, more debilitated in their general condition and presenting more frequent episodes of infectious exacerbation [39].

Table 3. – Clinical trials involving macrolides in adults suffering acute exhacerbations of chronic bronchitis (AECB)

Author	Year	Population	Valid cases	Regimen	Clinical response	Bacterial erradication
HOSIE et al. [31]	1995	AECB in adults	191	C 250 mg b.i.d. 7 days. D 500 mg od 5 days.	C=D	C=D
BEGHI et al. [32]	1995	Purulent AECB in adults	142	A 500 mg od 3 days A/C 875/125 mg b.i.d. 5–11 days	A/C>A	ND
ZACHARIAH et al. [33]	1996	AECB in adults	116	A 500 mg od 3 days A/C 375 mg t.i.d. 10 days	A=A/C	ND
CHODOSH et al. [34]	1998	Mild-to-moderate AECB in adults	190	C 500 mg b.i.d. 14 days Cipro 500 mg b.i.d. 14 days	Cipro>C	Cipro>C
ZIERING AND McELVAINE [35]	1998	AECB in adults	262	C 500 mg b.i.d. 7–14 days Cef 400 mg od 7–14 days	C=Cef	C=Cef
WASILEWSKI et al. [36]	1999	AECB in adults	690	E 250 mg q.i.d. 7 days D 500 mg od 5 days	E=D	E=D
WILSON et al. [37]	1999	AECB in adults	576	MX 400 mg od 5 days C 500 mg b.i.d. 7 days	MX=C	MX>C
DEABATE et al. [38]	2000	AECB in adults	567	MX 400 mg od 5 days A 500 mg q.i.d. 1 day; then 250 mg q.i.d. 4 days	MX=A	MX=A

The table only includes prospective, randomised and comparative studies. A: amoxicilin; A/C: amoxicilin/ clavulanic acid; b.i.d.: twice a day; C: clarithromycin; Cef: cefixime; CFX: cefuroxime axetil; Cipro: ciprofloxacin; D: dirithromycin; E: erythromycin; HI: *Haemophilus influenzae*; IV: intravenous; MX: moxifloxacin; ND: no data available; od: once daily; PO: oral; q.i.d.: four times a day; R: roxithromycin; SP: *Streptococcus pneumoniae*; Spar: sparfloxacin; t.i.d.: three times a day.

Community-acquired pneumonia

Community-acquired pneumonia (CAP) is a common infection caused by different causative organisms resulting in various clinical symptoms ranging from a mild febrile respiratory infection to a fulminating disease. Depending upon its presentation and severity, it is managed by different physicians including general practitioners and various hospital specialists. The incidence of CAP notably varies during life, with the young, the elderly and nursing home residents those more prone to suffer this infection. Age, as well as the chronic debilitating diseases, modulate the etiological spectrum, increasing the risk of pneumonia caused by *L. pneumophila* and pyogenic bacteria other than the pneumococcus.

Some of the clinically presentation characteristics of CAP and particularly the severity of the episode seem to modulate the etiological spectrum. According to the studies carried out in the community, mild pneumonias are most likely caused by: *S. pneumoniae*, *M. pneumoniae*, respiratory viruses and *Chlamydia pneumoniae*. *C. burnetii* may be prevalent in some rural areas. All other organisms should be considered infrequent in this setting. Among the hospital admitted episodes, the etiological pattern shows that *S. pneumoniae* remains the most common pathogen, whereas *L. pneumophila*, *H. influenzae*, and enteric gram-negative bacilli increase somewhat their relative frequency, although *L. pneumophila* may show a considerable temporal variation. Other etiologies such as *M. pneumoniae*, *C. pneumoniae*, and respiratory viruses become less frequent. Finally, in severe CAP episodes requiring intensive care *L. pneumophila* and *S. pneumoniae* are the leading pathogens. *H. influenzae*, enteric Gram-negative bacilli, *P. aeruginosa*, and *S. aureus* also increase its relative importance.

The initial antibiotic treatment of CAP is usually empirical, according to different therapeutic guidelines [40–42] that propose antibiotic prescription according to algorisms based on the different factors that modulate the etiological spectrum *i.e.* age, underlying diseases and severity at presentation. Owing to its antimicrobial activity, the macrolides play a central role in these strategies. First, owing to its combined activity against *S. pneumoniae* and the atypical bacteria they are considered the treatment of choice for mild CAP episodes affecting young and healthy people, and can be managed in the outpatient setting. Second, they are recommended in association to β-lactams for the treatment of the more severe CAP episodes that require hospitalisation in order to cover an eventual infection caused by *L. pneumophila*.

The validity of the aforementioned classical approach is nowadays under discussion because of the development of the pneumococcal macrolide resistance, and due to the introduction of other antibiotics *e.g.* the new quinolones or the ketolides that may afford more effectively this threat.

Clinical trials involving macrolides in the treatment of CAP [43–52] are summarised in table 4. Again, methodological flaws such as small or inhomogeneous populations, inadequate comparators and/or low dosages, poor microbiological data and the characteristics of the study designs, aimed to show equivalence rather than superiority, often make it very difficult to draw any conclusion.

Considering mild-to-moderate CAP, to be managed in an outpatient context, the macrolides seems to display similar activity when compared between themselves. This is also true when a 3-day azitromycin regimen were compared with other macrolide compounds at standard dosage [44, 45]. Finally, when compared with other nonmacrolide antibiotics *e.g.* β-lactams, quinolones, or ketolides, their clinical efficacy appear to be similar, although in some studies their efficacy was lower than those of quinolones [47]. However, it is important to note that there are a lack of well designed studies comming from areas which are known to have a high prevalence of high-level pneumococci macrolide resistance, therefore the use of macrolides as the treatment of choice remains open to question in these areas.

Among CAP presenting hospital admission criteria, the treatment of choice has been the association between a β-lactam *e.g.* a third generation parenteral cephalosporin or amoxicillin/clavulanate plus a macrolide by the IV route. The recent development of parenteral new quinolones presenting high activity against the pneumococcus appears a potential monotherapy alternative to the classical combination. Recently, a comparative trial comparing IV moxifloxacin for at least 3 days, then moved to oral administration, against the combination amoxicillin/clavulanate plus carithromycin concluded that moxifloxacin was associated with a lower mortality rate [52].

So far, the macrolides remain the basic alternative for the treatment of mild-to-moderate CAP to be managed in an outpatient context in areas where high-level macrolide resistance is not prevalent. The need of alternative regimens in countries where this type of resistance is important could be solved by the prescription of ketolides such as telithromycin or new quinolones active against the pneumococcus. In severe CAP more studies are needed to compare the classical association β-lactam plus macrolide and monotherapy with a parenteral new quinolone.

Nonantimicrobial properties of macrolides

Most of the clinical and therapeutical data on the anti-inflammatory properties of the macrolides comes from two original works by Japanese authors, one concerning the description of diffuse panbronchiolitis (DPB) [53], and the other describing the first clinical results using erythromycin [54]. Shortly after publication of the different series of patients with DPB succesfully treated with long term macrolide therapy, other authors used macrolides to treat patients presenting other bronchial diseases with similar clinical and pathological patterns, namely bronchiectasis associated with cystic fibrosis (CF). Consequently an increasing number of patients are now being empirically treated with macrolides.

DPB is a chronic disease presenting diffuse inflammation affecting initially the

Table 4. – Clinical trials involving macrolides in adults suffering from community-aquired pneumonia (CAP)

Author	Year	Population	Valid cases	Regimen	Clinical response	Bacterial erradication
LIIPPO et al. [43]	1994	Bacterial CAP in adults	241	E 250 mg q.i.d. 10–14 days		
				D 500 mg od 10–14 days	E=D	E=D
SCHÖNWALD et al. [44]	1994	Atypical pneumonia (Mycoplasma pneumoniae, Chlamidia spp., and Coxiella burnetti) in adults	142	A 500 mg od 3 days R 150 mg b.i.d.	A=R	ND
BOTHE et al. [45]	1995	Adults with CAP were in 2 groups: Pneumococcal pneumonia	104	A 500 mg b.i.d. 1 day; then 500 mg od 2–5 days BPEN 1x10^6 IU q.i.d. IV until afebrile for 5 days	A=BPEN	ND
		nonpneumococcal pneumonia		A 500 mg b.i.d. 1 day; then 500 mg od 2–5 days E 500 mg q.i.d. 10 days	A=E	ND
LODE et al. [46]	1995	CAP in adults	644	E 1000 mg b.i.d. 7–14 days	E 85%	SP 84%– HI 93%
				Spar 400 mg loading dose then 200 mg od 7–14 days	Spar 87%	SP 85%– HI 96%
				A/C 500/125 mg t.i.d. 7–14 days	A/C 80%	SP 80%– HI 90%
ORTQVIST et al. [47]	1996	CAP in adults	260	R 150 mg b.i.d. 10–14 days Spar 400 mg od 1 day then 200 mg od 9–13 days	Spar>R (95/80%)	R>Spar (95/80%)
HERNÁNDEZ et al. [48]	1996	CAP and bacteraemic pneumonia in adults	1108	E 250 mg q.i.d. D 500 mg od	E=D	E=D
GENE et al. [49]	1997	CAP in adults	112	C 500 mg IV b.i.d. (3–5 days) then 500 mg PO b.i.d. for at least 10 days. A/C 1.2 g IV q.i.d. (3–5 days) then 625 mg PO t.i.d. at least 10 days.	C=A/C	C=A/C
TELLIER et al. [50]	2000	CAP in adults		T 800 mg od 10 days C 500 mg t.i.d. 10 days	T=C	ND
HOEFFKEN et al. [51]	2001	CAP in adults	675	MX 200 mg od 10 days MX 400 mg od 10 days C 500 mg b.i.d.	MX=C	MX>C
FINCH et al. [52]	2002	CAP in adults	538	MX 400 mg IV od then 400 mg od PO for 7–14 days A/C 1.2 g t.i.d. EV; then 625 mg t.i.d. with or without C 500 mg t.i.d. (IV or PO) for 7–14 days	MX>A/C±C	ND

The table only includes prospective, randomised and comparative studies. A: amoxicilin; A/C: amoxicilin/clavulanic acid; b.i.d.: twice a day; BPEN: benzyl penicillin; C: clarithromycin; Cef: cefixime; CFX: cefuroxime axetil; D: dirithromycin; E: erythromycin; HI: Haemophilus influenzae; IV: intravenous; MX: moxifloxacin; ND: no data available; od: once daily; PO: oral; q.i.d.: four times a day; R: roxithromycin; SP: Streptococcus pneumoniae; Spar: sparfloxacin; T: telithromycin; t.i.d.: three times a day.

respiratory bronchioli and adjacent centrilobular areas and the later involving the more proximal bronchi creating associated bronchiectasis. The clinical presentation of DPB is characterised by chronic cough productive of abundant mucopurulent sputum, accompanied by a frequent purulent nasal discharge. Diffuse and bibasal reticulonodular opacities as well as hyperinflation are seen in the chest radiograph. In most of the advanced cases, *P. aeruginosa* is observed in the bronchial secretions instead of the common *H. influenzae*, seen in the initial phases of the disease. After the observation in 1987 of an isolated case successfully treated with erythromycin, an open trial prospectively demonstrated the favourable effect of a long term treatment with 400–600 mg·day^{-1} in most of the patients. This effect was observed even in patients with persistent *Pseudomonas* infection. Thereafter several double-blind, placebo-controlled trials have confirmed this preliminary results. Finally other macrolides, such as clarythromycin, azithromycin are also reported to be of benefit for this condition.

The effect of macrolides in DPB has to be related to mechanisms other than its antimicrobial properties, because the maximum serum and sputum concentration of erythromycin at the conventional dosage used is well below its minimum inhibitory concentration for *P. aeruginosa* and *H. influenzae*. The persistent observation of both microorganisms in the respiratory secretions of the treated patients supports this hypothesis, and additional evidence comes from retrospective data showing that erythromycin is more effective than fluoroquinolones in patients with DPB. Previously the classical observation shown during the long-term high-dose use of amoxycillin to treat bronchiectasis with mixed infection was the decrease of the bronchial load of *H. influenzae* associated with antibiotic resistant *P. aeruginosa*. Suggesting that the reduction of sensible organisms modified the local inflammatory response and permitted some recovery of the host's local clearance mechanisms.

Since the publication of these clinical studies a large amount of literature has appeared trying to demonstrate cellular, biological or immunological mechanisms by which macrolides could effectively control the clinical course of this disease. Presently different hypotheses are under discussion. The bronchoalveolar lavage (BAL) obtained before and after treatment demonstrates a decrease in the neutrophilic content of the bronchi and erythromycin has also been shown *in vitro* to suppress the neutrophilic influx into the alveoli in response to different interleukines and bacterial agents. It has been observed that *P. aeruginosa* when exposed to erythromycin are more susceptible to the bactericidal activity of polymorphonuclear leucocytes, by increasing the bacterial susceptibility to the neutrophil oxygen dependent killing mechanism. Furthermore, *in vitro* and in a milieu containing small concentrations of macrolides, *P. aeruginosa* loses its pili, thereby decreasing its adherence to the tracheal epithelium of the rat.

Immunological studies have shown that a long term treatment with macrolides modifies the CD4/CD8 pulmonary ratio and increase the percentages of CD4, CD8 and CD3 in the peripheral blood in patients with DPB. Alternatively other *in vitro* studies have confirmed that erythromycin accelerates apoptosis of cultured neutrophils in a dose dependent manner.

Erythromycin and other macrolides also inhibit the secretion of respiratory glycoproteins by human airways. The restoration of a regular chloride channel function observed in patients with CF treated with macrolides supports the hypothesis that these drugs favourably affect the rheology of bronchial secretions. Therefore both observations suggest another possible mechanism of action of macrolides, the modification of the quality and characteristics of the bronchial secretions.

In summary, the hypothetical nonantimicrobial mechanisms of action of erythromycin may be several fold: 1) modulation of the lymphocyte function changes the course of the disease without influencing the bacteria of the bronchial tree; 2) modification of the characteristics of the bronchial secretions; and 3) reduction of the inflammation of the bronchial tree by changing the functional activities of the polimorphonuclear present in the lung. It must be noted however, that there is a marked discrepancy between *in vitro* results of the effect of macrolides reducing inflammatory mediators, and the negative data observed in clinical trials. This difference may be due in part, to different factors *e.g.* the number of patients studied, the pharmacodymanics, dosage, time, *etc.* Further studies are needed to evaluate the role of such parameters in order to confirm *in vivo* the biological response observed *in vitro*. Meanwhile, Japanese epidemiological data seems to demonstrate that the survival of DPB, since the introduction of erythromycin therapy, has increased dramatically and the number of reported incidences is declining.

Bronchiectasis in CF usually shows *P. aeruginosa* growing characteristically forming biofilms. The gene expression of a community of microorganisms is coordinated by small molecules called, quorum sensors, consisting in lactones highly diffusible in and outside of the microorganism. In bronchiectasis where the bacterial load is high, the quorum sensors secreted by bacteria diffuse freely within the community creating a biofilm structure [55]. In this structure, these lactones interact with transcription activators expressing several factors that facilitate the penetration of bacteria in the lung (proteases, pyocianin, catalase, superoxide dismutase, etc,), thus, enabling the bacteria to resist the effects of antibiotics. Briefly, biofilm formation has been associated with bacterial drug resistance and persistence of infection in patients with CF.

The use of macrolides in cystic fibrosis stands has been based two facts: 1) the importance of clinical inflammation as demonstrated by the presence of abundant proinflammatory cytocines in BAL, bronchial biopsies and bronchial secretions of patients with CF; and 2) the *in vitro* evidence that macrolides disrupt and block diffusion of the quorum sensors, interfering the progression of biofilms and therefore, the appearance *in situ* of various proinflammatory molecules that negativelly disrupt the local anatomic and bacteriological defense mechanisms.

There are at least eight clinical studies (number of patients ranging from 7–60) confirming the beneficial effect of the long term use of macrolides (clarithromycin, azithromycin) during periods ranging from 6 weeks to 1.8 yrs [56]. The favourable effects are observed in terms of quality of life, number of clinical exacerbations, use of antibiotics and number of hospital admissions. Lung function changes are rather poor, and the effect of long term use of macrolides on the normal oropharyngeal flora has to be evaluated. These preliminary data on DPB and CF need confirmation with larger, double blind clinical studies, but strongly suggest the potential use of macrolides in this clinical context.

With the clinical evidence accumulated on these two suppurative bronchial diseases it is possible that pulmonologists will try to use macrolides in the treatment of "idiopathic", "non-CF" bronchiectasis, chronically colonised by *P. aeruginosa*, and nonresponding (or resistant) to the conventional combined antipseudomonal antibiotherapy. Anecdotal evidence exists on the positive effect of long term clarithromycin or azithromycin (500 mg·day^{-1}) on the volume of expectoration, quality of life, and number of exacerbations in this subgroup of bronchiectatic patients [57]. There is little doubt patients a presently receiving macrolides, however only well designed studies will provide the adequate confirmation of the validity of this understandable clinical interest.

Conclusions

The development of pneumococcal macrolide antibiotic resistance in some geographical locations and the introduction of new antibiotics that display higher than normal activity against certain specific pathogens, has challenged the central role of macrolides in the management of LRTIs. To date, this group of antibiotics and particularly azithromycin and clarithromycin remain valid alternatives, although there is a need for well-designed studies aimed to evaluate their efficacy with the different LRTIs in areas with high prevalence of pneumococcal macrolide resistance and in comparison with other potential new alternatives. Finally, in addition to its antimicrobial activity, the macrolides display some unique anti-inflammatory properties that could be of practical use in the management of chronic bronchial infection affecting cystic fibrosis and bronchiectasis.

Summary

During recent decades the macrolides have occupied a central position in the management of different types of lower respiratory tract infections. This is due in some part to their excellent activity and safety both in the adult and in the paediatric population. Recently, however, the development of pneumococcal macrolide antibiotic resistance in some geographical locations, in combination with the introduction of new antibiotics displaying higher activity against certain specific pathogens, has challenged this role.

In acute bronchitis, where antibiotics are not systematically needed, macrolides have the potential to be the alternative choice in selected cases, considering the different pathogens involved, due to its simplistic dosage regimen and relative safety. Considering the acute exhacerbations of chronic bronchitis, azithromycin and clarithromycin may be useful in patients with mild to moderate chronic obstructive pulmonary disease (COPD). Other alternatives such as amoxicillin/clavulanate or quinolones, which are more active against *Haemophilus influenzae*, should be preferred for the treatment of bronchial infection in the group of COPD patients with the poorest lung function, more debilitated in their general condition and presenting frequent episodes of infectious exacerbation.

Owing to their combined activity against the pneumococcus and the atypical bacteria, the macrolides have been the cornerstone for the management of community-acquired pneumonia (CAP). Today, the macrolides remain as a basic alternative for mild-to-moderate CAP managed in an outpatient context in areas where high level macrolide resistance is low. However, the ketolides and new quinolones should be preferred in countries where this type of resistance is important. In the more severe CAP, more studies are needed comparing the classical association β-lactam plus macrolide against monotherapy with a parenteral new quinolone.

Finally, in addition to its antimicrobial activity, the macrolides display some unique anti-inflammatory properties that could be of practical use in the management of chronic bronchial infections affecting cystic fibrosis and bronchiectasis.

Keywords: Antibiotic resistance, anti-inflammatory, community-acquired pneumonia, bronchiectasis, bronchitis, pneumococcus.

References

1.   Kirst HA. New macrolides: expanded horizons for and old class of antibiotics. *J Antimicrob Chemother* 1991; 28: 787–790.

2. Mazzei T, Mini E, Novelli A, *et al.* Chemistry and mode of actino of macrolides. *J Antimicrob Chemother* 1993; 31: Suppl. C, 1–9.

3. Charles L, Segreti J. Choosing the right macrolide antibiotic: a guide to selection. *Drugs* 1997; 53: 349–357.

4. Leclerq R, Courvalin P. Bacterial resistance to macrolide, lincosamide, and strptogramin antibiotics by target modification. *Antimicrob Agents Chemother* 1991; 35: 1267–1272.

5. Roberts MC, Sutclife J, Courvalin P, *et al.* Nomenclature for macrolide-lincosamide-streptogramin B resistance determinants. *Antimicrob Agents Chemother* 1999; 43: 2823–2830.

6. Sutcliffe J, Tait-Kamradt A, Wondrack L. *Streptococcus pneumoniae* and *Streptococcus pyogenes* resistant to macrolides but sensitive to clindamycin: a common resistance pattern mediated by an efflux syste. *Antimicrob Agents Chemother* 1996; 40: 1817–1824.

7. Kirst HA, Sides GD. New directions for macrolides antibiotics: pharmacokinetics and clinical efficacy. *Antimicrob Agents Chemother* 1989; 33: 1419–1422.

8. Langtry HD, Brogden RN. Clarithromycin. A review of its efficacy in the treatment of respiratory tract infections in immunocompetent patients. *Drugs* 1997; 53: 973–1004.

9. Dunn CJ, Barradell LB. Azithromicyn. A Review of its pharmacological propierties and use as 3-day therapy in respiratory tract infections. *Drugs* 1996; 51: 483–505.

10. Carbon C. Pharmacodynamics of macrolides, azalides, and streptogramins: effect on extracellular pathogens. *Clin Infect Dis* 1998; 27: 28–32.

11. Bahal N, Nahata MC. The new macrolides antibiotics: azithromycin, clarithromycin, dirithromycin and roxithromycin. *Ann Pharmacother* 1992; 26: 46–55.

12. Sturgill MG, Rapp RP. Clarithromycin: review of a new macrolide antibiotic with improved microbiologic spectrum and favorable pharmacokinetic and adverse effect profiles. *Ann Pharmacother* 1992; 26: 1099–1008.

13. Zhanel GG, Karlowsky JA, Palatnick L, *et al.* Prevalence of antimicrobial resistance in respiratory tract isolates of *Streptococcus pneumoniae*: results of a Canadian national surveillance study. *Antimicrob Agents Chemother* 1999; 43: 2504–2509.

14. Barry AL, Fuchs PC, Brown SD. *In vitro* activities of the ketolide HMR 3647 against Gram-positive clinical isolates and *Haemophilus influenzae*. *Antimicrob Agents Chemother* 1998; 42: 2138–2140.

15. Hoban DJ, Zhanel GG, Karlowsky JA. *In vitro* activity of the novel ketolide HMR 3647 and comparative oral antibiotics against Canadian respiratory tract isolates of *Streptococcus pneumoniae, Haemophilus influenzae* and *Moraxella catarrhalis*. *Diagn Microbiol Infect Dis* 1999; 35: 37 44.

16. Reinert RR, Bryskier A, Lütticken R. *In vitro* activities of the new ketolides antibiotics HMR 3004 and HMR 3647 against *Streptococcus pneumoniae* in Germany. *Antimicrob Agents Chemother* 1998; 42: 1509–1511.

17. Zhanel GG, Duek M, Hoban DJ, *et al.* Review of macrolides and ketolides. Focus on respiratory Tract infections. *Drugs* 2001; 61: 443–498.

18. Appelbaum PC. Antimicrobial resistance in *Streptococcus pneumoniae*: an overview. *Clin Infet Dis* 1992; 15: 77–83.

19. Liñares J, Alonso T, Pérez JL, *et al.* Decreased susceptibility of penicillin-resistant pneumococci to twenty-four beta-lactam antibiotics. *J Antimicrob Chemoter* 1992; 30: 279–288.

20. Lefevre JC, Bertrand MA, Faucon G. Molecular analysis by pulsed-field gel electrophoresis of penicillin-resistant *Streptococcus pneumoniae* in Toulouse (France). *Eur J Microbiol Infect Dis* 1995; 14: 491–497.

21. Shortridge VD, Doern GV, Brueggemann AB, *et al.* Prevalence of macrolide resistance mechanisms in *Streptococcus pneumoniae* isolates from a multicenter antibiotics resistance surveillance study conducrte in the USA (1994–5). *CID* 1999; 29: 1186–1188.

22. Baquero F, García Rodriguez JA, García de Lomas J, Aguilar L. Antimicrobial resistance of 1.113 Streptococcus pneumoniae isolates from patients with respiratory tract infections in Spain: results a multicenter surveillance study. *Antimicrob Agents Chemother* 1999; 43: 357–359.

23. Amsden GW. Pneumococcal macrolide resistance – myth or reality? *J Antimicrob Chemother* 1999; 44: 1–6.

24. Perez Trallero E. Pneumococcal macrolide resistance –not a myth. *J Antimicrob Chemother* 2000; 45: 401–402.

25. Lonks JR, Garau J, Gómez L, *et al.* Failure of macrolide antibiotic treatment in patients with bacteriemia due to erythromycin-resistant *Streptococcus pneumoniae*. *Clin Infect Dis* 2002; 35: 556–64.

26. Barry AL, Brown SD. Reconsideration of the interpretive criteria for clarithromycin against *Haemophilus influenzae*. Lisbon, 3rd International Conference on the macrolides, Azalides and Streptogramins, 1996; Abstract.

27. Odenholt-Tornqvist I, Löwdin E, Cars O. Postantibiotic effects and postantibiotic sub-MIC effects of roxithromycin, clarithromycin, and azithromycin on respiratory pathogens. *Antimicrob Agents Chemother* 1995; 39: 221–226.

28. Edeltein PH. Antimicrobial chemotherapy for Legionnaires' disease: A review. *Clin Infect Dis* 1995; 21: Suppl. 3, S265–S276.

29. Segreti J, Meyer P, Kepell K. *In vitro* activity of macrolides against intracellular *Legionella pneumophila*. *Diagn Microbiol Infect Dis* 1996; 25: 123–126.

30. Stout JE, Yu VL. Legionellosis. *N Engl J Med* 1997; 337: 682–687.

31. Hosie J, Quinn P, Smits P, *et al.* A comparasion of 5 days of dirithromycin and 7 days of clarithromycin in acute bacterial exacerbation of chronic bronchitis. *J Antimicrob Chemother* 1995; 36: 173–183.

32. Beghi G, Berni F, Carratu L, *et al.* Efficacy and tolerability of azithromycin versus amoxicillin/clavulanic acid in acute purulent exacerbation of chronic bronchitis. *J Chemoter* 1995; 7: 146–152.

33. Zachariah J. A randomized, comparative study to evaluate the efficacy and tolerability of a 3-day course of azithromycin *versus* a 10-day course of co-amoxiclav as treatment of adult patients with lower respiratory tract infections. *J Antimicrob Chemother* 1996; 37: Suppl. C, 103–113.

34. Chodosh S, Schreurs A, Siami G, *et al.* Efficacy of oral ciprofloxacin vs. clarithromycin for treatment of acute bacterial exacerbations of chronic bronchitis. *Clin Infect Dis* 1998; 27: 730–738.

35. Ziering W, McElvaine P. Randomized comparison of once-daily ceftibuten and twice-day clarithromycin in the treatment of acute exacerbations of chronic bronchitis. *J Antimicrob Chemoter* 1995; 36: 173–183.

36. Wasilewski MM, Johns D, Sides GD. Five-day dirithromycin therapy is as effective as seven-day erythromycin therapy for acute exacerbations of chronic bronchitis. *J Antimicrob Chemother* 1999; 43: 541–548.

37. Wilson R, Kubin R, Ballin I, *et al.* Five-day moxifloxacin therapy compared with 7 day clarithromycin therapy for the treatment of acute exacerbations of chronic bronchitis. *J Antimicrob Chemoter* 1999; 44: 501–513.

38. Deabate CA, Mathew CP, Warner JH, *et al.* The safety and efficacy of short course (5-day) moxifloxacin vs. azithromycin in the treatment of patients with acute exacerbation of chronic bronchitis. *Resp Med* 2000; 94: 1029–1037.

39. Grossman RF. Cost-effective therapy for acute exacerbations of chronic bronchitis. *Semin Respir Infect* 2000; 15: 71–81.

40. Niederman MS, Mandell MA, Anzueto A, *et al.* Guidelines for the management of adults with community-acquired pneumonia: diagnosis, assessment of severity, antimicrobial therapy and prevention. *Am J Respir Crit Care Med* 2001; 163: 1730–1754.

41. Bartlett JG, Dowell SJ, Mandell LA, *et al.* Practice guidelines for the management of community-acquired pneumonia in adults. *Infectious Diseases Society of America CID* 2000; 31: 347–382.

42. Huchon G, Woodhead M, Gialdoni-Grasi G, *et al.* Guidelines for management of adult community-acquired lower respiratory tract infections. *Eur Respir J* 1998; 11: 986–991.

43. Liippo K, Tala E, Puolijoki H, *et al.* A comparative study of dirithromycin and erythromycin in bacterial pneumonia. *J Infect* 1994; 28: 131–139.

44. Schönwald S, Barsi B, Klinar I, *et al.* Three-day azithromycin compared with ten-day roxithromycin treatment of atypical pneumonia. *Scand J Infect Dis* 1994; 26: 706–710.

45. Bothe R, van't Wout JW, Lobatto S, *et al.* Efficacy and safety of azithromycin versus benzylpenicillin or erythromycin in community-acquired pneumonia. *Eur J Clin Microbiol Infect Dis* 1995; 14: 182–187.

46. Lode H, Garau J, Grassi C, *et al.* Treatment of community-acquired pneumonia: a randomized comparison of sparfloxacin, amoxycilin-clavulanic acid and erythromycin. *Eur Respir J* 1995; 8: 1999–2007.

47. Örtqvist A, Valtonen M, Cars O, *et al.* Oral empiric treatment of community-acquired pneumonia: a multicenter, double-blind, randomized study comparing sparfloxacin with roxithromicyn. *Chest* 1996; 110: 1499–1506.

48. Hernández Jm, Sides gd, Conforti PM, *et al.* Clinical afficacy of dirithromycin in patients with bacteremic pneumonia. *Clin Ther* 1996; 18: 1128–38.

49. Genné D, Siegrist HH, Humair L, *et al.* Clarithromycin versus amoxicillin-clavulanic acid in the treatment of community-acquired pneumonia. *Eur J Clin Microbiol Infect Dis* 1997; 16: 783–788.

50. Tellier G, Hassman J, Leroy B, *et al.* Oral telithromycin (HMR 3647) 800 mg once daily is well tolerated and as effective as oral clarithromycin 500 mg twice daily in community-acquired pneumonia (CAP) in adults. Toronto, 40th Interscience Conference on Antimicrobial Agents and Chemotherapy, 2000; 2227.

51. Hoeffken G, Meyer HP, Winter J, *et al.* The efficacy and safety of two oral moxifloxacin regimens compared to oral clarithromycin in the treatment of community-acquired pneumonia. *Resp Med* 2001; 95: 553–64.

52. Finch R, SchÜrmann D, Collins O, *et al.* Randomized controlled trial of sequential IV (i.v.) and oral moxifloxacin compared with sequential *i.v.* and oral co-amoxiclav with or without clarithromycin in patients with community-acquired pneumonia requiring initial parenteral treatment. *Antimicrob Agents Chemother* 2002; 46: 1746–1754.

53. Homma H, Yamanaka A, Tanimoto S, *et al.* Diffuse panbronchiolitis- a disease of the transitional zone of the lung. *Chest* 1983; 83: 63–69.

54. Kudoh S, Uetake T, Hagiwara M, *et al.* Clinical effect of low dose log-term erythromycin chemotherapy on diffuse panbronchiolitis. *Jpn J Thorac Dis* 1987; 25: 632–634.

55. Prince AS. Biofilms, antimicrobial resistance and airway infection. *N Engl J Med* 2002; 347: 1110–1111.

56. Nguyen T, Louise SG, Beringer P, Gill MA. Potencial role of macrolides antibiotics in the management of cystic fibrosis lung disease. *Curr Opin Pulm Dis* 2002; 8: 521–528.

57. Equi A, Balfour-Lynn M, Bush A, Rosenthal A. Long term azithromycin in children with cystic fibrosis: a randomized, placebo controlled crossover trial. *Lancet* 2002; 360: 978–984.

CHAPTER 6

Fluoroquinolones and lower respiratory tract infections

A. Kuhnke, H. Lode

Dept of Chest and Infectious Diseases, Chest Hospital Emil Behring, Affil. Free University of Berlin, Berlin, Germany.

Correspondence: H. Lode, Dept of Chest and Infectious Diseases, City Hospital Emil Behring, Affil. Free University of Berlin, Zum Heckeshorn 33, 14109 Berlin, Germany.

Lower respiratory tract infections (LRTIs) are a major cause of morbidity and mortality. The efficacy of the antibiotics traditionally used in the treatment of these infections is increasingly compromised by the emergence of penicillin and macrolide resistant bacteria. This has resulted in a search for alternative treatment options. Currently marketed available newer fluoroquinolones are levofloxacin, gatifloxacin, moxifloxacin and very soon gemifloxacin. These agents offer many advantages such as excellent bioavailability, longer serum half-lives, infrequent dosing and achieving of high respiratory tissue concentrations. They provide a broad antibacterial spectrum incorporating penicillin and macrolide resistant pneumococci and also anaerobes, while retaining good Gram-negative coverage. However, they are inferior to ciprofloxacin in their antipseudomonal activity. The efficacy of the new fluoroquinolones in community-acquired respiratory tract infections has been confirmed in several clinical trials and therefore resulted in the inclusion in recent therapy guidelines.

Introduction

Respiratory infections are a major cause of morbidity and mortality and their impact is even growing in the aging population. LRTIs include acute exacerbations of chronic bronchitis (AECB), community-acquired pneumonia (CAP) as well as hospitalised-acquired pneumonia (HAP). Of these three conditions AECB is the most prevalent.

Community-acquired respiratory tract infection (RTIs) are commonly caused by Gram-positive organisms (predominantly *Streptococcus pneumoniae*), Gram-negative pathogens (*Haemophilus influenzae* and *Moraxella catarrhalis*) and "atypical" bacteria (*e.g. Chlamydia pneumoniae, Legionella pneumophila* and *Mycoplasma pneumoniae*). The emergence of penicillin resistant *S. pneumoniae* as well as increasing β-lactamase production among *H. influenzae, M. catarrhalis* and many Gram-negative bacteria has resulted in a widespread use of the new fluoroquinolones in the therapy of community-acquired respiratory infections. Due to the excellent activity of levofloxacin, gatifloxacin, moxifloxacin and gemifloxacin against Gram-negative pathogens and improved Gram-positive activity over ciprofloxacin they are first line antibiotic treatment options. Gatifloxacin and moxifloxacin also display improved activity against anaerobes.

Microorganisms responsible for HAP differ from that of community acquired RTIs. Predominant organisms are *Staphylococcus aureus, Pseudomonas aeruginosa* and Enterobacteriaceae. However potential pathogens differ according to the population

Eur Respir Mon, 2004, 28, 94–112. Printed in UK - all rights reserved. Copyright ERS Journals Ltd 2004; European Respiratory Monograph; ISSN 1025-448x. ISBN 1-904097-32-4.

of patients in the intensive care unit (ICU), the duration of stay in ICU and the hospital as well as the prior antimicrobial therapy that may have been given. Amongst the available fluoroquinolones, ciprofloxacin is the most active against Gram-negative bacteria, including *P. aeruginosa*, whereas activity against Gram-positive cocci and many anaerobes is limited. Therefore ciprofloxacin is a widely recommended antibiotic for the treatment of Gram-negative bacteria especially when *P. aeruginosa* is considered.

The new fluoroquinolones offer many advantages over currently recommended antibiotic regimes for serious bacterial infections in the lower respiratory tract. The combination of their excellent bioavailability with longer serum half-lives, infrequent dosing, high concentrations in respiratory tissue and broad spectrum antibacterial activity can hardly be matched by other available antibiotics.

Resistance to fluoroquinolones is still low, although emergence of resistance, especially by *S. pneumoniae*, has risen. [1, 2] That should lead to reconsiderations about widespread and indiscriminate use of these agents for trivial respiratory infections.

Antibacterial spectrum

Although the class of quinolones has been in existence since 1962, only when the molecule was fluorinated in 1983 was the class considered to be a major antibacterial group. The classic fluoroquinolones *e.g.* ciprofloxacin, norfloxacin and ofloxacin exert a strong activity against Gram-negative bacteria, but their effectiveness has been questioned when Gram-positive bacteria are involved. The new fluoroquinolones developed during the 1990s exhibit an enhanced activity against Gram-positive bacteria. Widely used fluoroquinolones are given in table 1 according to the Paul-Ehrlich-Gesellschaft für Chemotherapie (PEG) classification [3].

The most important causes of bacterial LRTIs are predominantly *S. pneumoniae*, *H. influenzae* and *M. catarrhalis*. The percentage of macrolide and β-lactam-resistant strains among these species is continuously increasing and therefore a worldwide problem. The *in vitro* activity of the new fluoroquinolones against clinical important respiratory pathogens is excellent and summarised in table 2. The given minimal inhibitory concentration (MIC) values were gathered by ZHANEL *et al.* [4] from reviews and synthesis of recently reported values for each drug. The table displays the effective concentration of the fluoroquinolones in order to inhibit 50 and 90% of the bacterial isolates, MIC_{50} and MIC_{90}, respectively. Based on the MIC_{90} values the order of activity of the fluoroquinolones against *S. pneumoniae* is approximately gemifloxacin (MIC_{90} 0.03 $\mu g \cdot mL^{-1}$)>moxifloxacin (MIC_{90}/0.25 $\mu g \cdot mL^{-1}$)>gatifloxacin (MIC_{90} 0.5 $\mu g \cdot mL^{-1}$)> levofloxacin (MIC_{90} 1 $\mu g \cdot mL^{-1}$)>ciprofloxacin (MIC_{90} 2 $\mu g \cdot mL^{-1}$). Concluding gemifloxacin is currently the most effective fluoroquinolone agent against *S. pneumoniae*.

Table 1. – Widely used fluoroquinolones grouped according to their Paul-Ehrlich-Gesellschaft für Chemotherapie (PEG) classification [3]

Group	Fluoroquinolone	Spectrum/therapeutic use
I	Norfloxacin	Mainly active against Gram-negative pathogens Used for urinary tract infections
II	Ciprofloxacin Ofloxacin	Broad indications for systemic use, Moderate activity against Gram-positive pathogens
III	Levofloxacin	Improved activity against Gram-positive and "atypical" pathogens Infections of the respiratory tract and others
IV	Gatifloxacin Gemifloxacin Moxifloxacin	Improved activity against Gram-positive and "atypical" pathogens as well as anaerobes, Infections of the respiratory tract and others

Table adapted from NADER and ADAM [3].

Table 2. – *In vitro* activity of the fluoroquinolones against major respiratory pathogens adapted from ZHANEL *et al.* [4]

Bacteria	Ciprofloxacin		Levofloxcacin		Gatifloxacin		Gemifloxacin		Moxifloxacin	
MIC	MIC50	MIC90	MIC50	MIC90	MIC50	MIC90	MIC50	MIC90	MIC50	MIC90
Streptococcus pneumoniae	1	2	1	1	0.25	0.5	0.03	0.03	0.12	0.25
Haemophilus influenzae	0.004	0.008	0.015	0.03	0.008	0.015	0.004	0.008	0.03	0.03
Moraxella catarrhalis	0.03	0.03	0.06	0.06	0.03	0.03	0.015	0.015	0.06	0.06
Staphylococcus aureus (MS)	0.5	1	0.12	0.5	0.12	0.12	0.015	0.03	0.06	0.12
Mycoplasma pneumoniae	1	2	0.5	0.5	0.06	0.12	0.06	0.12	0.12	0.12
Chlamydia pneumoniae	1	2	0.5	1	0.12	0.25	0.25	0.25	0.5	1
Legionella pneumophila	0.03	0.03	0.008	0.015	0.015	0.015	0.015	0.03	0.015	0.015
Escherichia coli	0.015	0.25	0.03	0.12	0.02	0.1	0.015	0.015	0.06	0.5
Klebsiella pneumoniae	0.03	0.06	0.06	0.12	0.06	0.12	0.03	0.12	0.12	0.5
Pseudomonas aeruginosa	0.25	4	0.5	16	2	8	0.25	8	2	8

All data presented as $mg \cdot L^{-1}$. MIC50: minimal inhibitory concentration of 50% of bacteria; MIC90: minimal inhibitory concentration of 90% of bacteria; MS: methicillin sensitive.

Overall the MIC90 values for all of the new fluoroquinolones against the majority of Gram-negative bacteria (except *P. aeruginosa*) are generally <1 $\mu g \cdot mL^{-1}$. However, ciprofloxacin continues to be comparable or superior to most of the new fluoroquinolones in Gram-negative pathogens. Against *H. influenzae* the new fluoroquinolones are highly active with MIC90 values ranging between 0.008 and 0.03 $\mu g \cdot mL^{-1}$.

For *M. catarrhalis* all of the new fluoroquinolones and ciprofloxacin display exceptional activity with MIC90 ranges from 0.015–0.06 $\mu g \cdot mL^{-1}$. Any atypical pathogens are also well covered. The MIC90 values against *C. pneumoniae* are usually ≤ 1.0 $\mu g \cdot mL^{-1}$, *versus L. pneumophila* ≤ 0.03 $\mu g \cdot mL^{-1}$ and *versus M. pneumoniae* ≤ 0.5 $\mu g \cdot mL^{-1}$.

Mechanism of actions and resistance

Intracellular accumulation of the fluoroquinolone molecule is essential for its antimicrobial activity and has been shown to occur by simple diffusion across the cell membrane into bacteria [5] and with some uptake through the porin pathway in the outer membrane of Gram-negative organism [6]. Once inside the bacterium the fluoroquinolones target two essential enzymes of bacterial cells. These are topoisomerase II (deoxyribosnucleic acid: DNA gyrase) and topoisomerase IV. Topoisomerases are essential enzymes in controlling the topological state of DNA by catalysing supercoiling, relaxing, knotting, and catenation reactions which are vital for DNA replication, transcription, recombination and repair. DNA gyrase is composed of two A and two B subunits, which are encoded by gyrA and gyrB genes. The A subunits cause strand breaks in the bacterial chromosome and reseal the chromosome after supercoiling. The subunits B are responsible for introducing negative supercoils into the DNA strands. The topoisomerase IV is composed of two ParC and two ParE subunits, encoded by the parC and parE genes. These enzymes play an essential role in partitioning replicated chromosomal DNA during cell division and in DNA relaxation. Furthermore it is important for decatenation reactions, the separation of the bacterial daughter chromosomes [7].

Resistance is mediated chiefly through two main mechanisms. Firstly mutations in the bacterial genes that encode the DNA gyrase and topoisomerase IV and secondly by active efflux pumps leading to decreased intracellular drug concentration.

The most important mechanism is mediated through alteration in genes that encode for the enzymes, occurring in an area called the "quinolone resistance determining region" (QRDR). The resistance arises stepwise. In some species, first step mutants occur in gyrA and occacionally in gyrB, while in others they occur in parC and less common in parE. Furthermore there seems to be a target preference: in Gram-positive pathogens, mutations occur more often in topoisomerase IV whereas alterations in DNA gyrase are more common in Gram-negative bacteria [8].

Fluoroquinolone resistance in *S. pneumoniae* is based on mutations in the topoisomerase IV and also in DNA gyrase genes. Resistance, however, is primarily mediated by mutations in QRDR of parC and gyrA genes. [9] The most frequent mutations that contributed resistance in gyrA and parC are Ser-81 Phe or Tyr and Ser-79 Tyr. It has also been demonstrated that the highest level of resistance occurs when there are double mutations in both parC and gyrA genes. The presence of these mutations raises the MIC for fluoroquinolones [10]. However there is a big heterogeneity of mutations. The position of amino acid changes within the genes affected resistance more than the total number of QRDR mutations [11].

The second resistance mechanism is mediated through active drug efflux by the overexpression of certain efflux pumps. These pumps are multidrug transporters and driven by the proton motive force. Until now several genes and mutations encoding for efflux pumps have been identified. For example Pmr A in *S. pneumoniae* [12], NorA in *S. aureus* [13], and MexAB-OprM in *P. aeruginosa* [14]. A possible strategy to lower fluoroquinolone resistance is the therapeutic use of efflux inhibitors and the development of new fluoroquinolones, which are not substrates for these pumps [15]. A third lesser important resistance mechanism is the impermeability of the outer bacterial cell wall for fluoroquinolones.

There is abundant evidence now that bacteria with acquired fluoroquinolone resistance are able to disseminate clonally and causes global spread of resistant strains. [16] The Pneumococcal Molecular Epidemiology Network has defined the nomenclature of antimicrobial-resistant pneumococcal clones and therefore facilitated the documentation of resistance among global clones [17]. Extensive molecular typing studies from various regions in the world have identified a number of clones of highly penicillin-resistant pneumococci. Predominant among these clones are the Spanish multidrug-resistant serotype 23F and 6B as well as the major penicillin-resistant serotype 9V. Due to the emergence of fluoroquinolone-resistance it became interesting to determine the clonality of fluoroquinolone resistance in pneumococci. Several studies have identified the Spain 23F-1 and Spain 9V-3 strain as predominant strains accounting for fluoroquinolone resistance. Mc Gee *et al.* [18] investigated 29 fluoroquinolone-resistant clinical isolates of *S. pneumoniae* from the Alexander Project (1992–1997) and from a collection of strains in Northern Ireland (1997). In this study 56% of fluoroquinolone-resistant strains belonged to the Spain 23F and Spain 9V strains. Another study conducted in Hong Kong in 2000 investigated the susceptibility of 180 pneumococcal isolates to antimicrobial [19]. The overall fluoroquinolone nonsusceptibility was 13.3%. Molecular analyses demonstrated in all strains the genetically relation to the Spain 23F-1 clone. Meanwhile this clone has also been found in the US [16]. In conclusion fluoroquinolone resistance has arisen in multidrug resistant clones. Further spread and selection of such resistance could compromise the utility of fluoroquinolones, a point that also emphasises the importance for the careful use of these agents in appropriate patients.

Pharmacokinetics and pharmacodynamics

The pharmacokinetic parameters of a drug define the rate and extent of drug delivery into blood and various extravascular sites, as well as the rate and extent of drug elimination. These parameters are quantified by characterising drug concentrations over a given period. Pharmacodynamic parameters define the relationship between drug concentration and effects that may be beneficial (therapeutic) or adverse (toxic). Pharmacodynamic parameters may be quantified *in vivo*, but in the case of antimicrobial agents, they are more often measured *in vitro*. The most common antibiotic pharmacodynamic parameters are the MIC and the minimal bactericidal concentrations (MBC). By appropriately combining pharmacokinetic and pharmacodynamic parameters of a specific antibiotic, an approximation of the drug's activity *in vivo* may be made.

All new fluoroquinolones have a bactericidal activity and a postantibiotic effect. Compared with ciprofloxacin, all new fluoroquinolones have a longer elimination half-life that allows once daily dosing (table 3). In addition, these antibiotics have excellent penetration into respiratory tissues, with the highest concentrations found in the epithelial lining fluid and alveolar macrophages (table 4). Both locations are important for extracellularly and intracellularly growing pathogens. The newer fluoroquinolones gatifloxacin, levofloxacin and moxifloxacin are currently available, or will be in the near future, in both intravenous (IV) and oral formulations. Gatifloxacin and moxifloxacin reach similar plasma concentrations with both formulations when administered in equivalent doses to levofloxacin. Physicians may therefore have greater flexibility in the use of all formulations in seriously ill patients, who would normally have to exclusively receive IV therapy [22].

With regard to the pharmacodynamic characteristics, the new fluoroquinolones cause concentration-dependent killing. For this category of antibiotics, peak serum concentrations, *i.e.* C_{max} and area under the curve (AUC), are important parameters for assessing clinical response. *In vitro* studies have shown that C_{max}/MIC ratio of >10 prevents the emergence of antimicrobial-resistant microorganisms and also favours

Table 3. – Pharmacokinetic and pharmacodynamic parameters of fluoroquinolones *versus Streptococcus pneumoniae*

Fluoroquinolone	$t_{1/2}$ h	C_{max} µg·mL^{-1}·70 kg^{-1}	AUC24 µg·mL^{-1}·70 kg^{-1}	MIC µg·mL^{-1}	AUC24/MIC
Ciprofloxacin 500 mg *b.i.d.*	3.5	2.3	20	2	10
Levofloxacin 500 mg od	6.95	5.1	48	1	48
Gatifloxacin 400 mg od	6.52	3.9	34	0.5	68
Moxifloxacin 400 mg od	9.15	3.3	34	0.25	136
Gemifloxacin 320 mg od	8.0	1.2	10	0.03	333

$t_{1/2}$: elimination half-life; C_{max}: concentration maximum; AUC24: area under the curve in 24 h; MIC: minimal inhibitory concentration. Table adapted from ZHANEL *et al.* [4] and LUBASCH *et al.* [20].

Table 4. – Antimicrobial concentrations in various sites of respiratory tract following standard doses of fluoroquinolones

	MIC90 µg·mL^{-1} Streptococcus pneumoniae	Concentrations in µg·mL^{-1} or µg·g^{-1}		
		Serum	Epithelial lining fluid	Alveolar macrophages
Ciprofloxacin[#]	2	1.9±0.16	3.0±1.05	13.39±3.53
Levofloxacin[¶]	1	4.1	10.9	27.7
Gatifloxacin[+]	0.5	3.22 (2.1–4.5)	6.16 (1.7–18.3)	77.32 (48.9–138.5)
Moxifloxacin[§]	0.25	3.2	20.7	56.7
Gemifloxacin[f]	0.03	1.4±0.44	2.69±1.96	107±77

MIC90: minimal inhibitory concentration of 90% of bacteria; [#]: 250 mg *b.i.d.* for 4 days, bronchoscopy performed at a mean of 288.25 min after final dose data presented as mean and mean±SD; [¶]: single dose 500 mg, bronchoscopy performed 4 h after dosing; [+]: single dose 400 mg, bronchoscopy performed 4 h after dosing (data as mean and range); [§]: single dose 400 mg, bronchoscopy performed 2.2 h after dosing; [f]: single dose 320 mg (mean±SD). Table adapted from LODE and ALLEWELT [21].

a positive clinical outcome. The ratio of the AUC over 24 h above the MIC90 (AUIC) also reflects a good clinical response when these values are >125. However, lower values, *e.g.* with levofloxacin in chronic bronchitis (CB) and pneumococcal pneumonia treatment, have also been demonstrated to be efficacious [23].

Clinical treatment

Acute exacerbations of chronic bronchitis

AECB is a frequent complication of chronic obstructive pulmonary disease (COPD). Infection has been identified as the cause of ~80% of these episodes. Bacterial pathogens can be isolated in ~50% [24]. Commonly associated with AECB are *H. influenzae*, *S. pneumoniae*, *M. catarrhalis* and *Haemophilus parainfluenzae*. Antibacterial therapy usually starts empirically, therefore it is important that the choice of agents and dosing regimen covers the most common pathogens. The antibacterial spectrum of the new fluoroquinolones encompasses the bacteria responsible for most pathogens in AECB.

The therapeutic efficacy of the newer fluoroquinolones levofloxacin, gatifloxacin, moxifloxacin and gemifloxacin has been evaluated in a number of randomised, multicenter trials. Table 5 shows the recent clinical comparative trials with marketed

Table 5. – Recent clinical multicentre comparative trials of newer fluoroquinolones in acute exacerbations of chronic bronchitis

Reference	Fluoroquinolone and comparator	Dosage and duration days	Response rate %	
			Clinical	Bacteriological
Wilson *et al.* [25]	Gemifloxacin	320 mg od×5	82.6[#]	89.6
	Ceftriaxone IV/Cefuroxime	1g od×3/500 mg *b.i.d.*×7	72.1	86.3
Wilson *et al.* [26]	Gemifloxacin	320 mg od×5	79.5	86.0
	Clarithromycin	500 *b.i.d.*×7	78.2	74.2
File *et al.* [27]	Gemifloxacin	320 mg od×5	93.6	90.9
	Amoxicillin/clavulanic acid	500/125 mg *t.i.d.*×7	93.2	79.5
Soler *et al.* [28]	Gatifloxacin	200 mg od×5	86.2	87.5
	Gatifloxacin	400 mg od×5	79.4	87.3
	Amoxicillin/clavulanic acid	500/125 mg *t.i.d.*×10	81.7	79.1
Gotfried *et al.* [29]	Gatifloxacin	400 mg od×5	89.0	98
		400 mg od×7	88.0	94
	Clarithromycin	500 mg *b.i.d.*×10	89	98%
Grassi *et al.* [30]	Moxifloxacin	400 mg od×5	90.6	91.7
	Ceftriaxone	IM×7	89.0	93.3
Schaberg *et al.* [31]	Moxifloxacin	400 mg od×5	96.2	87.7
	Co-amoxiclav	625 mg *t.i.d.*×7	91.6	89.6
Deabate *et al.* [32]	Moxifloxacin	400 mg od×5	88.0	95.0
	Azithromycin	500 mg od×1/250 mg od×4	88.0	94.0
Wilson *et al.* [33]	Moxifloxacin	400 mg od×5	89	77[#]
	Clarithromycin	500 mg *b.i.d.*×7	88	62
Amsden *et al.* [34]	Levofloxacin	500mg od×7	86	76
	Azithromycin	500 mg od×1/250 mg od×4	82	93
Weiss [35]	Levofloxacin	500 mg od×10	87.4	
	Clarithromycin	500 mg *b.i.d.*×10	87.9	
	Cefuroxime axetil	250 mg *b.i.d.*×10	79.8	
Shah *et al.* [36]	Levofloxacin	250 mg od×7–10	70	69
		500 mg od×7–10	70	77
	Cefuroxime axetil	250 mg *b.i.d.*×7–10	61	60

od: once daily, *b.i.d.*: twice daily; *t.i.d.*: three times daily; *q.i.d.*: four times daily; All study medications were given orally unless if specially signed, IV: intravenous, IM: intra muscular, [#]: significant.

newer fluoroquinolones in AECB, which were published between 1999–2003. Results of the cited studies are not completely comparable due to varying primary efficacy parameters, study settings and patient populations.

Gemifloxacin once daily 320 mg *per os* was compared with either: 1) 10 days sequential therapy of IV ceftriaxone and oral cefuroxime [25]; 2) 7 days clarithromycin *per os* [26]; and 3) 7 days amoxicillin/clavulanic acid *per os* [27]. However, the clinical response rates in recipients of gemifloxacin were 79.5%, 82.6% in the intention-to-treat (ITT) population and 93.6% in the per protocol (PP) population. Evaluation of clinical responses was performed with clarithromycin 13–24 days, with ceftriaxone/cefuroxime 21–28 days and with amoxicillin/clavulanic acid 14 days after the treatment had ended. In these studies the clinical success rate of gemifloxacin was at least as effective and as well tolerated as the comparative regime. Only one study showed a significant superiority of gemifloxacin when compared to ceftriaxone at follow up. In this study the mean time to hospital discharge was additionally significantly lower in gemifloxacin recipients. Bacteriological success was defined as eradication of the initial pathogen in a repeated sputum culture or presumed eradication in absence of sputum production. Bacteriological failure means persistence of the original pathogen or appearance of a new one. Bacteriological response rates at the end of therapy were evaluated for gemifloxacin with 89.6%, 86.0% and 90.9%.

In two trials comparing gatifloxacin with: 1) 10 days clarithromycin [29]; and 2) 10 days amoxicillin/clavulanic acid, the clinical success rates showed equivalence to comparators. In both studies bacteriological eradication rates were without any statistical difference. However it is important to note that SOLER *et al.* [28] evaluated the clinical and bacteriological efficacy for two dosing regiments these were 200 mg and 400 mg gatifloxacin, without statistically differences in their outcomes. Furthermore GOTFRIED *et al.* [29] demonstrated identical clinical and bacteriological success rates for 5 and 7 day duration of gatifloxacin therapy. These results were determined 7–14 days after completion of the study treatment and suggest that high clinical and bacteriological success rates can be achieved with short-course gatifloxacin therapy. Similar results were found for cephalosporins *e.g.* cefuroxime and cefibuten [37, 38].

Short-course therapy in AECB had been established and investigated for moxifloxacin in several clinical trials. Administration of 5 days moxifloxacin was compared with: 1) 7 days of ceftriaxione [30]; 2) 7 days of amoxicillin/clavulanic acid [31]; 4) 5 days of azithromycin [32]; and 5) 7 days of clarithromycin [33]. All these studies demonstrated at least equivalent clinical and bacteriological efficacy in addition. Data for clinical success ranged from 88–96.2% in clinical evaluable patients. Bacteriological success was determined between 77–95% for moxifloxacin. One study demonstrated a superior efficacy of moxifloxacin compared with 7 days of clarithromycin therapy [33].

A treatment of 7 or 10 days levofloxacin was compared with: 1) 5 days of azithromycin [34]; 2) with 10 days of cefuroxime axetil or clarithromycin in a three armed study [35]; and 3) with 7–10 days of cefuroxime axetil [36] treatment. In these studies the clinical success rate with fluoroquinolones was >86% in the clinical evaluable population, except in SHAH *et al.* [36] This study evaluated the clinical success rate for levofloxacin 250 mg or 500 mg with 70% in the ITT population and with 78% and 79% respectively in the PP population. This study was accompanied by relative high protocol violations. However, evaluation of patient subgroups revealed that the 250 mg dose of levofloxacin was less effective than the 500 mg dose in those patients who were hospitalised or revealed concomitant theophylline or corticosteroids medication.

To summarise in all these studies the fluoroquinolones demonstrated at least equivalent clinical success to standard regimen. But there are several facts to take in consideration. The major end points of clinical success were measured at different time points after completion of antibacterial therapy. Severity of AECB in enrolled patients was heterogeneous. Some studies only enrolled outpatients, whereas other investigated hospitalised patients. And furthermore these trials were performed for regulatory approval of these fluoroquinolones in AECB and were planned to demonstrate therefore equivalence rather than differences. However, reasons not to use these agents indiscriminately in AECB include concerns about emergence of resistance, frequent comparable efficacy of nonfluoroquinolone-comparators and higher costs. Alternatively once daily dosing regimens and short treatment duration of fluoroquinolones do not appear to compromise the therapeutic efficacy and may in fact be expected to promote patient compliance with the treatment regimen, potentially reducing the risk of development of resistance in the target pathogens. Furthermore the fluoroquinolones displayed good tolerability and safety profile.

Patients with AECB are a heterogeneous group and should therefore be stratified in low and high risk patients for a poor outcome. Factors that predict a poorer outcome include exacerbations characterised by multiple symptoms (increased dyspnoea, sputum production and sputum purulence), >65 yrs of age, underlying severe obstructive lung disease, frequent exacerbations in the previous year and presence of coexisting cardiac disease [39] Other important factors to take into account are prior use of antibiotics or residence in a long-term care facility. A study conducted by ELLER et al. [40] found that a compromised lung function in patients with COPD is correlated by a higher rate of Enterobacteriaceae and *Pseudomonas spp.* In contrast patients with better lung function had significantly more Pneumococci, *H. influenzae* and *M. catarrhalis* strains in sputum cultures. That means if *P. aeruginosa* is the anticipated or cultured pathogen, ciprofloxacin is the recommended fluoroquinolone due to its limited activity of newer fluoroquinolones in these cases [41].

The use of the new fluoroquinolones as first line therapy should be restricted for patients who have risk factors for a poor outcome or who are severely ill or require admission to intensive care units. Then the expected benefit to the patients justifies the higher costs and general concerns about resistance.

Community-acquired pneumonia

In CAP the causative organism remains unidentified in ~40–60% of the cases [42]. In those cases where a pathogen is identified, the most common aetiological agent is *S. pneumoniae*. Other bacteria include *H. influenzae* and atypical respiratory pathogens *i.e. M. pneumoniae*, *C. pneumoniae* and *L. pneumophila*. Atypical pathogens are not susceptible to β-lactam antibiotics, but are covered well by the newer fluoroquinolones and macrolides.

Similar to AECB the clinical efficacy of new fluoroquinolones has been evaluated in several comparative prospective trials, these are shown in table 6. In respect to clinical treatment guidelines comparators in these studies included β-lactams and macrolides.

Three clinical comparative trials investigating levofloxacin in ambulatory and hospitalised patients with CAP have been published since 1998. Levofloxacin in sequential IV/*per os* of levofloxacin was compared with: 1) azithromycin/ceftriaxione [43]; 2) clarithromycin [44]: and 3) ceftriaxone [45]. Clinical response rates for levofloxacin ranged in the clinical evaluable and per protocol population between 86–94% and bacteriological success were identified from 83–89.5%. The results showed that levofloxacin was as effective as the comparator in outpatients as well as hospitalised patients with moderate-to-severe pneumonia. Since levofloxacin is in *per os* and IV formulation available switch therapy is possible without changing the treatment drug [43, 45].

Similar results have been recently published in two studies comparing the efficacy of gatifloxacin with: 1) clarithromycin [46]; and 2) amoxicillin/clavulanic acid [47]. Clinical

Table 6. – Recent clinical comparative trials of newer fluoroquinolones in community-acquired pneumonia

Reference	Fluoroquinolone and comparator	Dosage and duration days	Response rate in %	
			Clinical	Bacteriological
FRANK E et al. [43]	Levofloxacin	500 mg IV/per os od×10	94.1	89.5
	Azithromycin	500 mg od IV/per os×10	92.3	92.3
	Ceftriaxone	1 g IV od×2		
GOTFRIED et al. [44]	Levofloxacin	500 mg od×7	86	88
	Clarithromycin ER	1000 mg od×7	88	86
NORRBY et al. [45]	Levofloxacin	500 mg IV/per os b.i.d.×≥5	87	83
	Ceftriaxone	4 g IV od×≥5	86	84
LODE et al. [46]	Gatifloxacin	400 mg od×5-14	92.2	96.7
	Clarithromycin	500 mg b.i.d.×5-14	93.1	87.5
LODE et al. [47]	Gatifloxacin	400 mg od×5-10	86.8	83.1
	Amoxicillin/ Clavulanic acid	500/125 mg t.i.d.×5-10	81.6	78.7
FINCH et al. [48]	Moxifloxacin	400 mg od IV/per os ×7-14	93.4[#]	93.7[#]
	Amoxicillin/clavulanic acid with or without clarithromycin	1,2 g mg t.i.d. IV/ 500/125 mg t.i.d. per os+500 mg b.i.d. IV/per os×7-14	85.4	81.7
HOEFFKEN et al. [49]	Moxifloxacin	200 mg od×10	93.9	72.5
	Moxifloxacin	400 mg od×10	94.4	78.7
	Clarithromycin	500 mg b.i.d.×10	94.3	70.7
PETITPRETZ et al. [50]	Moxifloxacin	400 mg od×10	91.5	89.7
	Amoxicillin	1 g t.i.d.×10	89.7	82.4
LODE et al. [51]	Gemifloxacin	320 mg od×7-14	92.2	90.6
	Ceftriaxone/Cefuroxime with or without a macrolide	2 g IV×1-7 500 mg b.i.d. per os×1-13	93.4	87.3
FILE et al. [52]	Gemifloxacin	320 mg od×7-14	87.6*	84.2
	Trovafloxacin	200 mg od×7-14	81.1	80.4

[#]: significant; ER: extended release; All study medication were given orally, unless if specially signed, IV: intravenous; od: once daily, b.i.d.: twice daily; t.i.d.: three times daily, q.i.d.: four times daily.

response rates of 86.8% and 92.2% confirmed the high effectiveness in CAP. Bacteriological success was also seen in high figures of 83.1% and 96.7%.

Moxifloxacin was compared either with: 1) clarithromycin [49]; 2) amoxicillin [50]; and 3) amoxicillin/clavulanic acid plus variable clarithromycin [48]. Clarithromycin was administered when atypical pathogens were considered. Results of these three trials are generally consistent with those of previous discussed studies. Interestingly, however, sequential IV and oral therapy of moxifloxacin displayed statistical significant higher clinical (93.4%) and bacteriological success (93.7%) over the regimen amoxicillin/ clavulanic acid with or without clarithromycin. These superiorities were irrespective of severity of pneumonia and whether or not the treatment regime included a macrolide [48] These findings are consistent with data published by LODE et al. [53] This trial also demonstrates equivalent effectiveness of sequential IV/per os moxifloxacin compared to amoxicillin/clavunalate with or without clarithromycin in patients with severe pneumonia. Although these studies are designed to show equivalence of treatment regimen, superiority has also been demonstrated comparing sequential therapy of levofloxacin with sequential therapy of ceftriaxone/cefuroxime axetil with or without erythromycin or doxycycline [54], whereas FRANK et al. [43] demonstrated equivalence again.

Gemifloxacin used to treat CAP was compared with trovafloxacin [52] and sequential therapy of IV ceftriaxone and per os cefuroxime axetil with or without a macrolide [51]. Meanwhile the use of trovafloxacin has, due to hepatotoxicity, been withdrawn from the market, however it was considered to be one of the most potent quinolones against pneumococci and a very effective antimicrobial for therapy of CAP. Currently gemifloxacin is the most potent member of the fluoroquinolones against *S. pneumoniae* with further excellent activity against other respiratory pathogens. Correspondingly oral gemifloxacin exhibited clinical success rates of 87.6% and 92.2% in these studies and high bacteriological success rates of 84.2% and 90.6% [51, 52].

In all these studies high rates of clinical and bacteriological efficacy were accompanied by good drug safety and tolerance. The frequency of drug-related adverse events was in generally comparable to standard regimen comparators in these studies. Most adverse events were generally mild or moderate in severity and mostly related to the digestive system.

Criteria for the use of such a highly effective and broad spectrum antibacterial therapy should assess the severity of infection, reconsider the anticipated pathogens and stratify patients by demographical and epidemiological features. A risk stratification that predict clinical outcome of pneumonia has been developed by FINE *et al.* [55]. The prediction rule assigns points based on age, the presence of coexisting diseases, abnormal physical and abnormal laboratory findings. According to a point score patients were assigned to five risk classes and classes IV and V are related to a higher mortality. Therefore newer fluoroquinolones offer major therapeutic advances especially in these risk classes.

A number of national society guidelines have been published; some of them are summarised in table 7. The British Thoracic Society guidelines [56] recommend the use of aminopenicillin in patients with simple community-treated pneumonia who are ambulatory, with erythromycin recommended as an alternative choice. In view of the fact that the greatest cause of mortality is due to *S. pneumoniae*, aminopenicillins are probably adequate in the treatment of the majority of patients with mild CAP. However, the emergence of penicillin and macrolide resistance in Southern and Eastern Europe, has led to the inclusion of newer fluoroquinolones with enhanced pneumococcal activity in guidelines of the European Respiratory Society as choices for first line management, even for ambulatory patients [57]. Similar concerns in the US have led to recommendations of newer fluoroquinolones in the guidelines of the Infectious Diseases Society of America. [58, 60] The American Thoracic Society (ATS) has developed a set of guidelines in which the likelihood of involvement of penicillin resistant *S. pneumoniae* or relatively unusual pathogens in certain patients groups is acknowledged. These guidelines also recommend newer fluoroquinolones as alternative choices for outpatients who have pulmonary and cardiac comorbidities, or other risk factors such as old age [59].

Due to the emerging worldwide resistance in pneumococci new fluoroquinolones became a preferential option for treatment. On the other hand fluoroquinolone-resistant bacteria had emerged in several parts of the world. Although currently resistance is very low, it is a major concern for the future. Despite national society guidelines, experts of the drug-resistant-*S. pneumoniae* Therapeutic Working Group recommend new fluoroquinolones for outpatients only in documented highly penicillin drug-resistant pneumococci infections (penicillin MIC ≥ 4 $\mu g \cdot mL^{-1}$), in patients who are allergic to alternative agents or in whom alternative regimens already have failed [61]. In reality this means that physicians working in regions with high frequency of drug-resistant pneumococci should consider fluoroquinolones as first-line therapy, whereas physicians who practise in regions with low penicillin resistant *S. pneumoniae* prevalence should consider fluoroquinolones in certain groups of CAP, such as elderly and patients with comorbidities in whom unusual and resistant pathogens might be involved.

Hospital-acquired pneumonia

Ciprofloxacin is used widespread in the treatment of HAP and is recommended as empirical therapy in the ATS guidelines [62]. This guideline stratifies cases of nosocomial

Table 7. – International guidelines for the management of community-acquired pneumonia

Society	Mild (outpatients)	With risk factors (outpatients)	Community-acquired pneumonia Hospitalisation (normal ward)	Hospitalisation severe (ICU)
British Thoracic Society [56]	Amoxicillin Erythromycin		Amoxicillin *per os* plus erythromycin OR Ampicillin IV plus clarithromycin IV Or Fluoroquinolone IV plus penicillin IV	Amoxicillin/clavulanic acid Or Cephalosporin And Clarithromycin±rifampicin Or Fluoroquinolone plus penicillin IV
European Respiratory Society [57]	Aminopenicillin Or New Tetracycline Or New fluoroquinolones Or Macrolide		2nd or 3rd generation cephalosporin IV Or β-lactam/β-lactamase IV Or aminopenicillin and macrolide IV	2nd or 3rd generation cephalosporin and A newer fluoroquinolone Or Macrolide±Rifampicin
Infectious Diseases Society of America [58]	Doxycycline Or Macrolide Or New Fluoroquinolone	Suspected DRSP or elderly or underlying disease Newer fluoroquinolone	Macrolide plus either extended spectrum cephalosporin Or β-lactam/β-lactamase inhibitor Or Newer fluoroquinolone	either extended spectrum cephalosporin or β-lactam/β-lactamase inhibitor plus Either a new fluoroquinolone Or Macrolide
American Thoracic Society [59]	Macrolide Or Doxycycline	Cardiopulmonary diseases: β-lactam *per os* Or ceftriaxone IV/cefpodoxime *per os* And Macrolide Or Doxycycline Or Antipneumococcal fluoroquinolone	Cardiopulmonary diseases or nursing home: β-lactam IV plus macrolide Or Doxycyclin Or Antipneumococcal fluoroquinolone IV Or Doxycycline plus β-lactam Or Antipneumococcal fluoroquinolone	β-lactam IV plus azithromycin IV Or Fluoroquinolone Risk of Pseudomonas: Antipseudomonal β-lactam IV and ciprofloxacin IV Or Antipseudomonal β-lactam IV plus aminoglycoside IV plus Azithromycin IV Or Fluoroquinolone IV

ICU: intensive care unit; IV: intravenous; DRSP: drug resistant *Streptococcus pneumoniae*.

pneumonia according to presence of risk factors and severity of illness. Of particular importance is the length of hospital stay. Nonpseudomonal Gram-negative bacteria (*e.g.* *Escherichia coli*, Proteus, Serratia, Klebsiella and *Enterobacter spp*), methicillin-sensitive *S. aureus*, *H. influenzae* and *Streptococcus ssp*. are the most likely causative pathogens in patients who present with mild-to-moderate HAP or in severe HAP of early onset. In addition *P. aeruginosa*, *Legionella spp*. and anaerobes should also be considered in mild–to–moderate HAP with concomitant risk factors, whereas in severe HAP more resistant and virulent Gram-negative bacteria such as Acinetobacter, *Stenotrophomonas maltophila* and *P. aeruginosa* can be found.

According to the ATS guidelines [62] ciprofloxacin is currently the only recommended fluoroquinolone and should be used as a part of a combination regimen. Recommendations include suspected *P. aeruginosa* as causative pathogen, severe early onset HAP with risk factors and late onset HAP. Ciprofloxacin monotherapy can be used as an alternative regimen for mild-to-moderate HAP in special clinical situations and in de-escalating initially broad-spectrum therapy. FINK *et al.* [63] investigated IV ciprofloxacin 400 mg every 8 h compared with imipenem 1,000 mg every 8 h in patients with severe pneumonia. 79% of the study population had nosocomial pneumonia. The patients who received ciprofloxacin had a significantly higher clinical response rate than the imipenem treated patients (69 *verus* 56%) and also had a significantly higher bacteriological eradication rate (69 *versus* 59%) especially in the Enterobacteriaceae group (93 *versus* 65%). However, in *P. aeruginosa* infections the study demonstrated development of resistance during monotherapy. In summary this study confirmed that initial ciprofloxacin monotherapy was effective in nonpseudomonal HAP, but therapy needed to be modified if *P. aeruginosa* is suspected or recovered from patients.

TORRES *et al.* [64] confirmed the efficacy of ciprofloxacin compared with imipenem in severe HAP, although he found no statistical differences between both treatment arms. Although comparing to FINK *et al.* [63] patients had microbiological confirmed severe HAP and required mechanical ventilation.

Recently data were published investigating the efficacy of sequential IV and *per os* levofloxacin 750 mg once daily compared with imipenem/cilastatin 500–1000 mgIV followed by oral ciprofloxacin 750 mg *b.i.d.* [65]. Levofloxacin demonstrated equivalent clinical success (58.1 *versus* 60.6%) and bacteriological eradication rates (66.7 *versus* 60.6%) to the comparator regimen. In suspected or documented *P. aeruginosa* infections the study population received according to ATS guidelines [62] adjunctive antipseudomonal antibiotics (*e.g.* amikacin or ceftazidime) and in cases of methicillin-resistant *S. aureus* (MRSA) infections additionally vancomycin.

Newer fluoroquinolones are also effective against *L. pneumophila* and EDELSTEIN [65] recommends these agents for empirical therapy in highly likely Legionnaires Disease in hospitalised and immunocompromised patients.

In summary the efficacy of the new fluoroquinolones in HAP is not yet established. However their use will be restricted in severe HAP due to limited efficacy against Gram-negative bacteria and MRSA.

Tolerance

Although fluoroquinolones are associated with a number of class-related adverse events, the potential for these differs greatly between individual agents. Several of the fluoroquinolones have been withdrawn from the market or had their use severely restricted because of adverse effects (clinafloxacin because of phototoxicity and hypoglycaemia; grepafloxacin because of prolongation of the cardiac output (QT) interval corrected for heart rate (QTc) and resultant Torsades de pointes; sparfloxacin because of phototoxicity; and trovafloxacin because of hepatotoxicity). However, currently available newer fluoroquinolones levofloxacin, gatifloxacin, moxifloxacin and gemifloxacin are generally well tolerated. The most common side effects known from phase III clinical trials and postmarketing surveillance studies are gastrointestinal disturbances, central nervous system (CNS) complaints and allergic reactions. (table 8) Other adverse events associated with fluoroquinolone treatment include phototoxicity, hepatotoxicity, tendonitis or tendon rupture, cardiovascular disturbances (QT-prolongation) and hypoglycaemia. Most events are mild-to-moderate in severity.

Nausea and diarrhea are the most frequent gastrointestinal complaints in treatment with newer fluoroquinolones. Diarrhea was observed with the newer fluoroquinolones at rates of ~4% and 6%, indicating that gastrointestinal tolerability is comparable to older fluoroquinolones [67]. It should be mentioned that *Clostridium difficile* associated pseudomembranous colitis has been very rare in fluoroquinolones-treated patients. This is consistent with published data on several fluoroquinolones that show considerable changes in the aerobic intestinal microflora, while effects on the anaerobic bacteria were less pronounced [68]. Nausea was the most common reported adverse event upto 8% in clinical trials. Vomiting occurred in ~2%.

Adverse CNS effects can include headache, dizziness, tiredness, insomnia, disturbed vision, nightmares and more rarely seizures, psychotic reactions and hallucinations. Most important are dizziness and headache with reported values of 3 and 6.4% [67] Some fluoroquinolones, such as levofloxacin have increased seizure potential when they are coadmistered with probenecid, or with nonsteroidal anti-inflammatory drugs. After all the elderly are at a hightened risk for CNS toxicity and should therefore be carefully monitored for symptoms of excitation such as insomnia, hallucinations and others [67].

In comparison to β-lactam-antibiotics fluoroquinolones cause less commonly allergic skin reactions. This has been considered as an advantage; nevertheless skin reactions such as phototoxicity have received attention. Rash and pruritus have been reported in <1% of patients treated with levofloxacin, gatifloxacin and moxifloxacin. However, it is noteworthy that gemifloxacin exhibits higher potential and causes a rash in up to 4.8% of patients, especially in young females [4]. Phototoxicity has not been reported with gatifloxacin and moxifloxacin and occurs very infrequently with levofloxacin and gemifloxacin. Mild symptoms present as erythema, oedema and desquamation of sun exposed areas, whereas painful blistering occurs in more severe cases. In generally phototoxicity is strongly related to treatment with 8-halogenated fluoroquinolones, *e.g.* clinafloxacin or sparfloxacin; whereas fluoroquinolones with a methoxy substituent at position 8, *e.g.* gatifloxacin and moxifloxacin, exhibit increased stability to ultra violet light [69].

Table 8. – Commonly reported adverse events with newer fluoroquinolones

Adverse event	Incidence % of patients
Gastrointestinal tract	
Nausea	7.1–8
Diarrhoea	4–5.9
Vomiting	1.7–2.2
Abdominal pain	2–2.6
Dyspepsia	1.4–2.5
CNS	
Dizziness	2.9–3
Headache	2–6.4
Insomnia	<1–4

CNS: central nervous system. Table adapted from STAHLMANN and LODE [67].

Serious hyper- and hypoglycaemic episodes are mainly associated with coadministration of gatifloxacin plus antihyperglycaemic agents. [70]. Therefore gatifloxacin should be used with cautions in diabetic patients and in the elderly.

Fluoroquinolones can cause mild and reversible elevations of transaminases and alkaline phosphatase without any clinical symptoms of liver disease. This occurs in ∼1–3% of fluoroquinolones recipients and usually does not require cessation of therapy [67] For ciprofloxacin, one of the most widely prescribed fluoroquinolones, only sporadic cases of patients developing hepatitis, liver necrosis, hepatic insufficiency or failure have been reported. In contrast trovafloxacin is known to induce fatal hepatotoxicity [71] Regarding gatifloxacin, moxifloxacin and levofloxacin elevations of liver enzymes are uncommon, whereas mild and reversible elevations of asparate aminotransferase and alanine aminotransferase were observed with high doses of gemifloxacin (640 mg) [72].

Many drugs in common use may cause prolongation of the QTc which is associated with risk of developing potentionally life-threatening ventricular tachyarrhythmias. The potential for QTc prolongation is considered as a potential class effect, but the capability is not equal for all fluoroquinolones [73]. The severity can vary from nonsignificant QT-prolongation to development of torsades de pointes, a polymorphic ventricular tachycardia that can lead to ventricular fibrillation and sudden cardiac death. These events have been especially reported in patients receiving grepafloxacin and sparfloxacin. With respect to the mechanism it is known that fluoroquinolones affect the human cardiac potassium channel HERG. This is of great interest, because drug-induced blockade of this channel provides a mechanistic explanation for QT interval prolongation and arrhythmias [74]. The normal QT interval is 450–470 msec including a considerable intraindividual variation (15–70 msec). The Committee of Proprietary Medicinal Products has defined criteria for significant QTc prolongations. These include any QT interval >500 msec, any QT interval changes of >60 msec, QT prolongation >30 msec above the normal value or changes of >15% [67]. In regard to the newer fluoroquinolones sporadic events of ventricular tachycardia caused by QTc prolongation have been published in treatment with levofloxacin [75], gatifloxacin [76] and moxifloxacin [73]. Gemifloxacin has been reported to demonstrate small nonsignificant QTc-prolongations, but there were no documented reports about Torsades de pointes. [4] In clinical practice, fluoroquinolones should generally be closely monitored and avoided in patients with known prolongation of the QT interval, patients with uncorrected hypokalaemia or hypomagnesaemia and patients receiving class Ia and III antiarrhythmic agents. Special attention should be paid to patients with significant cardiovascular diseases and a history of an arrhythmia, concurrent administration of other drugs capable of causing prolonged QTc interval or inhibiting metabolism of QTc -prolonging drugs. The potential to cause QT-prolongation is known for class I and III antiarrhythmics, macrolides, cotrimazole, the antihistamines (*e.g.* astemizole, terfenadine), antiprotozoals (*e.g.* chloroquine, mefloquine, quinine), some psychoactive agents (*e.g.* haloperidol, lithium, tricycic antidepressants) and vasopressin [4].

Fluoroquinolones have the potential to damage cartilage and tendon disorders, such as tendonitis and tendon ruptures. Implicated fluoroquinolones were mainly ciprofloxacin and pefloxacin. In ∼90% the achilles tendon is affected and ruptures can occur up to 120 days after start of treatment. The earliest sign is often an inflammatory and/or congestive oedema. The manifestation can persist for several weeks and result in significant functional impairment. Little is known about risk factors apart from male gender, aged >60 yrs and coadministration of corticosteroids. There exist sporadic reports about possible levofloxacin-related tendonitis, but the incidence appears to be very low [77]. For gatifloxacin, moxifloxacin and gemifloxacin cases of tendon rupture have not been recorded.

Drug interactions have been observed between all new fluoroquinolones and metal-ion containing drugs, such as antacids. These drugs reduce the bioavailability of concomitantly administered fluoroquinolones. Therefore fluoroquinolones should be administered at least 2 h prior to metal-ion containing drugs. Another potentially serious drug-interaction can occur in theophyllin recipients. Especially older fluoroquinolones have been shown to inhibit hepatic oxidative cytochrome P450 enzymes, leading to corresponding increases of theophyllin concentrations. Neglible or no effects have been reported for the newer fluoroquinolones, nevertheless patients receiving both agents should be observed. Neither levofloxacin, gemifloxacin or moxifloxacin have shown potentiated anticoagulation due to co-administration of warfarin until now [4].

Summary

The newer fluoroquinolones levofloxacin, gatifloxacin, moxifloxacin and gemifloxacin offer major therapeutic advances compared with previous antibacterial agents in the treatment of lower respiratory tract infections (LRTIs). They provide a broad antibacterial spectrum combined with pharmacokinetic advantages that include excellent penetration into respiratory tissue and high bioavailability with oral therapy. In overall they can be considered safe and well tolerated. Therefore current treatment guidelines for management of community-acquired LRTIs recommend these agents for empirical therapy in several clinical situations. In guidelines for management of hospital-acquired pneumonia (HAP) only ciprofloxacin is recommend, although efficacy of levofloxacin has been recently evaluated in one clinical trial. However the use of the newer fluoroquinolones will be restricted in severe (HAP) due to limited efficacy against Gram-negative bacteria and methicillin-resistant Staphylococcus aureus.

Keywords: Acute exacerbations of chronic bronchitis, community-acquired pneumonia, fluoroquinolones, hospital-acquired pneumonia, lower respiratory tract infections.

References

1. Chen DK, McGeer A, de Azavedo JC, Low DE. Decreased susceptibility of *Streptococcus pneumoniae* to fluoroquinolones in Canada. Canadian Bacterial Surveillance Network. *N Engl J Med* 1999; 341: 233–239.
2. Sahm DF, Jones ME, Hickey ML, Diakun DR, Mani SV, Thornsberry C. Resistance surveillance of *Streptococcus pneumoniae*, *Haemophilus influenzae* and *Moraxella catarrhalis* isolated in Asia and Europe, 1997–1998. *J Antimicrob Chemother* 2000; 45: 457–466.
3. Naber KG, Adam D. Classification of fluoroquinolones. *Int J Antimicrob Agents* 1998; 10: 255–257.
4. Zhanel GG, Ennis K, Vercaigne L, *et al*. A critical review of the fluoroquinolones: focus on respiratory infections. *Drugs* 2002; 62: 13–59.
5. Piddock LJ, Jin YF, Ricci V, Asuquo AE. Quinolone accumulation by Pseudomonas aeruginosa, *Staphylococcus aureus* and *Escherichia coli*. *J Antimicrob Chemother* 1999; 43: 61–70.
6. Bryan LE, Bedard J, Wong S, Chamberland S. Quinolone antimicrobial agents: mechanism of action and resistance development. *Clin Invest Med* 1989; 12: 14–19.
7. Schmitz FJ, Higgins PG, Mayer S, Fluit AC, Dalhoff A. Activity of quinolones against gram-

positive cocci: mechanisms of drug action and bacterial resistance. *Eur J Clin Microbiol Infect Dis* 2002; 21: 647–659.

8.   Drlica K, Zhao X. DNA gyrase, topoisomerase IV, and the 4-quinolones. *Microbiol Mol Biol Rev* 1997; 61: 377–392.

9.   Jones ME, Sahm DF, Martin N, *et al.* Prevalence of gyrA, gyrB, parC, and parE mutations in clinical isolates of *Streptococcus pneumoniae* with decreased susceptibilities to different fluoroquinolones and originating from Worldwide Surveillance Studies during the 1997–1998. *Antimicrob Agents Chemother* 2000; 44: 462–466.

10.   Varon E, Janoir C, Kitzis MD, Gutmann L. ParC and GyrA may be interchangeable initial targets of some fluoroquinolones in *Streptococcus pneumoniae. Antimicrob Agents Chemother* 1999; 43: 302–306.

11.   Dalhoff A, Schmitz FJ. *In vitro* antibacterial activity and pharmacodynamics of new quinolones. *Eur J Clin Microbiol Infect Dis* 2003; 22: 203–221.

12.   Gill MJ, Brenwald NP, Wise R. Identification of an efflux pump gene, pmrA, associated with fluoroquinolone resistance in Streptococcus pneumoniae. *Antimicrob Agents Chemother* 1999; 28: 187–189.

13.   Kaatz GW, Seo SM, Ruble CA. Efflux-mediated fluoroquinolone resistance in *Staphylococcus aureus. Antimicrob Agents Chemother* 1993; 37: 1086–94.

14.   Kohler T, Michea-Hamzehpour M, Plesiat P, Kahr AL, Pechere JC. Differential selection of multidrug efflux systems by quinolones in *Pseudomonas aeruginosa. Antimicrob Agents Chemother* 1997; 41: 2540–2543.

15.   Markham PN, Westhaus E, Klyachko K, Johnson ME, Neyfakh AA. Multiple novel inhibitors of the NorA multidrug transporter of *Staphylococcus aureus. Antimicrob Agents Chemother* 1999; 43: 2404–2408.

16.   Klugman KP. The role of clonality in the global spread of fluoroquinolone-resistant bacteria. *Clin Infect Dis* 2003; 36: 783–785.

17.   McGee L, McDougal L, Zhou J, *et al.* Nomenclature of major antimicrobial-resistant clones of *Streptococcus pneumoniae* defined by the pneumococcal molecular epidemiology network. *J Clin Microbiol* 2001; 39: 2565–2571.

18.   McGee L, Goldsmith CE, Klugman KP. Fluoroquinolone resistance among clinical isolates of *Streptococcus pneumoniae* belonging to international multiresistant clones. *J Antimicrob Chemother* 2002; 49: 173–176.

19.   Ho PL, Yung RW, Tsang DN, *et al.* Increasing resistance of *Streptococcus pneumoniae* to fluoroquinolones: results of a Hong Kong multicentre study in 2000. *J Antimicrob Chemother* 2001; 48: 659–665.

20.   Lubasch A, Keller I, Borner K, Koeppe P, Lode H. Comparative pharmacokinetics of ciprofloxacin, gatifloxacin, grepafloxacin, levofloxacin, trovafloxacin, and moxifloxacin after single oral administration in healthy volunteers. *Antimicrob Agents Chemother* 2000; 44: 2600–2603.

21.   Lode H, Allewelt M. Role of newer fluoroquinolones in lower respiratory tract infections. *J Antimicrob Chemother* 2002; 50: 151–154.

22.   Wise R, Honeybourne D. Pharmacokinetics and pharmacodynamics of fluoroquinolones in the respiratory tract. *Eur Respir J* 1999; 14: 221–229.

23.   Preston SL, Drusano GL, Berman AL, *et al.* Levofloxacin population pharmacokinetics and creation of a demographic model for prediction of individual drug clearance in patients with serious community-acquired infection. *Antimicrob Agents Chemother* 1998; 42: 1098–1104.

24.   Sethi S. Infectious etiology of acute exacerbations of chronic bronchitis. *Chest* 2000; 117: 380S–385S.

25.   Wilson R, Langan C, Ball P, Bateman K, Pypstra R. Oral gemifloxacin once daily for 5 days compared with sequential therapy with *i.v.* ceftriaxone/oral cefuroxime (maximum of 10 days) in the treatment of hospitalized patients with acute exacerbations of chronic bronchitis. *Respir Med* 2003; 97: 242–249.

26. Wilson R, Schentag JJ, Ball P, Mandell L. A comparison of gemifloxacin and clarithromycin in acute exacerbations of chronic bronchitis and long-term clinical outcomes. *Clin Ther* 2002; 24: 639–652.

27. File T, Schlemmer B, Garau J, Lode H, Lynch S, Young C. Gemifloxacin versus amoxicillin/ clavulanate in the treatment of acute exacerbations of chronic bronchitis. The 070 Clinical Study group. *J Chemother* 2000; 12: 314–325.

28. Soler M, Lode H, Baldwin R, *et al.* Randomised Double-Blind Comparison of Oral Gatifloxacin and Co- amoxiclav for Acute Exacerbation of Chronic Bronchitis. *Eur J Clin Microbiol Infect Dis* 2003; 22: 144–150.

29. Gotfried MH, DeAbate CA, Fogarty C, Mathew CP, Sokol WN. Comparison of 5-day, short-course gatifloxacin therapy with 7-day gatifloxacin therapy and 10-day clarithromycin therapy for acute exacerbation of chronic bronchitis. *Clin Ther* 2001; 23: 97–107.

30. Grassi C, Casali L, Curti E, Tellarini M, Lazzaro C, Schito G. Efficacy and safety of short course (5-day) moxifloxacin vs 7-day ceftriaxone in the treatment of acute exacerbations of chronic bronchitis (AECB). *J Chemother* 2002; 14: 597–608.

31. Schaberg T, Ballin I, Huchon G, Bassaris H, Hampel B, Reimnitz P. A multinational, multicentre, non-blinded, randomized study of moxifloxacin oral tablets compared with co-amoxiclav oral tablets in the treatment of acute exacerbation of chronic bronchitis. *J Int Med Res* 2001; 29: 314–328.

32. DeAbate CA, Mathew CP, Warner JH, Heyd A, Church D. The safety and efficacy of short course (5-day) moxifloxacin vs. azithromycin in the treatment of patients with acute exacerbation of chronic bronchitis. *Respir Med* 2000; 94: 1029–37.

33. Wilson R, Kubin R, Ballin I, *et al.* Five day moxifloxacin therapy compared with 7 day clarithromycin therapy for the treatment of acute exacerbations of chronic bronchitis. *J Antimicrob Chemother* 1999; 44: 501–513.

34. Amsden GW, Baird IM, Simon S, Treadway G. Efficacy and safety of azithromycin vs levofloxacin in the outpatient treatment of acute bacterial exacerbations of chronic bronchitis. *Chest* 2003; 123: 772–7.

35. Weiss LR. Open-label, randomized comparison of the efficacy and tolerability of clarithromycin, levofloxacin, and cefuroxime axetil in the treatment of adults with acute bacterial exacerbations of chronic bronchitis. *Clin Ther* 2002; 24: 1414–1425.

36. Shah PM, Maesen FP, Dolmann A, Vetter N, Fiss E, Wesch R. Levofloxacin versus cefuroxime axetil in the treatment of acute exacerbation of chronic bronchitis: results of a randomized, double-blind study. *J Antimicrob Chemother* 1999; 43: 529–539.

37. Guest N, Langan CE. Comparison of the efficacy and safety of a short course of ceftibuten with that of amoxycillin/clavulanate in the treatment of acute exacerbations of chronic bronchitis. *Int J Antimicrob Agents* 1998; 10: 49–54.

38. Henry D, Ruoff GE, Rhudy J, *et al.* Effectiveness of short-course therapy (5 days) with cefuroxime axetil in treatment of secondary bacterial infections of acute bronchitis. *Antimicrob Agents Chemother* 1995; 39: 2528–2534.

39. Obaji A, Sethi S. Acute exacerbations of chronic bronchitis: what role for the new fluoroquinolones? *Drugs Aging* 2001; 18: 1–11.

40. Eller J, Ede A, Schaberg T, Niederman MS, Mauch H, Lode H. Infective exacerbations of chronic bronchitis: relation between bacteriologic etiology and lung function. *Chest* 1998; 113: 1542–1548.

41. Sethi S. Infectious exacerbations of chronic bronchitis: diagnosis and management. *J Antimicrob Chemother* 1999; 43: Suppl. A, 97–105.

42. Bartlett JG, Breiman RF, Mandell LA, File TM Jr. Community-acquired pneumonia in adults: guidelines for management. The Infectious Diseases Society of America. *Clin Infect Dis* 1998; 26: 811–838.

43. Frank E, Liu J, Kinasewitz G, *et al.* A multicenter, open-label, randomized comparison of levofloxacin and azithromycin plus ceftriaxone in hospitalized adults with moderate to severe community-acquired pneumonia. *Clin Ther* 2002; 24: 1292–308.

44. Gotfried MH, Dattani D, Riffer E, *et al.* A controlled, double-blind, multicenter study comparing clarithromycin extended-release tablets and levofloxacin tablets in the treatment of community-acquired pneumonia. *Clin Ther* 2002; 24: 736–751.

45. Norrby SR, Petermann W, Willcox PA, Vetter N, Salewski E. A comparative study of levofloxacin and ceftriaxone in the treatment of hospitalized patients with pneumonia. *Scand J Infect Dis* 1998; 30: 397–404.

46. Lode H, Aronkyto T, Chuchalin A, *et al.* A randomised, double-blind, double-dummy comparative study of gatifloxacin with clarithromycin in the treatment of community acquired pneumonia. *Clin Microbiol Infect* 2004; (in press)

47. Lode H, Magyar P, Muir J, Loos U, Kleutgens K, International gatifloxacin study group. Once-daily oral gatifloxacin versus three-times-daily co-amoxiclav in the treatment of patients with community-acquired pneumonia. *Clin Microbiol Infect* 2004; (in press)

48. Finch R, Schurmann D, Collins O, *et al.* Randomized controlled trial of sequential intravenous (i.v.) and oral moxifloxacin compared with sequential i.v. and oral co-amoxiclav with or without clarithromycin in patients with community-acquired pneumonia requiring initial parenteral treatment. *Antimicrob Agents Chemother* 2002; 46: 1746–1754.

49. Hoeffken G, Meyer HP, Winter J, Verhoef L. The efficacy and safety of two oral moxifloxacin regimens compared to oral clarithromycin in the treatment of community-acquired pneumonia. *Respir Med* 2001; 95: 553–564.

50. Petitpretz P, Arvis P, Marel M, Moita J, Urueta J. Oral moxifloxacin vs high-dosage amoxicillin in the treatment of mild- to-moderate, community-acquired, suspected pneumococcal pneumonia in adults. *Chest* 2001; 119: 185–195.

51. Lode H, File TM Jr, Mandell L, Ball P, Pypstra R, Thomas M. Oral gemifloxacin versus sequential therapy with intravenous ceftriaxone/oral cefuroxime with or without a macrolide in the treatment of patients hospitalized with community-acquired pneumonia: a randomized, open-label, multicenter study of clinical efficacy and tolerability. *Clin Ther* 2002; 24: 1915–1936.

52. File TM Jr, Schlemmer B, Garau J, Cupo M, Young C. Efficacy and safety of gemifloxacin in the treatment of community- acquired pneumonia: a randomized, double-blind comparison with trovafloxacin. *J Antimicrob Chemother* 2001; 48: 67–74.

53. Lode H, Grossmann C, Choudhri S, *et al.* Sequential iv/po moxifloxacin treatment of patients with severe community-acquired pneumonia. *Respir Med* 2003; 10: 1134–1142.

54. File TM Jr, Segreti J, Dunbar L, *et al.* A multicenter, randomized study comparing the efficacy and safety of intravenous and/or oral levofloxacin versus ceftriaxone and/or cefuroxime axetil in treatment of adults with community-acquired pneumonia. *Antimicrob Agents Chemother* 1997; 41: 1965–1972.

55. Fine MJ, Auble TE, Yealy DM, *et al.* A prediction rule to identify low-risk patients with community-acquired pneumonia. *N Engl J Med* 1997; 336: 243–250.

56. BTS Guidelines for the Management of Community Acquired Pneumonia in Adults. *Thorax* 2001; 56: Suppl. 4, IVI–164.

57. ERS Task Force Report. Guidelines for management of adult community- acquired lower respiratory tract infections. European Respiratory Society. *Eur Respir J* 1998; 11: 986–991.

58. Bartlett JG, Dowell SF, Mandell LA, File Jr TM, Musher DM, Fine MJ. Practice guidelines for the management of community-acquired pneumonia in adults. *Infectious Diseases Society of America Clin Infect Dis* 2000; 31: 347–382.

59. Niederman MS, Mandell LA, Anzueto A, *et al.* Guidelines for the management of adults with community-acquired pneumonia. Diagnosis, assessment of severity, antimicrobial therapy, and prevention. *Am J Respir Crit Care Med* 2001; 163: 1730–1754.

60. Bernstein JM. Treatment of community-acquired pneumonia IDSA guidelines. Infectious Diseases Society of America. *Chest* 1999; 115: 9S–13S.

61. Heffelfinger JD, Dowell SF, Jorgensen JH, *et al.* Management of community-acquired pneumonia in the era of pneumococcal resistance: a report from the Drug-Resistant *Streptococcus pneumoniae* Therapeutic Working Group. *Arc Intern Med* 2000; 160: 1399–1408.

62. Hospital-acquired pneumonia in adults: diagnosis, assessment of severity, initial antimicrobial therapy, and preventive strategies. A consensus statement, American Thoracic Society, November 1995. *Am J Respir Crit Care Med* 1996; 153: 1711–1725.

63. Fink MP, Snydman DR, Niederman MS, *et al.* Treatment of severe pneumonia in hospitalized patients: results of a multicenter, randomized, double-blind trial comparing intravenous ciprofloxacin with imipenem-cilastatin. The Severe Pneumonia Study Group. *Antimicrob Agents Chemother* 1994; 38: 547–557.

64. Torres A, Bauer TT, Leon-Gil C, *et al.* Treatment of severe nosocomial pneumonia: a prospective randomised comparison of intravenous ciprofloxacin with imipenem/cilastatin. *Thorax* 2000; 55: 1033–1039.

65. West M, Boulanger BR, Fogarty C, *et al.* Levofloxacin compared with imipenem/cilastatin followed by ciprofloxacin in adult patients with nosocomial pneumonia: a multicenter, prospective, randomized, open-label study. *Clin Ther* 2003; 25: 485–506.

66. Edelstein PH. Antimicrobial chemotherapy for Legionnaires disease: time for a change. *Ann Intern Med* 1998; 129: 328–330.

67. Stahlmann R, Lode H. Fluoroquinolones in the elderly: safety considerations. *Drugs Aging* 2003; 20: 289–302.

68. Edlund C, Nord CE. Effect of quinolones on intestinal ecology. *Drugs* 1999; 58: Suppl. 2, 65–70.

69. Stahlmann R, Lode H. Toxicity of quinolones. *Drugs* 1999; 58: Suppl. 2, 37–42.

70. Baker SE, Hangii MC. Possible gatifloxacin-induced hypoglycemia. *Ann Pharmacother* 2002; 36: 1722–1726.

71. Lucena MI, Andrade RJ, Rodrigo L, *et al.* Trovafloxacin-induced acute hepatitis. *Clin Infect Dis* 2000; 30: 400–401.

72. Allen A, Bygate E, Vousden M, *et al.* Multiple-dose pharmacokinetics and tolerability of gemifloxacin administered orally to healthy volunteers. *Antimicrob Agents Chemother* 2001; 45: 540–545.

73. Ball P. Quinolone-induced QT interval prolongation: a not-so-unexpected class effect. *J Antimicrob Chemother* 2000; 45: 557–559.

74. Kang J, Wang L, Chen XL, Triggle DJ, Rampe D. Interactions of a series of fluoroquinolone antibacterial drugs with the human cardiac K+ channel HERG. *Mol Pharmacol* 2001; 59: 122–126.

75. Samaha FF. QTC interval prolongation and polymorphic ventricular tachycardia in association with levofloxacin. *Am J Med* 1999; 107: 528–529.

76. Bertino JS Jr, Owens RC Jr, Carnes TD, Iannini PB. Gatifloxacin-associated corrected QT interval prolongation, torsades de pointes, and ventricular fibrillation in patients with known risk factors. *Clin Infect Dis* 2002; 34: 861–863.

77. Hurst M, Lamb HM, Scott LJ, Figgitt DP. Levofloxacin: an updated review of its use in the treatment of bacterial infections. *Drugs* 2002; 62: 2127–2167.

CHAPTER 7

Treatment of difficult Gram-positive infections

R. Cosentini*, P. Tarsia*, M. Cazzola#, F. Blasi¶

*Emergency Medicine Department, ¶Institute of Respiratory Diseases, University of Milan, IRCCS Ospedale Maggiore Milano, Milan, and #Dept of Respiratory Medicine, Unit of Pneumology and Allergology, A. Cardarelli Hospital, Naples, Italy.

Correspondence: R. Cosentini, Emergency Medicine Department, IRCCS Ospedale Maggiore di Milano, Via F. Sforza 35, 20122 Milan, Italy.

From the 1980s onwards, bacterial resistance to antibiotics has steadily compromised the standard therapy used for bacterial lower respiratory tract infections (LRTIs). The spread of methicillin-resistant staphylococci, and penicillin- and macrolide-resistant pneumococci alongside the emergence of glycopeptide-resistant staphylococci and erythromycin-resistant strains of *Streptococcus pyogenes* underline the need for therapeutic alternatives. Although the rational use of antibiotics can limit the development of future resistances, this is not sufficient to abate currently resistant bacteria. Therefore, it is now necessary to design new drugs with these emerging needs in mind, specifically in regards to resistant and hard-to-treat organisms. However, difficulties in developing truly innovative drugs are a major problem. The only drugs that can be truly regarded as structurally novel drugs are the oxazolidinones, which have recently been launched in several countries, the cationic peptides and the lipopeptide antibiotics. However, in conjuction with these the peptide deformylase inhibitors and, possibly, the pleuromutilins may also be considered as potential advancements within this field. Other agents that are under development or have just been marketed are analogues of existing compounds, which have been in use for many years [1].

The approach to community- and hospital-acquired LRTI's sustained by difficult-to-treat Gram-positive pathogens will be discussed will be discussed in this chapter.

Relevant multiresistant Gram-positive bacteria

Staphylococcus aureus

Infections caused by resistant Gram-positive bacteria, particularly methicillin-resistant *Staphylococci aureus* (MRSA), have increased dramatically over the past two decades world wide [2]. These pathogens are now among the most common causes of nosocomial infections, with an extremely high incidence in intensive care units (ICU). Recent reports indicate that $\geq 50\%$ of nosocomial infections in ICU patients are due to MRSAs, with a 37% increase from 1994–1998 [2]. Among *S. aureus* infections, the presence of methicillin resistance represents a risk factor for mortality. In a review of community- and nosocomial-acquired *S. aureus* infections in New York city hospitals, MRSAs caused 29% of all infections and 48% of overall mortality. Moreover, the mortality rate due to a MRSA infection was significantly higher than particularly methicillin-susceptible *S. aureus* (MSSA) infection (21 *versus* 8%) [3]. A recent meta-analysis comparing mortality

Eur Respir Mon, 2004, 28, 113–130. Printed in UK - all rights reserved. Copyright ERS Journals Ltd 2004; European Respiratory Monograph; ISSN 1025-448x. ISBN 1-904097-32-4.

associated with MRSA bacteremia showed a significant increase in mortality associated with MRSA bacteremia compared with MSSA with a pooled odds ratio of 1.93 (95% CI, 1.54–2.42, p<0.001) [4].

Methicillin resistance is not due to the production of hydrolytic enzymes (β-lactamase) but to the acquisition of a gene (mecA) that encodes expression of a penicillin-binding protein 2a (PBP2a) penicillin binding protein that determines extremely low affinity for all β-lactam antibiotics [5]. Moreover, these strains of staphylococci harbour conjugative plasmids and trasposones determining further resistance.

MRSA may colonise both patients and health personnel, person-to-person spread within wards may be facilitated principally through the hands of nurses or physicians and in a more restricted number of cases, through the use of contaminated materials (e.g. gloves, medical equipment, detergents etc.). Nosocomial risk factors for an MRSA infection includes prolonged or recurrent antibiotic exposure, prolonged hospitalisation, and hospitalisation in an intensive care unit. Among outpatients, MRSA infection is generally observed in chronically ill patients, nursing home residents, intravenous drug abusers and patients with repeated parenteral pharmacological administrations (e.g. diabetics and dialysis patients) [6], although recent reports indicate infections by this agent has occurred in previously healthy subjects with no obvious risk factors [7].

Coagulase-negative staphylococci

A variety of species of coagulase-negative staphylococci (CNS) inhabit the human skin, the most common being *Staphylococcus epidermidis*. These pathogens were previously regarded as insignificant pathogens, however they are now increasingly being recognised as important causative agents of infections. CNS produce an extracellular "slime" that allows them to adhere to artificial surfaces within a protective biofilm. With the increasing use of plastics and prostheses in medical practice these bacteria are now among the most common isolates identified in blood cultures. Among these microrganisms, methicillin resistance is even more frequent than amongst *S. aureus*, and is reported to be steadily increasing over the last decade [8]. CNS have a pronounced tendency to colonise orthopaedic or vascular prostheses in addition to the skin and nasal airways of both patients and health personnel.

Enterococci

Enterococci are normal flora of the human bowel. *Enterococcus faecalis* and particularly, *Enterococcus faecium* have recently attracted much attention due to their multidrug resistance. *E. faecalis* is responsible for ~90% of enterococcal infections. Most infections are endogenous, arising from the patient's own bowel, but cross-infection does occur. These bacteria are generally less virulent than staphylococci but are particularly daunting for several reasons. Firstly they are intrinsically poorly susceptible to most antimicrobial agents and secondly they have acquired relevant resistance even towards the limited number of originally active drugs [9]. Specifically, *E. faecium* is intrinsically resistant to β-lactams, aminoglucosides, and lincosamides, and has acquired a high-level of resistance to many other compounds, including vancomycin [10]. Studies on vancomycin resistant enterococci report a 24% resistance rate for *E faecium* and 5% resistance rate to *E. faecalis* in 1998, reaching 27% and 11%, respectively in the year 2000 [11, 12]. To date, the therapeutic options towards these highly resistant organisms are extremely limited.

Streptococcus pneumoniae

Streptococcus pneumoniae is naturally sensitive to β-lactams, tetracyclines, erythromycin, chloramphenicol, rifampicin, and sulfonamides. Resistance to all these agents has been described since the 1960s. Multiple resistant strains are now common around the world. Resistance to penicillin is the result of alterations in the PBPs of the cell wall. PBP2b appears as the most important protein involved in structural alterations associated with resistance [13]. Although many penicillin-resistant isolates are sensitive to newer β-lactams, some strains have developed resistance by producing simultaneous changes in more than one PBP. Identified factors associated with increased risk for infection with penicillin-resistant pneumococcal infection are of age >65 yrs, alcoholism, recent β-lactam use, multiple medical co-morbidities, therapy with corticosteroids, and exposure to a child in a day care centre [14]. Throughout the world, penicillin-resistant strains of pneumococci are usually also resistant to tetracycline, erythromycin and chloramphenicol.

Oxazolidinones

DuPont (Wilmington, DE, US) researchers reported on the first oxazolidinones in 1987. These compounds had limited activity against *Mycobacterium tuberculosis* [15]. The introduction of the fluorine substituent afforded oxazolidinones with excellent activity against resistant Gram-positive cocci. They possess a unique mechanism of bacterial protein-synthesis inhibition [16]. The mechanism of action for this class of drug involves interference with the binding of messenger ribonuleic acid (mRNA) to the ribosomes at the initiation phase of translation. Oxazolidinones inhibit the initiation of protein synthesis by binding to the 50S ribosomal subunit and preventing it from complexing with the 30S subunit, mRNA and initiation factors. This stage of protein biosynthesis has not been exploited previously as an antimicrobial target [17]. In particular, oxazolidinones arrest the formation of the initiation complex in bacterial translation systems by preventing formation of the N-formylmethionyl-transcriptional RNA-ribosome-mRNA ternary complex. The susceptibility of Gram-positive organisms to oxazolidinones can also be attributed to a lack of Gram-positive transmembrane pumps with oxazolidinone specificity.

Antibacterial spectrum

The most advanced agents in this class, such as eperezolid (formerly U-100592) and linezolid (formerly U-100766), have bacteriostatic activity against a number of important Gram-positive pathogens including MRSA, and penicillin-resistant *S. pneumoniae*, although a bactericidal effect has been described for strains of *S. pneumoniae*. They present a uniform susceptibility in sensitive bacteria independent of resistance to other antibiotics. Extremely rare resistance has been associated with amino acid substitutions in the 23S ribosomal RNA. They are also active against the atypical bacteria. Both eperezolid and linezolid appear to be efficacious and well tolerated both orally and parenterally at doses that produce plasma concentrations in excess of the levels predicted to be necessary for efficacy [18]. Linezolid has superior pharmacokinetics to eperezolid, and its development has been continued. In particular, linezolid demonstrated 100% bioavailability after oral dosing [19]. Linezolid shows good activity against MRSA and CNS, with minimal inhibitory concentrations of 90% of bacteria (MIC90) of 4 mg·L^{-1} and no differences in activities against methicillin-resistant and methecillin-susceptible

strains. Interestingly, all teicoplanin-resistant coagulase-negative staphylococci are inhibited by 2 mg·L^{-1} of linezolid (table 1). The *in vitro* activity of linezolid against *S. pneumoniae* appears to be independent of penicillin and cefotaxime resistance, and in all cases the MICs of linezolid are >2 mg·L^{-1}. Linezolid also exhibits excellent activity against erythromycin-resistant *S. pneumoniae*. This effect suggests a potential therapeutic option for the treatment of infections due to multiple resistant pneumococci [20]. It must be highlighted that neither the presence of modifying enzymes (LinA, LinA', LinB, Vgb, Vat, SatA, ANT(4') (4")-I, AAC(6')-APH(2"), APHA-3 and Cat), nor the presence of an efflux mechanism (MsrA, MefE, MefA, MreA, Vga, TetK and TeL), nor the modification or protection of antimicrobial target (because of ribosomal methylases or TetM and TetO) affect linezolid activity as demonstrated by similar *in vitro* activity

Table 1. – *In vitro* activity of linezolid compared with vancomycin, teicoplanin and other antimicrobial agents against 450 Gram-positive clinical isolates

Organism(s) and type	No. of organims tested	Antimicrobial agent	MIC mg·L^{-1}			%[#]			
			MIC50	MIC90	Range	S	I	R	≤4 mg·L^{-1}
Staphylococcus aureus methicillin susceptible	31	Linezolid	2	2	1–2				100
		Vancomycin	1	2	0.5–2	100			
		Teicoplanin	0.5	2	0.12–4	100			
S. aureus methicillin resistant	50	Linezolid	2	2	0.5–4				100
		Vancomycin	1	2	0.5–4	100			
		Teicoplanin	2	2	0.25–2	100			
Coagulase-negative staphylococcus methicillin susceptible	28	Linezolid	1	1	0.25–2				100
		Vancomycin	1	2	0.25–2	100			
		Teicoplanin	0.5	2	0.03–4	100			
Coagulase-negative staphylococcus methicillin resistant	46[¶]	Linezolid	0.5	2	0.5–4				100
		Vancomycin	2	2	0.5–4	100			
		Teicoplanin	2	64	0.06–64	67		33	
Strptococcus. pneumoniae penicillin susceptible	19	Linezolid	1	1	0.5–2				100
		Vancomycin	0.25	0.25	0.5	100			
		Teicoplanin	≤0.01	≤0.01	≤0.01	100			
		Erythromycin	≤0.25	≤0.25	≤0.25–>4	90		10	
		Cefotaxime	≤0.06	≤0.06	≤0.06	100			
		Penicillin	≤0.03	0.06	≤0.03–0.06	100			
S. pneumoniae penicillin intermediate	27	Linezolid	0.5	1	0.25–1				100
		Vancomycin	0.25	0.25	0.5	100			
		Teicoplanin	≤0.01	≤0.01	≤0.01	100			
		Erythromycin	4	>4	≤0.25–>4	41		59	
		Cefotaxime	0.5	1	≤0.06–1	81	19		
		Penicillin	0.5	1	0.12–1		100		
S. pneumoniae penicillin resistant	45	Linezolid	0.5	1	0.12–1				100
		Vancomycin	0.25	0.5	0.5	100			
		Teicoplanin	≤0.01	≤0.01	≤0.01–012	100			
		Erythromycin	>4	>4	>4	27	4	69	
		Cefotaxime	1	2	0.5–2	13	53	34	
		Penicillin	4	4	2–4			100	

[#]: Percentage of isolates that were susceptible (S) intermediate (I) and/or resistant (R) to the agent or inhibited with ≤4 mg·L^{-1}of the agent. [¶]: Includes 15 teicoplanin-resistant strains. Table adapted from CERCENADO *et al.* [20].

against resistant isolates and sensitive control isolates [21]. The SENTRY Antimicrobial Surveillance Program monitored linezolid before, during and after its release by various regulatory agencies. Among staphylococci, linezolid was active against all isolates (MICs ≤ 4 g·L^{-1}) regardless of susceptibility patterns of other antimicrobial agents. It was also consistently active against streptococci (MIC90, 1 g·L^{-1}). Linezolid remained active (MIC, ≤ 4 g·L^{-1}) against all Gram-positive species strains tested in the SENTRY Program (1998–2000) [22]. However, sporadic *in vitro* resistance has been described in clinical isolates of MRSA in patients who have received linezolid therapy [23].

Point mutations in the gene encoding for the 23S bacterial ribosome appear to be the mechanism culminating in acquired resistance to linezolid in MRSA [24]. At present this phenomenon remains extremely uncommon.

It must be highlighted that linezolid exerts postantibiotic effects (PAEs). Mean maximal PAEs against strains of *S. aureus*, *S. epidermidis*, *E. faecalis*, *E. faecium* and *S. pneumoniae* are 2.2, 1.8, 2.8, 2.0 and 3.0 h, respectively [25].

Resistance to methicillin or vancomycin (for staphylococci), and penicillin (for pneumococci) have no effect on the duration of the PAE.

Pharmacokinetics and pharmacodynamics

In general, linezolid produces a higher plasma concentration profile for a given dose in comparison to eperezolid. The mean concentration maximum (Cmax) of linezolid (600 mg every 12 h for a total of five doses) in plasma was 18.3 g·L^{-1}, with a time maximum (tmax) of 0.7 h after the administration of the fifth oral dose (table 2) [26]. The mean $t_{1/2}$ from plasma was 4.9 h (range, 2.9–7.9 h). The area under the time curve at the last measured concentration (AUClast) and area under the time curve from 0–infinity (AUC0–∞) were 107.5 and 140.3 g·h^{-1}·L^{-1}, respectively. Linezolid penetrated into the inflammatory fluid rather rapidly, the mean tmax being 3 h (range, 2–4 h). The mean Cmax in the inflammatory fluid was 16.4 g·L^{-1} (range, 6.8–36.8 g·L^{-1}). The mean $t_{1/2}$ of linezolid from the inflammatory exudate was 5.7 h, slightly greater than that from plasma. The mean percentage of penetration of linezolid into inflammatory fluid was 104% (range, 80–130%). The degree of protein binding of an antimicrobial can play a major role in determining the level of tissue penetration [27]. The plasma protein binding of linezolid is relatively low at 31% [28]. The degree of drug penetration into well-perfused areas of the body is also related to the volume of distribution (Vd). The steady-state Vd for linezolid has been shown to be approximately 50 L.

In healthy adult male subjects, after a treatment with linezolid (600 mg every 12 h for a total of five doses), concentrations in plasma, epithelial lining fluid (ELF), and alveolar cells (AC), respectively, were 7.3, 64.3, and 2.2 g·L^{-1} at the 4-h bronchoalveolar lavage (BAL) time point and 7.6, 24.3, and 1.4 g·L^{-1} at the 12-h BAL time point [29].

Linezolid concentrations in plasma, ELF, and AC declined monoexponentially, with half-lives of 6.9, 7.0, and 5.7 h, respectively. For an MIC of 4, the 12-h plasma AUC/

Table 2. – Pharmacokinetic parameters for linezolid in plasma and inflammatory fluid after five doses of 600-mg tablets at 12-h intervals.

Source of fluid	Mean±SD					
	Cmax g·L^{-1}	tmax h	$t_{1/2}$ h	AUClast g·h^{-1}·L^{-1}	AUC0–∞ g·h^{-1}·L^{-1}	% Penetration
Plasma	18.3±6.0	0.7±0.3	4.9±1.8	107.5±40.6	140.3±73.1	
Blister	16.4±10.6	3.0±0.6	5.7±1.7	101.6±63.0	155.3±80.1	104±20.7

Cmax: concentration maximum; tmax: time maximum; $t_{1/2}$: half life; AUClast: area under the time curve the last measured concentration; AUC0–∞: area under the time curve from 0–infinity. Table adapted from GEE *et al.* [26].

MIC and maximum concentration/MIC ratios were 34.6 and 3.9, respectively, and the percentage of time the drug remained above the MIC for the 12-h dosing interval was 100%. The corresponding ratios in ELF were 120 and 16.1, respectively, and the percentage of time the drug remained above the MIC was 100%.

The AUC serum concentration-time curve to the MIC (AUC24/MIC) ratios of linezolid for *S. aureus* and *S. pneumoniae* are 215 and 107.5, respectively. Cmax/MIC ratio is 9.1. The time period in which the concentrations of the drug in the plasma remain >MIC is at least 12 h, which is ~100% of the dosing interval when a *b.i.d.* regimen is employed [26]. It has been demonstrated that the free-fraction pharmacodynamic parameters, predictive of the outcome in a rat model of pneumococcal pneumonia were >39% for the percentage of time in the experimental dosing interval in which the linezolid concentration exceeded the MIC and a value of >147 for the ratio of the AUC24/MIC [30].

Clinical and bacteriological experience

Linezolid is effective in patients with community-acquired pneumonia (CAP) requiring hospitalisation, and significantly better when patients were bacteremic. In particular, empirical intravenous (IV)/oral linezolid was more effective than ceftriaxone/cefpodoxime in patients hospitalised with CAP, with comparable cure rates in *S. pneumoniae* pneumonia and higher cure rates in pneumonia complicated by bacteremia [31]. Linezolid has also been evaluated for the treatment of CAP in 66 hospitalised children. A total of 61 patients (92.4%) were considered cured, including all the patients with proven pneumococcal pneumonia, one failed (MRSA) and four were considered indeterminate [32].

Hospitalised adults with known or suspected MRSA-induced pneumonia were treated with linezolid (600 mg *b.i.d.*) or vancomycin (1 g *b.i.d.*). At the test-of-cure visit, among evaluable patients with MRSA, there was no statistical difference between the two treatment groups with respect to clinical cure rates or microbiological success rates. Both regimens were well tolerated, with similar rates of adverse events [33].

A recent study evaluated the efficacy and safety of linezolid in combination with aztreonam compared with vancomycin combined with aztreonam in the treatment of suspected nosocomial pneumonia due to a Gram-positive organism in adult patients [34]. The combination with linezolid demonstrated clinical cure and microbiological success rates equivalent to those reported with that including vancomycin in the intended-to-treat, clinically evaluable, and microbiologically evaluable populations. Eradication rates of MRSA and safety evaluations were similar between treatment groups. As expected, patients in both treatment groups at risk for a concomitant or subsequent Gram-negative infection, including those who underwent intubation at baseline (~57% of patients per treatment group) and/or who had high APACHE II scores, demonstrated lower cure rates.

Side effects

Data accrued from 1,498 patients who received the drug in five randomised, comparative clinical trials have shown that the overall frequency of adverse events was 58.6% (878 of 1,498) in the linezolid group and 52.4% (767 of 1,464) in the comparator group [35]. Disturbances of gastrointestinal function, such as diarrhoea (8.3%), nausea (6.6%), and vomiting (4.3%), were the most commonly observed side effects. Less common adverse events included headache, taste alterations, vaginal moniliasis and other fungal infections, tongue discolouration, and abnormal findings on liver function tests. The incidence of these side effects was not significantly greater than in those patients treated with the standard comparator agent(s) no serious or irreversible sequelae were observed. Discontinuation of linezolid because of the above symptoms occurred in fewer than 4% of cases. Thrombocytopenia (<75% of lower limit of normal and/or baseline platelet count), which occurred in 2.4% of patients in comparative trials and 2.6% of compassionate-use patients, associated with linezolid therapy for >10 days has also been reported as a side effect of linezolid [36, 37]. Anaemia, due to reversible red blood cell hypoplasia and bone marrow changes showing vacuolated erythroblasts in patients receiving longer courses of linezolid have been reported since linezolid was approved by the Food and Drug Administration [35]. Therefore, even patients who are not considered to be at risk for development of thrombocytopenia or anaemia should be monitored closely if linezolid therapy is continued for >10 days [37].

Pharmacoeconomic studies

Oxazolidinones are very expensive. Therefore their use is only justified when they offer a distinct advantage over the cheaper treatment vancomycin. No formal cost-efficacy analyses have been published, but the direct cost impact must be considered in light of the considerable aggregate morbidity and associated costs of serious Gram-positive infection and the cost of other efficacious antimicrobial options. A recent randomised multicentre trial comparing linezolid with vancomycin for the treatment of patients with known or suspected MRSA species infections showed that patients treated with linezolid had a moderately shorter median length stay in hospital (LOS) when compared with the vancomycin group. These were 1 day in the total intent-to-treat sample or 2 days in the clinically evaluable sample (neither was statistically significant) [38]. It must be highlighted that LOS typically represents ~70–90% of the total cost for treating serious infections. A further analysis of this trial documented that when the antibiotic treatment started 27.1% of patients treated with linezolid were in ICU or step-down unit compared with 20.5% treated with vancomycin [38]. The median LOS was 21 days for patients whose treatment began in the ICU or step-down unit, whereas the median LOS was only 13 days for patients whose treatment began in the general ward. Such an imbalance may have biased the treatment effect on LOS. Moreover, linezolid-treated patients also had a higher than average number of concomitant medical conditions. The median LOS was longer for those with (18 days) compared with those without (13 days) seven or more comorbid conditions. Using more appropriate but less commonly used methods, such as the log-logistic model and multivariate survival analysis, it was possible to reveal that across several measures linezolid-treated patients had significant LOS reductions that otherwise would be masked. The average reduction in LOS associated with linezolid treatment, based on the log-logistic model after correction for covariate effects, was 18.1% or 2.53 days at the median. This treatment effect on LOS may be important for economic analysis. The higher cost of linezolid (versus vancomycin) may partially or completely be offset by shorter stay in hospital, given the option to convert to oral linezolid when patients rapidly respond to parenteral treatment.

Glycopeptides

Vancomycin and teicoplanin are the two glycopeptides currently used. Vancomycin and teicoplanin are natural antibiotics produced by *Amycolatopsis orientalis* and *Actinoplanes teichomyceticus*, respectively. Both drugs are large polar molecules and cannot penetrate the lipid membrane of Gram negative bacteria and are selectively used against Gram-positive microorganisms.

Vancomycin and teicoplanin have a similar mechanism of action that interferes with the second stage of cell wall synthesis. They interact with the C-terminal D-alanyl-D-alanine residue of peptidoglycan precursors and formation of these complexes blocks the transglycosylation and transpeptidation reactions and thus incorporation of the precursors into the bacterial cell wall [39].

Antibacterial spectrum

Teicoplanin and vancomycin inhibit essential tranglycosylation reactions during bacterial cell wall synthesis and their antimicrobial activity is therefore largely restricted to Gram-positive organisms. They exert an effect on aerobic and anaerobic Gram-positive microrganisms. Both drugs are slowly bactericidal for most susceptible bacteria.

Teicoplanin is partially more active than vancomycin against S. aureus (both methicillin-susceptible and-resistant strains) [40]. Activity towards CNS is generally similar between both compounds, although certain strains of S. haemolyticus are more susceptible to vancomycin. Teicoplanin is generally more active towards Streptococcus spp, including S. pneumoniae [41]. Likewise, teicoplanin is more active than vancomycin against enterococci.

Glycopeptide resistance to enterococci has a broad geographical distribution and has become an increasing problem in clinical practice. It is due to the presence of an alternative pathway for peptidoglycan synthesis allowing the formation of low-affinity precursors, and the elimination of precursors normally produced by the host. Ther are five types of acquired resistance and an intrinsic mechanism that have been described in the literature. VanC-type resistance is an intrinsic property of some enterococci displaying low-level resistance to vancomycin. The VanA-type is associated with high-level resistance to both vancomycin and teicoplanin and is transposon mediated [42]. VanB-type strains possess variable degrees of resistance to vancomycin only. VanD-type enterococci are variably resistant to both glycopeptides, whereas VanE and VanG are characterised by low-level resistance to vancomycin and susceptibility to teicoplanin.

Reports are emerging from some countries (particularly the US and Japan) on the emergence of glycopeptide-resistant S. aureus (so called GISA: glycopeptide-intermediate S. aureus and VISA: vancomycin-intermediate S. aureus) associated with clinical failures [43]. The apparent mechanism is related to the over production of penicillin-binding proteins which trap the antibiotics before they reach their targets at the surface of the cell.

Pharmacokinetics and pharmacodynamics

Although vancomycin and teicoplanin share a common glycopeptide structure built around a linear heptapeptide chain, specific characteristics of each drug determine different pharmacokinetic properties. Whereas vancomycin is a single moiety, teicoplanin is a mixture of closely related components. The latter is 50–100 times more lipophilic than the former. It therefore possesses good cellular and tissue penetration with a prolonged half-life. Teicoplanin enters tissues rapidly and is then released slowly back into the bloodstream [44]. Vancomycin is used as vancomycin-chloridrate, highly hydrosoluble and stable in acid solutions.

Both glycopeptides are poorly absorbed by the intestinal tract, but may be employed orally in complex intestinal infections (Clostridium difficile). The higher solubility of teicoplanin allows intramuscular (IM) or IV administration of this agent as opposed to strictly IV route for vancomycin.

Following IV administration of teicoplanin, maximum serum concentrations can be achieved within 30 min, whereas peak serum concentrations are attained 4 h after IM administration [42]. The half-life is extremely prolonged (83–168 h), with high fully reversible plasma-protein binding (>90%). This allows once-daily dosing of teicoplanin, although it is essential that a loading dose be administered (two doses at 12-h intervals during the first 24 h) [45]. Teicoplanin shows good penetration into lung, bone, and soft tissues.

Vancomycin requires slow (90 min) administration in order to minimise its side effects (hypotension or the "red man" syndrome). Peak serum concentrations are approximately half those exhibited by teicoplanin and vancomycin plasma half-life is also significantly lower (4–8 h). As a result, vamcomycin must be administered in either a *b.i.d.* or *t.i.d.* dosing schemes [46].

Both drugs are eliminated principally by glomerular filtration and elimination half-lives of teicoplanin and vancomycin increase substantially for patients with impaired renal function. In this circumstance lower doses are essential, particularly so for vancomycin, where dosage and safety are tightly linked. Similarly, drug elimination may be delayed in elderly patients [46].

Both glycopeptides are bactericidal towards susceptible bacteria. Once concentrations exceed MIC values, bactericidal activity is not significantly enhanced by further increases in drug concentration, making this class an example of time-dependent antibiotics. Therapy is best adjusted according to through concentration level.

Clinical and bacteriological experience

Glycopeptides are electively employed in all severe infections caused by methicillin-resistant *S. aureus* and *S. epidermidis*, and as an alternative to β-lactams in patients with hypersensitivity reactions to these agents.

Effective serum concentrations of both glycopeptides in critically ill patients are considered similar. Teicoplanin and vancomycin should be between 10–20 mg·L^{-1} at through and between 20–50 mg·L^{-1} at peak [47]. Comparative trials of vancomycin and teicoplanin failed to show consistent differences in clinical or bacteriological efficacy, regardless of methicillin susceptibility [48]. A meta-analysis of 11 combined studies revealed a positive clinical response in 78.8% of patients treated with teicoplanin and 77.2% of patients receiving vancomycin. In the same analysis, bacteriological cures were obtained in 83.7% of those receiving teicoplanin and 82.6% of patients given vancomycin [49].

Vancomycin has been in clinical use for almost 30 years before high-level resistant strains emerged. Such strains can naturally occur or develop through low-level mutational resistance. The Center for Disease Control and Prevention [50] provided recommendations in 1997 for the prudent use of vancomycin, to prevent the spread of vancomycin-resistant staphylococci.

Endocarditis is associated with a 30% mortality rate and is primarily caused by streptococci and staphylococci. Glycopeptides are commonly used when pathogens are resistant to β-lactams [51]. Due to their large molecular size, glycopeptides generally penetrate poorly in the endocardium, although teicoplanin has shown high penetration of vegetations. Treatment of staphylococcal endocarditis requires higher doses of teicoplanin than those commonly used (12 mg·kg^{-1}·day^{-1}), if this agent is to be employed in monotherapy.

S. aureus is among the leading causes of nosocomial pneumonia, and in some reports the rate of methicillin-resistant strains may reach 90% [52]. Associated mortality is ∼30%. The use of glycopeptides to treat multiresistant Gram-positive infections has therefore increased rapidly over the last years.

Clinical cure or improvement of septicaemia, when treated with teicoplanin has been reported in a mean of 82% of patients (range 65–100%) [53]. Similar clinical results have been described for skin and soft tissue infections (59–100%) and lower respiratory tract infections [53].

Side effects

A meta-analysis of 11 randomised clinical studies on teicoplanin *versus* vancomycin showed that there were significantly fewer adverse effects associated with teicoplanin than with vancomycin [49]. The lack of toxicity renders routine serum monitoring of teicoplanin unnecessary.

Nephrotoxicity

Increases in serum creatinine were commonly reported with early preparations of vancomycin, whereas with modern preparations it occurs less frequently [54]. Concomitant treatment with aminoglycosides is an important cofactor. The toxicity of vancomycin occurs particularly in the elderly if serum trough concentrations are >30 mg·L^{-1}, or if treatment is prolonged beyond 21 days. Several studies have found significantly more common occurrence of nephrotoxicity in patients treated with vancomycin compared to teicoplanin [55, 47].

Ototoxicity

Neither teicoplanin or vancomycin have been associated with ototoxicity in animals, and the evidence of vancomycin ototoxicity in humans has been designated as "confusing" and unrelated to vancomycin serum concentrations [56].

Hypersensitivity reactions and the "red man" syndrome

Hypersensitivity reactions are among the most common reasons for discontinuation of glycopeptide therapy. The degree of cross-reactivity between vancomycin and teicoplanin has not been specifically determined [57]. The "red man" syndrome consists of erythema and itching of the upper chest and neck often associated with rapid infusion of vancomycin. Hypotension and angio-edema can also sometimes occur. The syndrome was more frequent in earlier, relatively crude, preparations of IV vancomycin. The syndrome may be caused by histamine release, as suggested by the efficacy of preventive treatment with antihistamines. Teicoplanin-associated "red man" syndrome is extremely rare [58].

Haematological effects

Vancomycin-associated neutropaenia and thrombocytopenia (by antiplatelet mediated antibodies) have been described [57]. In most studies, no significant differences in the incidence of thrombocytopenia were observed between vancomycin and teicoplanin.

Thrombophlebitis

This is a very common problem following IV administration of vancomycin through a peripheral venous cannula, less commonly described for teicoplanin.

Glycopeptides under development

In order to overcome resistance to vancomycin, drug derivatives have been produced by introducing hydrophobic substituents on the vancosamine nitrogen. Alkyl modification of the disaccharide amino led to the production of several compounds, the most active of which is LY-333328 (oritavancin) [59]. Oritavancin and related compounds act at the same site in peptidoglycan synthesis as vancomycin, by blocking the transglycosylation step in a substrate-dependent manner. As for other glycopeptides, the effects of this drug on cell wall synthesis are attributable to interactions with dipeptidyl residues of peptidoglycan precursors. A hydrophobic side-chain in the glycopeptide structure allows anchoring of the agent at the membrane-associated target site, facilitating an intramolecular interaction [60]. The property of new glycopeptides associated with enhanced activity is not derived from a higher affinity to the D-Ala-D-Ala residues but rather from their propensity to form dimers and anchor to the cell membrane in a manner similar to that of teicoplanin [61]. Cooperative interactions derived from dimerisation and membrane anchoring may enable binding to peptidoglycan residues in vancomycin-resistant bacteria. Oritavancin is currently in phase III clinical trials for use in Gram-positive infections.

Streptogramins

Streptogramin antibiotics have been developed for the treatment of multi-drug resistant Gram-positive bacterial infections. They exert their activity by inhibiting protein synthesis [62]. Semisynthetic streptogramins consist of two molecules which are group A streptogramins (macrolactones) and group B streptogramins (cyclic hexadepsipeptides). These antibiotics are produced naturally by *Streptomyces sp.*, but the therapeutic use of the natural compounds is limited. The new semisynthetic derivative, the injectable streptogramin quinupristin/dalfopristin (30:70 mixture), which is water-soluble, offers promise for treating the rising number of infections that caused by multi-drug resistant bacteria [63]. Quinupristin/dalfopristin consists of two structurally unrelated compounds, group A (dalfopristin) and group B (quinupristin). The two groups bind to separate sites on the 50S subunit of the bacterial ribosome. In particular, attachment of dalfopristin to the peptidyl transferase domain of 23S rRNA in the bacterial 50S ribosomal subunit results in a conformational change which increases the ribosome's affinity for quinupristin [64]. Individually the two components are bacteriostatic *in vitro*. In combination, synergy occurs yielding an activity that is at least eight-fold higher than the sum of activities of the individual components [65]. The combination has bactericidal activity against most Gram-positive bacteria. They act synergistically not only against multi-drug-resistant Gram-positive strains, but also towards other respiratory pathogens, including *Moraxella catarrhalis, S pneumoniae, S. pyogenes*, and *Legionella pneumophila*, and are somewhat less active against *Haemophilus influenzae*. The most characteristic aspect of this class of drugs is that there is no cross-resistance with macrolides or lincosamides, although they all inhibit protein synthesis at the ribosomal level. Resistance to these agents may be determined by inactivating enzymes (*e.g.* vat), efflux mechanisms (*e.g.* lsa) or target modification (*e.g.* erm) [66]

Antibacterial spectrum

Quinupristin/dalfopristin's spectrum of activity includes *S. pneumoniae, S. aureus*, CNS and *E. faecium*. Almost all studied streptococci have been found to be susceptible to quinupristin/dalfopristin [67]. This agent is bactericidal towards *S. pneumoniae*, including penicillin-resistant strains. Pneumococci may be killed ≤ 3 h after exposure to the drug at MIC [68].

Most strains of *S. aureus* are susceptible to quinupristin/dalfopristin [69]. This includes methicillin- and erythromycin-resistant strains, in addition to CNS. Quinupristin/dalfopristin shows potent bactericidal activity towards methicillin-susceptible strains but is moderately active against some strains of methicillin-resistant staphylococci, and is only inhibitory towards erythromycin- and clindamycin-resistant strains [64, 70].

Quinupristin/dalfopristin is not active against *E. faecalis* but is bactericidal against most *clinical E. faecium* strains, even among vancomycin-resistant isolates [71]. Resistance to *E. faecalis* appears to be mediated by an efflux pump mechanism intrinsic to this species [72].

Clinical and bacteriological experience

Several studies have reported clinical experience with quinupristin/dalfopristin, particularly in severe infections caused by vancomycin-resistant *E. faecium* [73–76]. The overall success rate (clinical response plus bacterial eradication) in the evaluable patients was ~65%. The recommended dosage was 7.5 mg·kg^{-1} given every 8 h. Clinical success rates were similar for quinupristin/dalfopristin and comparators (oxacillin, cefazolin, and vancomycin). A recent trial on the treatment of Gram-positive nosocomial pneumonia prospectively compared quinupristin/dalfopristin with vancomycin [77]. The study demonstrated equivalence among the two drugs for the all-treated population, for patients intubated at inclusion, in early- and late-onset pneumonia, and by the type of causative agent (*S. aureus* and *S. pneumoniae*).

Side effects

Quinupristin/dalfopristin significantly interferes with the metabolism of agents cleared through the cytochrome P450 (3A4) system, with important drug interactions [63]. Venous intolerance is common when the antibiotic is administered *via* a peripheral vein. The drug is incompatible with saline, and is normally given in 5% dextrose. Variable numbers of patients treated with quinupristin/dalfopristin for infections due to vancomycin-resistant *E. faecium* have developed myalgias and/or arthralgias that may be severe. These symptoms were noted in 7–10% of patients in noncomparative studies, but are recorded less frequently in comparative trials [78].

Daptomycin

This is the first representative of a novel class of lipopetide drugs. The compound is derived from fermentation of *Streptomyces roseosporus*. Daptomycin was first discovered in the 1980s but clinical trials were suspended for concerns regarding muscle toxicity. New clinical data has now been gathered, prompted by the spread of resistant Gram-positive bacterial infections.

Daptomycin exerts its activity by disrupting bacterial membrane function in the presence of calcium ions. Membrane action potentials are dissipated, thus reducing cell viability [79].

Daptomycin is active exclusively towards Gram-positive bacteria. In recent studies this agent was active against all strains of *S. aureus*, β-haemolytic and viridans streptococci [80]. Furthermore, daptomycin exhibits rapid concentration-dependent bactericidal activity against enterococci [81].

Resistance to daptomycin is so far rare but increases on exposure of organisms to increasing antibiotic concentrations [80].

Two multicentre, international, randomised, prospective, double-blind studies are underway comparing daptomycin 4 mg·kg^{-1} once daily IV *versus* ceftriaxone IV once daily in patients with CAP.

As mentioned above, early development of daptomycin was interrupted for concerns regarding reversible muscle damage, but phase I and phase II trials on this drug have failed to identify serious adverse events [82].

Glycylcyclines

Glycylcyclines are derived from the class of tetracycline antibiotics by modification of position nine of chlorotetracycline, minocycline or doxycycline. These agents manifest the broad range of antibacterial activity that tetracyclines exhibited up to some years ago. The best studied member of the glycylcyclines is GAR-936, a new derivative of minocycline, active against tetracycline-resistant organisms [83].

Tetracyclines inhibit protein translation at the ribosomal level (30S subunit), preventing incorporation of amino acid residues into elongating peptides. The most important clinical mechanism of resistance to tetracyclines is mediated acquisition of genetically mobile tetracycline resistance (tet) genes. These genes encode proteins that confer efflux pump activity or ribosomal alteration mechanisms that diminish antibiotic binding [84]. To restore the potential of tetracyclines as useful antibiotics , a systematic search was conducted in the 1990s to discover new analogues. These new compounds retain antibacterial activity and display activity against bacteria containing tet genes. GAR-936 does not exhibit cross-resistance with other tetracyclines. This is probably due to the differences in action mechanism it uses, given that glycylcyclines bind to 70S ribosomal targets [85].

Unlike the strictly bacteriostatic properties of tetracyclines, GAR-936 possesses bactericidal activity towards some Gram-positive cocci (*e.g. S. pneumoniae*) [86]. This drug shows lower MIC values than all other tetracyclines towards *S. pneumoniae*. Importantly, as opposed to tetracyclines, its activity is independent of pneumococcal penicillin susceptibility [87]. GAR-936 shows *in vitro* activity towards minocycline-resistant strains of *S. aureus* and coagulase negative staphylococci, although overall potency of the drug against this agent is lower than that of the parent compound. *Enterococcus spp.* are generally sensitive to GAR-936, irrespective of tetracycline susceptibility [88].

Conclusion

The emergence of bacterial resistance to existing antibiotics is a serious medical issue that is complicating the chemotherapy of infectious diseases and adding to health-care costs. Whereas resistant Gram-negative bacteria were a major concern in previous years, over the last few years a dramatic increase in the problems associated with Gram-positive bacteria has occurred, these have included multidrug-resistant staphylococci, penicillin-resistant *S. pneumoniae*, and vancomycin-resistant enterococci. Based on the epidemiological trend observed during this last decade it is reasonable to assume that the near future will be associated with the continuing emergence of further antibiotic resistance among clinical isolates of Gram-positive bacteria. For example, high-level vancomycin resistance spread from enterococci to staphylococci and pneumococci would represent a dire prospect in the future control of bacterial infections. Highly resistant organisms might produce intractable infections similar to those observed in the pre-antibiotic era. Therefore, there is an urgent need to reduce antibiotic pressure on the multiresistant Gram-positive bacteria and prevent their dissemination. Nonetheless such strategies may simply delay the emergence of fully resistant organisms, therefore the development of new, effective drug therapies is also a priority. Recent efforts have focused both on the development of derivatives based on previously existing compounds, and the more complex creation of innovative antibiotic classes.

Summary

Over the past 20 yrs resistance has steadily compromised standard therapy of bacterial lower respiratory tract infections. The spread of methicillin-resistant staphylococci, and penicillin/macrolide-resistant pneumococci, the emergence of glycopeptide-resistant staphylococci, and the increasing emergence of erythromycin-resistant strains of *Streptococcus pyogenes* underline the need for therapeutic alternatives. There is an urgent need to reduce antibiotic pressure on the multiresistant Gram-positive bacteria and prevent their dissemination. Nonetheless, such strategies may simply delay the emergence of fully resistant organisms, so that the development of new, effective drug therapy is also a priority. Recent efforts have focused both on the development of derivatives based on previously existing compounds, and the more complex creation of innovative antibiotic classes. However, difficulties in developing truly innovative drugs are a major problem. Currently, oxazolidinones, novel glycopeptides, streptogramins, glycylcyclines, and lipopetides hold promises for the development of a new armamentarium of highly effective compound towards multiresistant Gram-positive bacteria.

Keywords: Antimicrobial resistance, glycylcyclines, glycopeptides, lipopeptides, oxazolidinones, streptogramins.

References

1. Cazzola M, Blasi F, Centanni S, *et al.* Advances in the research and development of chemotherapeutic agents for respiratory tract bacterial infections. *Pulm Pharmacol Ther* 2001; 14: 367–381.
2. National Nosocomial infections surveillance (NNIS) System report, data summary from January 1990–May 1999. *Am J Infect Control* 1999; 27: 520–532.
3. Rubin RJ, Harrington CA, Poon A, Dietrich K, Greene JA, Moidudd A. The economic impact of *Staphylococcus aureus* infections in New York city hospitals. *Emerg Infect Dis* 1999; 5: 9–17.
4. Cosgrove SA, Sakoulas G, Perencevich EN, Schwaber MJ, Karchmer AW, Carmeli Y. Comparison of mortality associated with methicillin resistant and methicillin susceptible *Staphylococcus aureus* bacteremia: a meta-analysis. *Clin Infect Dis* 2003; 36: 53–59.
5. Archer G, Niemeyer DM. Origin and evolution of DNA associated with resistance to methicillin in staphylococci. *Trends Microbiol* 1994; 2: 343–7.
6. Strausbaugh LJ, Jacobson C, Sewell DL, Potter S, Ward TT. Methicillin-resistant *Staphylococcus aureus* in extended care facilities: experience in Veterans Affair nursing home and a review of the literature. *Infect Control Hosp Epidemiol* 1991; 12: 36–45.

7. Bukharie HA, Abdelhadi MS, Saeed IA, Rubaish AM, Larbi EB. Emergence of methicillin-resistant *Staphylococcus aureus* as a community-acquired pathogen. *Diagn Microb Infect Dis* 2001; 40: 1–4.

8. Gerberding JL, McGowan JE Jr, Tenover FC. Emerging nosocomial infections and antimicrobial resistance. *Curr Clin Top Infect Dis* 1999; 19: 83–98.

9. Murray BE. The life and times of the enterococcus. *Clin Microbiol Rev* 1990; 3: 46–65.

10. Iwen PC, Kelly DM, Linder J, *et al.* Change in prevalence and antibiotic resistance to Enterococcus species isolated from blood cultures over an 8-year period. *Antimicrob Agents Chemother* 1995; 41: 494–495.

11. Reacher MH, Shah A, Livermore DM, *et al.* Bacteraemia and antibiotic resistance of its pathogens reported in England an Wales between 1990 and 1998: trend analysis. *Br Med J* 2000; 320: 213–216.

12. *Acinetobacter spp* and *Enterococcus spp* bacteremia, England and Wales: 1999 and 2000. *Commun Dis Rep CDR Wkly* 2001; 11:

13. Harwell JI, Brown RB. The antibiotic-resistant pneumococcus. *Chest* 2000; 117: 530–541.

14. Markiwicz Z, Tomasz A. Variation of penicillin-binding genes of penicillin-resistant clinical isolates of pneumococci. *J Clin Microbiol* 1989; 27: 405–10.

15. Slee AM, Wuonola MA, McRipley RJ, *et al.* Oxazolidinones, a new class of synthetic antibacterial agents: *in vitro* and *in vivo* activities of DuP 105 and DuP 721. *Antimicrob Agents Chemother* 1987; 31: 1791–1797.

16. Shinabarger DL, Marotti KR, Murray RW, *et al.* Mechanism of action of oxazolidinones: effects of linezolid and eperezolid on translation reactions. *Antimicrob Agents Chemother* 1997; 41: 2132–2136.

17. Swaney SM, Aoki H, Ganoza MC, Shinabarger DL. The oxazolidinone linezolid inhibits initiation of protein synthesis in bacteria. *Antimicrob Agents Chemother* 1998; 42: 3251–3255.

18. Dresser LD, Rybak MJ. The pharmacologic and bacteriologic properties of oxazolidinones, a new class of synthetic antimicrobials. *Pharmacotherapy* 1998; 18: 456–462.

19. Pawsey SD, Daley-Yates PT, Wajszczuk CP, *et al.* U-100766 safety, toleration and pharmacokinetics after oral and intravenous administration. *Program and abstracts of the 1st European Congress of Chemotherapy* 1996; F151

20. Cercenado E, García-Garrote F, Bouza E. *In vitro* activity of linezolid against multiply resistant Gram-positive clinical isolates. *J Antimicrob Chemother* 2001; 47: 77–81.

21. Fines M, Leclercq R. Activity of linezolid against Gram-positive cocci possessing genes conferring resistance to protein synthesis inhibitors. *J Antimicrob Chemother* 2000; 45: 797–802.

22. Mutnick AH, Biedenbach DJ, Turnidge JD, Jones RN. Spectrum and potency evaluation of a new oxazolidinone, linezolid: report from the SENTRY Antimicrobial Surveillance Program, 1998–2000. *Diagn Microbiol Infect Dis* 2002; 43: 65–73.

23. Tsiodras S, Gott HS, Sakoulas G, *et al.* Linezolid resistance in a clinical isolate of *Staphylococcus aureus*. *Lancet* 2001; 358: 207–208.

24. Prystowsky J, Siddiqui F, Chosay J, *et al.* Resistance to linezolid: characterization of mutations in rRNA and comparison of their occurrences in vancomycin-resistant enterococci. *Antimicrob Agents Chemother* 2001; 45: 2154–2156.

25. Munckhof WJ, Giles C, Turnidge JD. Post-antibiotic growth suppression of linezolid against Gram-positive bacteria. *J Antimicrob Chemother* 2001; 47: 879–883.

26. Gee T, Ellis R, Marshall G, Andrews J, Ashby J, Wise R. Pharmacokinetics and tissue penetration of linezolid following multiple oral doses. *Antimicrob Agents Chemother* 2001; 45: 1843–1846.

27. Hyatt JM, McKinnon PS, Zimmer GS, *et al.* The importance of pharmacokinetic/pharmacodynamic surrogate markers of outcome. Focus on antibacterial agents. *Clin Pharmacokinet* 1995; 28: 143–160.

28. Ford C, Hamel J, Stapert D, *et al.* Oxazolidinones: a new class of antimicrobials. *Infect Med* 1999; 16: 435–445.

29. Conte JE Jr, Golden JA, Kipps J, Zurlinden E. Intrapulmonary pharmacokinetics of linezolid. *Antimicrob Agents Chemother* 2002; 46: 1475–1480.
30. Gentry-Nielsen MJ, Olsen KM, Preheim LC. Pharmacodynamic activity and efficacy of linezolid in a rat model of pneumococcal pneumonia. *Antimicrob Agents Chemother* 2002; 46: 1345–1351.
31. San Pedro GS, Cammarata SK, Oliphant TH, Todisco T. Linezolid versus ceftriaxone/cefpodoxime in patients hospitalized for the treatment of *Streptococcus pneumoniae* pneumonia. *Scand J Infect Dis* 2002; 34: 720–728.
32. Kaplan SL, Patterson L, Edwards KM, Hunt JL, Batts DH, Hafkin B. Linezolid for the treatment of community-acquired pneumonia in hospitalized children. Linezolid Pediatric Pneumonia Study Group. *Pediatr Infect Dis J* 2001; 20: 488–494.
33. Rubinstein E, Cammarata S, Oliphant T, *et al.* Linezolid (PNU-100766) *versus* vancomycin in the treatment of hospitalized patients with nosocomial pneumonia: a randomized, double-blind, multicenter study. *Clin Infect Dis* 2001; 32: 402–412.
34. Stevens DL, Herr D, Lampiris H, Hunt JL, Batts, Haftkin B. Linezolid versus vancomycin for the treatment of methicillin-resistant *Staphylococcus aureus* infections. *Clin Infect Dis* 2002; 34: 1481–1490.
35. Linden P. Use of linezolid for Gram-positive infections. *Infect Med* 2002; 19: 25–32.
36. Green SL, Maddox JC, Huttenback ED. Linezolid and reversible myelosuppression. *JAMA.* 2001; 285: 1291.
37. Attassi K, Hershberger E, Alam R, *et al.* Thrombocytopenia associated with linezolid therapy. *Clin Infect Dis* 2002; 34: 695–698.
38. Li Z, Willke RJ, Pinto LA, Zervos MG. Comparison of length of hospital stay for patients with known or suspected methicillin-resistant *Staphylococcus* species infections treated with linezolid or vancomycin: a randomized, multicenter trial. *Pharmacotherapy* 2001; 21: 263–274.
39. Reynolds PE. Structure, biochemistry, and mechanism of action of glycopeptide antibiotics. *Eur J Clin Microbiol Infect Dis* 1989; 8: 943–950.
40. Parenti F, Schito GC, Courvalin P. Teicoplanin chemistry and microbiology. *J Chemother* 2000; 12: 5–14.
41. Spencer RC, Goering R. A critical review of the *in vitro* activity of teicoplanin. *Int J Antimicrob Agents* 1995; 5: 169–177.
42. Arthur M, Reynolds PE, Courvalin P. Glycopeptide resistance in enterococci. *Trends Microbiol* 1996; 4: 401–407.
43. Hiramatsu K, Hanaki H. Glycopeptide resistance in staphylococci. *Curr Opin Infect Dis* 1998; 11: 635–658.
44. Harding I, Sorgel F. Comparative pharmacokinetics of teicoplanin and vancomycin. *J Chemother* 2000; 12: 15–20.
45. Thompson GA, Smithers JA, Kenny MT, *et al.* Pharmacokinetics of teicoplanin upon multiple dose intravenous administration to normal healthy volunteers. *Biopharm Drug Dispos* 1992; 13: 213–220.
46. Rotschafer JC, Crossley K, Zaske DE, Mead K, Sawchuk RJ, Solem LD. Pharmacokinetics of vancomycin: observations in 28 patients and dosage recommendations. *Antimicrob Agents Chemother* 1982; 22: 391–394.
47. Charbonneau P, Harding I, Garaud JJ, Aubertin J, Brunet F, Domart Y. Teicoplanin: a well-tolerated and easily administered alternative to vancomycin for Gram-positive infections in intensive care patients. *Int Care Med* 1994; 20: S35–S42.
48. Wilson APR, Grüneberg RN, Neu H. A critical review of the dosage of teicoplanin in Europe and the USA. *Int J Antimicrob Agents* 1994; 4: S1–S30.
49. Wood MJ. The comparative efficacy and safety of teicoplanin and vancomycin. *J Antimicrob Chemother* 1996; 37: 209–222.
50. Center for Diseases Control: Interim guidelines for prevention and control of staphylococcal infection associated with reduced susceptibility to vancomycin. *MMWR Morb Mortal Wkly Rep* 1997; 46: 626–365.

51. Working Party of the British Society of Antimicrobial Chemotherapy. Antibiotic treatment of streptococcal and staphylococcal endocarditis. *Lancet* 1985; 2: 815–817.

52. Perrone C. Teicoplanin: its role in serious nosocomial chest infections. *Int J Antimicrob Agents* 1992; 1: S49–S51.

53. Schaison G. Graninger W, Bouza E. Teicoplanin in the treatment of serious infections. *J Chemother* 2000; 12: 26–33.

54. Chow AW, Azar RM. Glycopeptides and nephrotoxicity. *Int Care Med* 1994; 20: S23–29.

55. Wood MJ. Comparative safety of teicoplanin and vancomycin. *J Chemother* 2000; 12: 21–25.

56. Brummett RE, Fox KE. Vancomycin and erythromycin induced hearing loss in humans. *Antimicrob Agents Chemother* 1989; 33: 791–796.

57. Wilson APR. Comparative safety of teicoplanin and vancomycin. *Int J Antimicrob Agents* 1998; 10: 143–152.

58. Wallace MR, Mascola JR, Oldfield EC. Red man syndrome: incidence, aetiology and prophylaxis. *J Infect Dis* 1991; 164: 1180–1185.

59. Nicas TI, Mullen DL, Flokowitsch JE, *et al.* Semisynthetic glycopeptide antibiotics derived from LY264826 active against vancomycin-resistant enterococci. *Antimicrob Agents Chemother* 1996; 40: 2194–2199.

60. Allen NE, LeTorneau DL, Hobbs JN Jr. Molecular interactions of a semisynthetic glycopeptide antibiotic with D-alanyl-D-alanine and D-alanyl-D-lactate residues. *Antimicrob Agents Chemother* 1997; 41: 66–71.

61. Allen NE, Hobbs JN Jr, Nicas TI. Inhibition of peptidoglycan synthesis in vancomycin-susceptible and resistant bacteria by semisynthetic glycopeptide antibiotics. *Antimicrob Agents Chemother* 1996; 40: 2356–2362.

62. Cocito C, Di Giambattista M, Nyssen E, Vannuffel P. Inhibition of protein synthesis by streptogramins and related antibiotics. *J Antimicrob Chemother* 1997; 39: Suppl. A, 7–13.

63. Eliopoulos GM. Quinupristin/dalfopristin and linezolid: evidence and opinion. *Clin Infect Dis* 2003; 36: 473–481.

64. Bouanchaud DH. *In vitro* and *in vivo* antibacterial activity of quinupristin/dalfopristin. *J Antimicrob Chemother* 1997; 39: 15–21.

65. Bouanchaud DH. *In vitro* and in-vivo synergic activity and fractional inhibitory concentrations (FIC) of the components of a semisynthetic streptogramin, RP 59500. *J Antimicrob Chemother* 1992; 30: 95–100.

66. Thal LA, Zervos MJ. Occurrence and epidemiology of resistance to virginiamycin and quinupristin/dalfopristin. *J Antimicrob Chemother* 1999; 43: 171–176.

67. Gordon KA, Beach ML, Biedenbach DJ, *et al.* Antimicrobial susceptibility patterns of β-hemolytic and viridans group streptococci: report from the SENTRY antimicrobial surveillance program (1997–2000). *Diagn Microbiol Infect Dis* 2002; 43: 157–162.

68. Johnson CC, Slavoski L, Schwartz M, *et al.* In vitro activity of RP 59500 (quinupristin/dalfopristin) against antibiotic-resistant strains of *Streptococcus pneumoniae* and enterococci. *Diagn Microbiol Infect Dis* 1995; 21: 169–73.

69. Archer G, Auger P, Doern G, *et al.* RP 59500, a new streptogramin highly active against recent isolates of North American staphylococci. *Diagn Microbiol Infect Dis* 1993; 16: 223–226.

70. Fuchs PC, Barry AL, Brown SD. Bactericidal activity of quinupristin/dalfopristin against Staphylococcus aureus: clindamycin susceptibility as a surrogate indicator. *Antimicrob Agents Chemother* 2000; 44: 2880–2882.

71. Eliopoulos GM, Wennersten CB, Gold HS, *et al.* Characterization of vancomycin-resistant *Enterococcus faecium* isolates from the United States and their susceptibility in vitro to quinupristin/dalfopristin. *Antimicrob Agents Chemother* 1998; 42: 1088–1092.

72. Singh KV, Weinstock GM, Murray BE. An *Enterococcus faecalis* ABC homologue (Lsa) is required for the resistance of this species to clindamycin and quinupristin/dalfopristin. *Antimicrob Agents Chemother* 2002; 46: 1845–1850.

73. Winston DJ, Emmanouilides C, Kroeber A, *et al.* Quinupristin/dalfopristin therapy for infections due to vancomycin-resistant *Enterococcus faecium. Clin Infect Dis* 2000; 30: 790–797.

74. Moellering RC, Linden PK, Reinhardt J, *et al.* The efficacy and safety of quinupristin/dalfopristin for the treatment of infections caused by vancomycin-resistant *Enterococcus faecium. J Antimicrob Chemother* 1999; 44: 251–261.

75. Linden PK, Moellering RC Jr, Wood CA, *et al.* Treatment of vancomycin-resistant *Enterococcus faecium* infection with quinupristin/dalfopristin. *Clin Infect Dis* 2001; 33: 1816–23.

76. Nichols RI, Graham DR, Barriere SI, *et al.* Treatment of hospitalized patients with complicated Gram-positive skin and skin structure infections: two randomized, multicentre studies of quinupristin/dalfopristin versus cefazolin, oxacillin, or vancomycin. *J Antimicrob Chemother* 1999; 44: 263–73.

77. Fagon JY, Patrick H, Haas DW, *et al.* Treatment of Gram-positive nosocomial pneumnia, prospective randomized comparison of quinupristin/dalfopristin versus vancomycin. *Am J Respir Crit Care Med* 2000; 161: 753–762.

78. Rubinstein E, Prokocimer P, Talbot GH. Safety and tolerability of quinupristin/dalfopristin: administration guidelines. *J Antimicrob Chemother* 1999; 44: 37–46.

79. Alborn WE Jr, Allen NE, Preston DA. Daptomycin disrupts membrane potential in growing *Staphylococcus aureus. Antimicrob Agents Chemother* 1991; 35: 2282–2287.

80. Barry AL, Fuchs PC, Brown SD. *In vitro* activities of daptomycin against 2,789 clinical isolates from 11 North American medical centers. *Antimicrob Agents Chemother* 2001; 45: 1919–1922.

81. Snydman DR, Jacobus NV, McDermott LA, Lonks JR, Boyce JM. Comparative in vitro activities on daptomycin and vancomycin against resistant Gram-positive pathogens. *Antimicrob Agents Chemother* 2000; 44: 3447–3450.

82. Tally FP, DeBruin MF. Development of daptomycin for Gram-positive infections. *J Antimicrob Chemother* 2000; 46: 523–526.

83. Sum PE, Petersen P. Synthesis and structure-activity relationship of novel glycylcycline derivatives leading to the discovery of GAR-936. *Bioorg Med Chem Lett* 1999; 9: 1459–1462.

84. Chopra I, Roberts M. Tetracycline antibiotics: mode of action, applications, molecular biology and epidemiology of bacterila resistance. *Microbiol Mol Biol Rev* 2001; 65: 232–260.

85. Bergeron J, Ammirati M, Danley D, *et al.* Glycyclcyclines bind to the high-affinity tetracycline ribosomal binding site and evade Tet(M)- and (TetO)-mediated ribosomal protection. *Antimicrob Agents Chemother* 1996; 40: 2226–2228.

86. Hoellman DB, Pankuch GA, Jacobs MR, Appelbaum PC. Antipneumococcal activities of GAR-936 (a new glycylcycline) compared to those of nine other agents against penicillin-susceptible and –resistant pneumococci. *Antimicrob Agents Chemother* 2000; 44: 1085–1088.

87. Petersen PJ, Jacobus NV, Weiss WJ, Sum PE, Testa RT. *In vitro* and *in vivo* antibacterial activities of a novel glycylcycline, the 9-t-butylglycylamido derivative of minocycline (GAR-936). *Antimicrob Agents Chemother* 1999; 43: 738–744.

88. Boucher HW, Wennersten CB, Eliopopoulos GM. *In vitro* activities of the glycylcycline GAR-936 against Gram-positive bacteria. *Antimicrob Agents Chemother* 2000; 44: 2225–2229.

CHAPTER 8

The impact of antibiotic resistance in the management of lower respiratory tract infections

G.C. Schito, A. Marchese

Institute of Microbiology, University of Genoa, Genoa, Italy.

Correspondence: G.C. Schito, Institute of Microbiology, University of Genoa, Genoa, Italy.

Lower respiratory tract infections (LRTIs) have been the focus of much attention for almost two decades. Their importance lies in their frequency as a leading cause of morbidity and mortality in all age groups despite all the advances made by medical science. Respiratory tract infections (RTIs) account for >50 million deaths globally each year and acute RTIs are the third leading cause of morbidity and mortality worlwide [1]. Within the community they account for the majority of all antibiotics prescribed, impacting heavily on healthcare drug budgets [2]. In the case of LRTSs, diseases such as community-acquired pneumonia (CAP), acute exacerbations of chronic bronchitis (AECB), and increasingly, cystic fibrosis are the most prevalent.

The most common bacterial agents of CAP, AECB are *Streptococcus pneumoniae*, *Haemophilus influenzae* and *Moraxella catarrhalis*. The "atypical" bacteria *i.e. Chlamydia pneumoniae*, *Mycoplasma pneumoniae* and *Legionella pneumophila* are also known to play a role in these disorders [3].

While importance has been given recently to atypical infections caused by *M. pneumoniae*, *Coxiella burnetii*, *L. pneumophila* and *C. pneumoniae*, are relatively infrequent or epidemic in nature compared with conventional bacterial pathogens against which much antibiotic prescribing in the community is directed [4].

Diagnosis of the causative agents in community-acquired RTIs is often unreliable and usually slow to reach the clinician. The choice of antimicrobial therapy for the treatment of RTIs is, therefore, most frequently empirical. Accurate and local information on the bacterial aetiology of the infection concerned, the prevalence of antimicrobial resistance amongst those pathogens and the outcome analyses are needed to facilitate the development of optimal therapeutic guidelines.

Resistance to antibiotics is widespread among the bacteria commonly implicated CA LRTIs (table 1).

In *S. pneumoniae* alterations in penicillin-binding proteins (PBP), the targets for penicillin and remaining β-lactam agents, are responsible for resistance to these drugs. Low affinity PBP derived from "mosaic" PBP-encoding genes, which have acquired deoxyribonucleic acid from other *Streptococcus spp.* by transformation [6]. Depending on which PBP is altered, strains with different penicillin resistance levels and different phenotypes towards β-lactam resistance are produced. The National Committee for Clinical Laboratory Standards currently defines the susceptibility of pneumococcus isolates to penicillin as follows: susceptible minimal inhibitory concentration (MIC) <0.06 mg·L^{-1}; intermediate MIC 0.1–1 mg·L^{-1}; and resistant MIC>2 mg·L^{-1} [7]. Penicillin-intermediate and –resistant pneumococci are also referred to as low- and high-level resistant strains respectively.

Eur Respir Mon, 2004, 28, 131–145. Printed in UK - all rights reserved. Copyright ERS Journals Ltd 2004; European Respiratory Monograph; ISSN 1025-448x. ISBN 1-904097-32-4.

Concerning the macrolides, two main mechanisms are responsible for resistance in *S. pneumoniae*: target site modification and efflux [8]. Alteration of ribosomal ribonucleic acid by methylases confers resistance to the entire macrolide-lincosamide-streptogramin B (MLSB) group of antibiotics. This type of resistance is mediated by products of the *erm* genes (*erm*B and very rarely *erm*TR) and can be inducible or constitutive. Efflux-mediated resistance, whereby the antibiotic is pumped out of the cell has been recently described and it is conferred by the *mef* genes (*mef*A and *mef*E) [9]. This last mechanism results in resistance limited to the 14- and 15-membered macrolides (*e.g.* erythromycin, clarithromycin and azithromycin). Among pneumococci containing *mef* genes erythromycin MICs range 1–32 mg·L^{-1}, whereas among *erm*B mutants MIC typically exceeds 64 mg·L^{-1} [8, 9]. Both of these types of macrolide resistance have been also described in *Streptococcus pyogenes*.

In addition to erm and mef mutants, 1–3% of macrolide resistant pneumococci lack *mef* or *erm* genes, indicating that additional mechanisms are operative [10–12]. Novel mechanisms of macrolide resistance have been recently described in Eastern Europe and North America [10, 13].

Resistance to penicillin (intermediate) tetracycline, erythromycin, singly or in combination, appeared in *S. pneumoniae* in the 1960s [14], and resistance to chloramphenicol and cotrimoxazole in the 1970s [15]. Of special concern was the first description of multiresistant strains (including penicillin high-level resistant micro-organisms), which were initially reported in the 1970s in South Africa [16]. During the 1980s and the 1990s, *S. pneumoniae* has become resistant to cephalosporins and quinolones, and there has been a spread of penicillin-resistant and multiresistant pneumococci all worldwide [17–19]. Penicillin-resistant *S. pneumoniae* isolates seem to be prone to acquirinh resistance not only to other β-lactams, but also to non β-lactam antibiotics, including erythromycin and other macrolides, tetracycline, chloramphenicol and co-trimoxazole.

Clonal spread is an important mechanism for dissemination of resistant *S. pneumoniae* among day-care centres, hospitals and geographical regions [17]. The most remarkable example of these multidrug-resistant pneumococcal clones is the serotype 23F clone (Spain23F-1), which was initially identified in Spain in the early 1980s and is now found in most regions of the world [17].

Currently, the prevalence and patterns of antibiotic resistance in *S. pneumoniae* vary widely from one country to another (table 2) and the inability to extrapolate data from one location to another is a compelling argument for continued surveillance. At present,

Table 1. – Major mechanisms of antibiotic resistance in respiratory tract pathogens

Pathogen	Antibiotics	Major resistance mechanisms
Streptococcus pneumoniae	β-lactams	Mosaicism in DNA-encoding penicillin-binding proteins
	Macrolides	Modification (methylation) of ribosomal RNA targets by erm gene products. Efflux of 14- and 15-membered macrolides by *mef*A gene products
	Tetracyclines	Protection of target by genes encoding M protein
	Chloramphenicol	Inactivation by acetyltransferase
	Co-trimoxazole	Alterations in binding capacity of dihidropteroate synthetase and dihydrofolate reductase
	Fluoroquinolones	Mutations in genes encoding for DNA topoisomerase IV (parC and parE) and subsequently DNA gyrase (gyrA). Hyperexpression of endogenous multidrug efflux system
Haemophilus influenzae	β-lactams	β-lactamase production TEM-1 and ROB-1
Moraxella catarrhalis	β-lactams	β-lactamase production BRO-1 and BRO-2

DNA: deoxyribonucleic acid; RNA: ribonucleic acid; Modified from Felmingham *et al.* [5].

Table 2. – Percentages of *Streptococcus pneumoniae* strains by penicillin G and erythromycin A suceptibility interpretative category in several countries

Region/Country	Total isolates tested n	Penicillin susceptibility %			Erythromycin susceptibility %	
		S	I	R	S	R
Western Europe						
Austria	57	93	1.8	5.3	86	14.1
Belgium	28	82.1	3.6	14.3	67.9	32.1
Ireland	53	58.5	7.5	34	73.6	26.4
France	184	38	15.8	46.2	41.8	58.1
Germany	325	91.7	6.2	2.2	84.3	15.7
The Netherlands	51	96.1	3.9	0	92.2	7.8
Portugal	106	71.7	17.9	10.4	84	16
Spain	133	46.6	11.3	42.1	71.4	28.6
Sweden	64	90.6	1.6	7.8	95.3	4.7
Switzerland	111	87.4	8.1	4.5	91	9
UK	91	85.7	8.8	5.5	86.8	13.2
Eastern Europe						
Czech Republic[#]	99	92.9	6.1	1	99	1
Hungary	54	35.2	51.9	13	44.4	55.6
Poland	68	73.5	13.2	13.2	76.5	23.5
Turkey	77	63.6	22.1	14.3	84.4	15.6
Slovak Republic[#]	72	48.6	20.8	30.6	91.7	8.3
North America						
Canada	350	78.9	10.6	10.6	83.4	16.6
USA	337	57	10.4	32.6	69.1	30.9
Latin America						
Argentina	55	72.7	10.9	16.4	89.1	10.9
Brazil	260	66.2	25.8	8.1	93.1	6.9
Mexico	203	43.3	32.5	24.1	72.4	27.6
Australasia						
Australia	114	79.8	15.8	4.4	86.8	13.2
Indonesia	7	57.1	42.9	0	100	0
Asia						
Hong Kong	70	41.4	1.4	57.1	28.6	71.4
Japan	308	35.7	19.8	44.5	21.8	78.2
South Korea	137	19	9.5	71.5	12.4	87.6

S: sensitive; I: intermediate; R: resistence; [#]: data taken from Alexander Project 1998 SCHITO *et al.* [20] all the other data was taken from PROTEKT study 1999–2000 FELMINGHAM *et al.* [21].

the great majority of information concerning the prevalence of antibiotic-resistance among respiratory pathogens in different geographical areas have been obtained by several international surveillance studies (*e.g.* The Alexander Project, SENTRY and PROTEKT) [19–22] prompted by the increasing rate of resistance observed among these pathogens (mainly *S. pneumoniae*) during last two decades.

Generally, pneumococcal penicillin resistance occurs at a relatively low frequency in Northern Europe. A prevalence of penicillin nonsusceptible (PNSP) *S .pneumoniae* of <15% has been reported by FELMINGHAM *et al.* [5, 21] in The Netherlands (3.9%), the UK (14.3%) and Sweden (9.4%). In contrast, penicillin resistance is dominant in France and Spain, where its prevalence exceeds 50%. Importantly, high-level resistance predominates in these countries. However, in Northern Ireland and Ireland, penicillin nonsusceptibility has reached 25%.

Highly resistant isolates are also emerging in Germany, with point prevalence ranging from 0.3–3.9% [19, 20, 23]. In contrast to western Mediterranean countries penicillin-resistant *S. pneumoniae* has been isolated at low frequency in Italy during the Alexander Project study from 5.5% in 1993 to 9.1% in 1996 [19, 24]. Starting from 1997, in an attempt to obtain more detailed data some local surveys involving ~60 centres have been

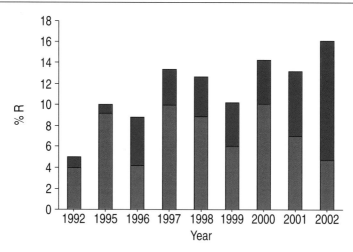

Fig. 1. – The evolution of penicillin-resistance in *Streptococcus pneumoniae* circulating in Italy. R: resistance; ■ high-level resistance; ■ low-level resistance.

established (The Italian Epidemiological Observatory, SEMPRE study, PROTEKT Italy) [25, 26] According to these studies the frequency of penicillin-resistant isolates appears to be still on the rise in this Country reaching 16.1% in 2002 (unpublished data). Highly-resistant pneumococci whose prevalence in the past was lower than that of intermediate strains and fixed at ∼4% during 1997–2001, has now reached 11.3% (unpublished data; fig. 1).

The highest prevalence rates of PNSP strains in Central and Eastern Europe have been reported from Hungary and Romania (>40%), followed by Croatia (38%), the Slovak Republic and Poland (>25%). The lowest prevalence rates have been found in the Czech Republic (<5%), [20–22].

Concerning North America the prevalence of PNSP in Canada (low in the 1980s) rose during the last two decades from 1.3% of intermediate strains between 1984 and 1986 [27] to10.6–12.4% (intermediate) and 5.8–10.6% (resistant) in 2000 [28]. Higher figures were found in the US among pneumococci isolated during the period 1999–2000. Of these isolates 43.0% were penicillin nonsusceptible and 32.6% resistant [20]. In Latin America high rates (>50%) of penicillin-resistance were observed in Mexico compared with Argentina and Brazil [21].

During the 1990s across Europe there was a steady increase in macrolide resistance in both penicillin-susceptible and –resistant *S. pneumoniae* isolates. Both the Alexander Project and the PROTEKT study reported an overall prevalence of erythromycin resistance of 25% in 1999–2000.

Macrolide resistance is most common in France, Spain and Italy, where the respective prevalences are 58.2%, 28.6–35% and 25.5–42.9% [21, 25, 29]. The rate of macrolide resistance exceeds 25% also in Ireland, Greece and Belgium, but is <10% in Finland, Germany, UK and Switzerland [21, 5]. The MLSB phenotype, which usually results in high-level resistance (MIC ≥ 64 mg·L^{-1}) is the dominant resistance phenotype in Europe [30, 31]. High rates of macrolide-resistance has been observed in Hungary (55.6%) and Poland (23.5%).

In Canada macrolide resistance in *S. pneumoniae* has increased from <3% in the early 1990s to 11% in 2000 [22, 28]. In the same year 16.0% of macrolide-resistance was recorded by the PROTEKT study for Canada [21]. In the US macrolides resistance rate is

~30% [21]. In North America macrolide-resistance is mainly dictated by *mef* genes [10, 32].

In South America macrolide resistance was also slightly more common in Mexico than in Argentina and Brazil.

Rates of antibiotic resistance in community-acquired RTI pathogens in some Countries (South Korea, Japan, Hong Kong) within the Asia-Pacific area are among the highest in the world (>75% of both penicillin- and macrolide-resistance).

In the early 1970s, resistance of *H. influenzae* to ampicillin began to emerge [33, 34] and has increased steadily thereafter. Production of β-lactamases (TEM-1 and ROB-1 types) is the primary mechanism of resistance to ampicillin and other β-lactam antibacterials by this species [35, 36]. In particular these enzymes confer resistance to penicillin and the aminopenicillins and to some cephalosporins. Both TEM-1 and ROB-1 are inhibited by the β-lactamase inhibitor, clavulanate. Generally, any one isolate of *H. influenzae* produces only one of the two β-lactamases, although rare strains with both TEM-1 and ROB-1 have been reported. ROB-1 β-lactamase in *H. influenzae* is considerably less prevalent than TEM-1. Ampicillin resistance (MIC ≥ 4 mg·L^{-1}) has also been detected among non-β-lactamase-producing ampicillin-resistant (BLNAR) *H. influenzae*, although their global prevalence is very low (<0.1%) [37]. Resistance in BLNAR strains is mediated *via* altered PBPs or diminished permeability. Because of this mechanism of resistance BLNAR strains are resistant also to amoxicillin combined with clavulanate.

International and national studies showed that the prevalence of β-lactamase-positive *H. influenzae* varies considerably with geographical region (table 3). In Europe synthesis of β-lactamase occurs with higher rates in the, France (22–31%), Ireland (17–26%), Belgium (16–18%), UK (15–18%), and Romania (16%) and lower rates in Czech Republic (11%), Poland (8%), Slovak Republic (8.1%) Germany (3–7%), The Netherlands (3–6%) Austria (3–4%) and Hungary (33%). However, 17 and 26% have been reported for Hungary and Slovak Republic recently. In Italy, the proportion of β-lactamase-positive isolates increased from 5% in 1997 to 16% in 1999 [38]. Preliminary data from the PROTEKT Italy in 2002 show again a low figure of 6.6% in Northern Italy (unpublished results; fig. 2).

In the US β-lactamase-mediated resistance in *H. influenzae* has become increasingly prevalent with the percentages of resistance ranging from 24–34.6% 37, 39], a lower rate (~20%) has been observed recently in Canada [37]. In Latin America the rate of β-lactamase production rarely exceeds 20%.

Concerning the Asian area the rates of β-lactamase production is highly variable with the highest figure recorded for South Korea (64.7%) [37].

Production of β-lactamase is also the principal mechanism of antibacterial resistance among *M. catarrhalis*. Two different β-lactamases: BRO-1 and BRO-2 have been found and characterised in *M. catarrhalis*. It is thought that BRO-1 evolved from BRO-2 (at present predominant) [40]. The prevalence of *M. catarrhalis* strains producing β-lactamase has risen at an astounding rate globally over the last 30 yrs, such that >90% of this species are now β-lactamase positive in the world [37]. In view of the high prevalence of β-lactamase production, *M. catarrhalis* is invariably resistant to ampicillin and penicillin G.

Over the last 20 yrs multiple studies have documented the rapid rise in drug resistance among common community-acquired respiratory pathogens as well as treatment failures, although perhaps not on the scale predicted by susceptibility testing data.

In addition, there have been an extremely limited number of controlled studies documenting clinical failures as a result of this rapidly emerging drug resistance. Compelling evidence that drug-resistant pneumococci affect clinical outcomes in patients with meningitis and otitis media exist [41–46]. However, the clinical relevance of

Table 3. – Prevalence of β-lactamase positive and negative *Haemophilus influenzae* in several countries

Region/country	Total isolates tested n	β-lactamase-positive %	β-lactamase-negative %
Western Europe			
Austria	40	2.5	97.5
Belgium	73	17.8	82.2
Ireland	51	25.5	74.5
France	193	31.1	68.9
Germany	284	3.2	96.8
The Netherlands	35	2.9	97.1
Portugal	135	12.6	87.4
Spain	92	10.9	89.1
Sweden	42	9.5	90.5
Switzerland	52	13.5	86.5
UK	96	14.6	85.45
Eastern Europe			
Czech Republic[#]	98	14.3	85.7
Hungary	30	3.3	96.7
Poland	43	9.3	90.7
Turkey	12	8.3	91.7
Slovak Republic[#]	99	8.1	91.9
North America			
Canada	336	19.6	80.4
US	276	25.7	74.3
Latin America			
Argentina	52	19.2	80.8
Brazil	273	11.0	89.0
Mexico	195	24.6	75.4
Australasia			
Australia	193	27.5	72.5
Indonesia	2	50.0	50.0
Asia			
Hong Kong	41	17.1	82.9
Japan	281	8.5	91.5
South Korea	51	64.7	35.3

*: Data taken from the Alexander Project 1998 SCHITO *et al.* [20], all other data taken from the PROTEKT study 1999–2000 data FELMINGHAM *et al.* [21].

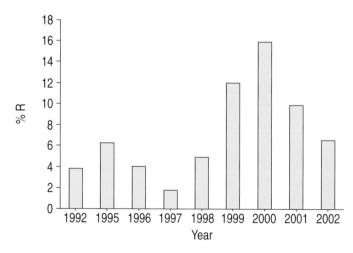

Fig. 2. – The evolution of β-lactamase production in *Haemophilus influenzae* circulating in Italy. R: resistance.

Table 4. – Impact of penicillin susceptibility on outcome and mortality for patients with nonmeningeal pneumococcal infections

Study	Subjects	Sample size	Relative risk of death for NS *versus* S infections	Risk of death	Relative improvement after 7 days of treatment
PALLARES *et al.* 1987 [47]	Bacteremic pneumococcal pneumonia	24 penicillin NS 48 penicillin S	2.2, (p=0.03)		
PALLARES *et al.* 1995 [48]	Pneumococcal pneumonia	145 penicillin NS 359 penicillin S	1.0[#] (95% CI 0.5–1.9)		
FRIEDLAND [49]	Pneumonia, occult bacteremia, peritonitis	35 penicillin NS 73 penicillin S			1.9 (95% CI 0.3–15.9)
CHOI AND LEE 1999 [50]	Bacteremia, pneumonia, peritonitis	18 penicillin R 11 penicillin I 40 penicillin S		11% (p=0.22) 7.1% (p=0.45) 2.5%	
WINSTON *et al.* 1999 [51]	Pneumococcal infection	65 penicillin NS 411 penicillin S	1.25 (p=0.82)		
DEEKS *et al.* 1998 [52]	Nonmeningeal pneumococcal infections	99 penicillin NS 175 penicillin S	Nonsignificant differences		
EWIG *et al.* 1999 [53]	Pneumococcal pneumonia	49 penicillin NS 52 penicillin S	1.2[¶] (95% CI 0.3–5.3)		
TURRET *et al.* 1999 [54]	Pneumococcal bacteremia	20 penicillin R[+] 429 penicillin S	6.0[#] (p<0.02)		
METLAY *et al.* 2000 [55]	Bacteremic pneumococcal pneumonia	44 penicillin NS 148 penicillin S	1.7[#] (95% CI 0.8–3.4)		
FEIKIN *et al.* 2000 [56]	Invasive pneumococcal pneumonia	183 penicillin R[§] 3452 penicillin S	7.1[f] (95% CI 1.7–30.0)		

A penicillin nonsusceptible isolate is defined as intermediate plus resistant (MIC>0.1 mg·L^{-1}); NS: nonsusceptible; S: susceptible; R: resistant; I: intermediate; CI: confidence interval; [#]: adjusted for severity of illness; [¶]: adjusted for discordance therapy; [+]: resistant defined as MIC>1.0 mg·L^{-1}; [§]: resistant defined as MIC$\geq$4 mg·L^{-1}; [f]: adjusted for severity of illness, deaths during first 4 days of hospitalisation excluded. Data was modified from METLAY and SINGER [57].

resistance in the therapy of nonmeningeal pneumonia infections remains controversial. By convention, resistance is usually defined on the basis of *in vitro* testing and, as described below, much of the controversy relates to the interpretation of the breakpoints for pneumococcus susceptibility and resistance.

Since1987, there have been a limited number of studies comparing outcomes and/or mortality for patients with predominantly infections caused by penicillin-resistant and penicillin-susceptible *S. pneumoniae* (table 4) [47–56]. Seven of these studies reported no significant impact of antimicrobial resistance on improvement of conditions and/or mortality following pneumococcal infection [48–53, 55]. Only one of these studies identified a significant 4.8-fold increase in the risk of suppurative complications (*i.e.* empyemas) among patients with penicillin-resistant compared to penicillin-susceptible pneumococcal pneumonia, even after adjusting for differences in baseline severity of illness [55].

The above mentioned studies suggest that the levels of penicillin resistance in *S. pneumoniae* have little effect on therapeutic outcome in pneumonia and bacteremia. However, a review from the Drug-Resistant *S. pneumoniae* Therapeutic Working Group argues for more caution [58]. The reportindicates that the majority of nonsusceptible isolates examined in the previous studies fell into the intermediate class (MIC

0.1–1 mg·L^{-1}). Although some reports of poor outcome among patients infected with intermediate susceptibility strains do exist in literature [59, 60], most evidence indicates standard treatment with β-lactam antimicrobials is effective against pneumococcal pneumonia caused by strains with penicillin MIC<2 mg·L^{-1}. The same may not be true for isolates with higher MICs.

Among the three studies that identified a significant impact on mortality, one study did not adjust for baseline differences in severity of illness [47]. A second study focused on patients with human immunodefincy virus infection and pneumococcal bacteremia and measured an increased mortality for those patients infected with resistant bacteria. The majority of isolates in this study demonstrated high-level resistance (MIC>1.0 mg·L^{-1}) [54]. Moreover it is likely that patients with immunodeficiencies represent a particular group at risk of adverse outcomes in settings where antimicrobial therapy has reduced efficacy. A third study of patients with invasive pneumococcal pneumonia did not find a significant impact of penicillin and cefotaxime resistance on overall mortality after adjusting for underlying severity of illness. However, after excluding deaths occurring during the first 4 days of hospitalisation, a significant risk of death was noted for pneumococcal infections with penicillin MIC$\geq$4.0 mg·L^{-1} or cefotaxime MIC$\geq$2.0 mg·L^{-1} [56]. The rationale for this conclusion was based on the observation that antibiotic therapy has had minimal impact on the early mortality rate from bacteremic pneumococcal pneumonia [61]. However, this study did not include data on antimicrobial therapy and therefore the impact of discordant therapy on mortality could not be assessed.

Few studies have evaluated the impact of drug resistance on outcomes other than mortality. In one study, length of stay and rates of complications were not significantly worse for patients with antimicrobial-resistant pneumococcal infections [53]. FRIEDLAND [49] found that the duration of respiratory distress, fever and oxygen requirement were similar in penicillin-susceptible and nonsusceptible infections.

No studies have analysed the impact of drug resistance on postdischarge outcomes, *e.g.* symptom resolution and return to usual activities.

Controlled studies measuring the impact of drug resistance on clinical outcomes of care for outpatients with CAP are not available. In part, this reflects the general principle that therapeutic failure and adverse outcomes are more likely to occur among severely ill patients than among lower-risk patients for whom the impact of adequate antimicrobial therapy is only marginal. Alternatively because most outpatients with CAP are treated with a course of a single antimicrobial agent and most inpatients are treated with multiple antimicrobial drugs, outpatients may be more likely to receive discordant therapy that may translate into significant number of therapeutic failures. This hypothesis seems to be supported by recently published case reports describing patients with CAP who failed outpatient therapy, required subsequent hospitalisation and had macrolide-resistant *S. pneumoniae* isolated from blood cultures at the time of hospitalisation [62]. The relatively small number of such case reports suggests that the current rate of treatment failures is low, but large-scale controlled studies of outpatient care are needed to measure more accurately the rates of treatment failure due to antimicrobial resistance.

Potentially, the most important issue for outpatient CAP management is penicillin and multidrug resistance in *S. pneumoniae*.

For clinical purposes, *in vitro* MIC breakpoints must be interpreted in relation to pharmacokinetic and pharmacodynamic parameters characterising the antibiotic at specific infection sites. The original breakpoints for β-lactam resistance in *S. pneumoniae* are of relevance in the context of the low cerebrospinal fluid penetration achieved by these agents in patients with meningitis, and middle-ear penetration in relation to otitis media. They have been of questionable relevance in the management of

RTIs because β-lactams reach far higher concentrations in blood and lung tissue. As a result, β-lactams can eradicate even nonsusceptible (although perhaps not highly resistant) strains from the lungs. Published studies described previously suggest that penicillin nonsusceptibility (MIC>0.1 mg·L^{-1}) does not significantly affect the clinical efficacy of penicillin, ampicillin, or amoxicillin in the treatment of pneumococcal pneumonia in hospitalised patients. Importantly, there are relatively few data from patients with CAP caused by pneumococci with higher-level resistance (MIC>4 mg·L^{-1}), which are more likely to produce clinical failure [54, 56]. Moreover, there are few data concerning the impact of resistance on the effectiveness of oral antibiotic treatment for outpatient CAP.

This discrepancy between *in vitro* resistance and clinical outcome is reflected in the guidelines of the British Thoracic Society (BTS) [63] and others [64], in which β-lactams remain recommended agents for the empirical outpatient treatment of CAP, but at an increased dosage Also according to the Infectious Diseases Society of America [65] guidelines β-lactams are recommended agents for the empirical outpatient treatment of CAP. Coverage against atypical organisms is also suggested when the aetiological agent is unknown. This underlines the fact that differences between the BTS and North American guidelines, regarding initial empirical therapy, are a result of differences in interpretation of the relative frequency and significance of aetiological agents and their susceptibility to recommended therapies, as well as the recognised difficulties of altering prescribing practices in primary care. It also emphasises the importance of severity assessment, for which resistance is only one of several possible causes in defining the choice of therapy.

Despite the high prevalence of *in vitro* macrolide resistance in *S. pneumoniae* in many areas of the world [20], few studies have evaluated the clinical impact of this phenomenon. Pharmacokinetic/pharmacodynamic analysis is more complex for macrolides than for β-lactams because of the intracellular concentration of the former [66]. Worlwide, *erm*B and *mef* genes account for >97% of macrolide resistance among pneumococci. The MIC differences between *erm*B and mef mutants are likely to be important *in vivo*. It has been suggested that the modest levels of resistance (MIC 1–32 mg·L^{-1}) associated with efflux-mediated macrolide resistanc, the dominant mechanism in North America [10, 67], might overcome by adequate macrolide doses [66]. However, high-level resistance (MIC≥64 mg·L^{-1}) caused by *erm*-mediated ribosomal alteration, which is dominant in Europe and South Africa, might not be surmountable using common clinical dosages. Reports of failure and breakthrough bacteremia during outpatient macrolide therapy for pneumococcal pneumonia have recently been published, although the numbers of cases are small [62, 68] Alternativley, recent data indicates that macrolide resistance is associated with clinical failure in a minority of documented infections [69]. It is foreseeable that more widespread reports of failure may occur as high-level macrolide resistance becomes more common [66].

Resistance to the newer "respiratory" fluoroquinolones (*e.g.* levofloxacin, gatifloxacin, moxifloxacin) has not yet greatly influenced prescribing guidelines for CAP. However, reports of fluoroquinolone resistance in Canada [70, 71] and Hong Kong [72–74], are cause of concern over the more widespread use of these agents. Evidence suggests that exposure to fluoroquinolones is associated with increased risk of subsequent infection or colonisation with fluoroquinolone-resistant *S. pneumoniae* [74]. Fluoroquinolone resistance has been linked to clinical failure of these agents in pneumococcal nosocomial LRTIs [74] and CAP [75].

Much more limited is the knowledge about the natural history of AECB and the impact of antibiotic therapy. The overall mortality associated with exacerbations requiring hospitalisation is 3–4%. However, among patients in intensive care units, rate of mortality can be as high as 11–24%. Functional respiratory decline after an acute exacerbation can be significant and re-admission is common [76].

The impact of antibiotic therapy on outcomes for patients with AECB has been assessed, employing a variety of measures, including duration of illness, symptom scores and forced expiratory breath in one second [76]. Systematic reviews have concluded that antibiotics do improve peak expiratory flow rates [77]. In general, the benefits of antibiotics are more apparent for patients with more severe exacerbations. For example, patients with more severe attacks have greater symptom reduction with antibiotics, but patients with mild attacks have similar outcomes with or without antibiotic therapy [76].

There is great interest in the use of alternatives more sensitive outcome measures than mortality to assess the adequacy of antimicrobial therapy in AECB. For example "time to next exacerbation" may be a parameter that has particular clinical meaningfulness and significant economic implications [57]. If this measure is significantly sensitive to differences in the adequacy of antimicrobial therapy, it should be used as an end-point in future studies. Regardless of this, future studies on the impact and adequacy of antimicrobial therapy on outcomes for patients with AECB are clearly needed due to all available data having been collected prior to the recent emergence of antimicrobial resistance among the relevant respiratory pathogens.

As experienced in the last two decades antimicrobial drug resistance among respiratory tract pathogens is a growing problem [78, 79]. In addition, clinical practice guidelines for the treatment of LRTIs, particularly CAP, are continually being revised, resulting in changing strategies to face resistance. Moreover, in contrast to the extraordinary number of microbiological studies documenting the patterns of antimicrobial drug susceptibility, very few studies have analysed the clinical relevance of antibiotic resistance and the extent of the challenge presented by this phenomenon remains unclear. Further research is required to establish the clinical impact of antibiotic resistance focused not only on mortaly but also on morbidity and costs [57, 78, 79]. Ideally, prospective studies comparing treatment outcomes in microbiologically documented infections by high-, low-level resistant and susceptible bacteria are required. Data are clearly important both in the management of individual patients and in the development of guidelines and other prescribing support systems.

Summary

In recent years one of the more alarming aspects in the field of clinical microbiology has been the dramatic increase in the incidence of resistance to antibacterial agents among pathogens causing nosocomial as well as community-acquired infections. Profound geographical differences exist in the incidence of resistance among pathogens causing community-acquired lower respiratory tract infections, only some of which can be explained by the local use of antibiotics. In some cases increased resistance has been shown to be caused by the spread of one or more resistant clone. *Streptococcus pneumoniae*, one of the main organisms implicated in respiratory tract infections, has developed multiple resistance mechanisms to fight the effect of the most commonly used antibiotics. Insusceptibility to both penicillin and macrolides among strains of *S. pneumoniae* is seen worldwide but is highly variable from country to country, with the eastern countries usually more affected. Increasing antibiotic resistance has been reported for other major respiratory tract pathogens, including *Haemophilus influenzae* and *Moraxella catarrhalis*. A high percentage of *M. catarrhalis* strains (>90%) produces β-lactamase, while β-lactamase production among strains of

H. influenzae rarely reaches more than 30% around the world.

In contrast to the extraordinary number of microbiological studies documenting the patterns of antimicrobial drug susceptibility, very few studies have analysed the clinical relevance of antibiotic resistance and the extent of the challenge presented by this phenomenon remains unclear. Further research is required to establish the clinical impact of antibiotic resistance in respiratory pathogens.

Keywords: Antibiotic resistance, antibiotic resistance and clinical outcome, *Haemophilus influenzae*, lower respiratory tract infections, *Moraxella catarrhalis*, *Streptococcus pneumoniae*.

References

1. World Health Organization. The World Health Organization Report: 1997: Conquering suffering, enriching humanity. *World Health Forum* 1997; 18: 240–260.
2. Mogyoros M. Challenges of managed care organizations in treating respiratory tract infections in an age of antibiotic resistance. *American J Managed Care* 2001; 7: Suppl. 6, 163–169.
3. Felmingham D. The need for antimicrobial resistance surveillance. *J Antimircob Chemother* 2002; 50: Suppl. S1, 1–7.
4. Finch RG, Wilcox MH, Wood MJ. Preface. *J Antimircob Chemother* 1996; 38: Suppl. A, V.
5. Felmingham D, Feldman C, Hryniewicz W, *et al*. Surveillance of resistance in bacteria causing community-acquired respiratory tract infections. *Clin Microbiol Infect* 2002; 8: Suppl. 2, 12–42.
6. Spratt BG. Resistance to antibiotics mediated by target alterations. *Science* 1994; 264: 388–93.
7. NCCLS. Performance Standards for Antimicrobial Susceptibility Testing: Twelfth Informational Supplement. NCCLS document M 100-S12. NCCLS, Pennsylvania, NCCLS, 2002: 19087–1898.
8. Leclercq R, Courvalin P. Resistance to macrolides and related antibiotics in *Streptococcus pneumoniae*. *Antimicrob Agents Chemother* 2002; 46: 2727–2734.
9. Tait-Kamradt A, Clancy J, Cronan M, *et al*. *mefE* is necessary for the erythromycin-resistant M phenotype in *Streptococcus pneumoniae*. *Antimicrob Agents Chemother* 1997; 41: 2251–2255.
10. Tait-Kamradt A, Davies T, Appelbaum PC, *et al*. Two new mechanisms of macrolide resistance in clinical strains of *Streptococcus pneumoniae* from Eastern Europe and North America. *Antimicrob Agents Chemother* 2000; 44: 3395–3401.
11. Shortridge VD, Doern GV, Brueggemann AB, Beyer JM, Flamm RK. Prevalence of macrolide resistance mechanisms in *Streptococcus pneumoniae* isolates from a multicenter antibiotic resistance surveillance study conducted in the United States in 1994–1995. *Clin Infect Dis* 1999; 29: 1186–1188.
12. Johnston NJ, De Azavedo JC, Kellner JD, Low DE. Prevalence and characterization of the mechanisms of macrolide, lincosamide, and streptogramin resistence in isolates of *Streptococcus pneumoniae*. *Antimicrob Agents Chemother* 1998; 42: 2425–2426.
13. Depardieu F, Courvalin P. Mutation in 23S rRNA responsible for resistance to 16-membered macrolides and streptogramins in *Streptococcus pneumoniae*. *Antimicrob Agents Chemother* 2001; 45: 319–23.
14. Finland M. Editorial. *N Engl J Med* 1970; 284: 212.
15. Appelbaum PC, Bhamjee A, Scragg JN, Hallett AF, Bowen AJ, Cooper RC, *et al*. *Streptococcus pneumoniae* resistant to penicillin and chloramphenicol. *Lancet ii* 1990; 995–997.
16. Jacobs MR, Koornhof HJ, Robins-Browne RM, *et al*. Emergence of multiply-resistant pneumococci. *N Engl J Med* 1978; 299: 735–740.
17. Dominguez MA, Pallares R. Antibiotic resistance in respiratory pathogens. *Curr Opin Infect Dis* 1998; 11: 139–145.
18. Tomasz A. The challenge of multiresistant *Streptococcus pneumoniae*: international initiatives

in day-care centers and the use of molecular epidemiologic techniques. *Clin Microbiol Infect* 1999; 5: Suppl. 4, 64–68.

19. Felmingham D, Gruneberg RN. The Alexander Project 1996–1997: latest susceptibility data from this international study of bacterial pathogens from community-acquired lower respiratory tract infections. *J Antimicrob Chemother* 2000; 45: 191–203.

20. Schito GC, Debbia EA, Marchese A. The evolving threat of antibiotic resistance in Europe: new data from the Alexander Project. *J Antimicrob Chemother* 2000; 46: Topic T1, 3–9.

21. Felmingham D, Reinert RR, Hirakata Y, Rodloff A. Increasing prevalence of antimicrobial resistance among isolates of *Streptococcus pneumoniae* from the PROTEKT surveillance study, and comparative *in vitro* of the ketolide, telithromycin. *J Antimircob Chemother* 2002; 50: Suppl. 1, 25–37.

22. Hoban DJ, Doern GV, Fluit AC, Roussel-Delvallez M, Jones RN. Worldwide prevalence of antimicrobial resistance in *Streptococcus pneumoniae, Haemophilus influenzae,* and *Moraxella catarrhalis* in the SENTRY Antimicrobial Surveillance Program 1997–1999. *Clin Infect Dis* 2001; 32: Suppl. 2, 81–93.

23. Reinert RR, Simic S, Al Lahham A, Reinert S, Lemperle M, Lutticken R. Antimicrobial resistance of *Streptococcus pneumoniae* recovered from out-patients with respiratory tract infections in Germany from 1998 to 1999: results of a national surveillance study. *J Clin Microbiol* 2001; 39: 1187–1189.

24. Goldstein FW, Acar JF, and The Alexander Project Collaborative Group. Antimicrobial resistance among lower respiratory tract isolates of *Streptococcus pneumoniae*: results of a 1992–1993 Western Europe and USA collaborative surveillance study. *J Antimicrob Chemother* 1996; 38: Suppl. A, 71–84.

25. Marchese A, Mannelli S, Tonoli E, *et al.* Prevalence of antimicrobial resistance in *Streptococcus pneumoniae* circulating in Italy: results of the Italian Epidemiological Observatory (1997–1999). *Microb Drug Resist* 2001; 7: 277–87.

26. Marchese A, Montanari M, Nicoletti G, *et al. S. pneumoniae* serotypes circulating in Italy during the year 2000: results of the Epidemiological Study aimed at surveying multiresistant pneumococci (SEMPRE) [Sierotipi di *S. pneumoniae* circolanti in Italia nel 2000: risultati dello Studio Epidemiologico per il monitoraggio dello Pneumococco Resistente (SEMPRE)]. *GIMMOC* 2002; VI: 139–151.

27. Jette LP, Lamothe F. Survaillance of invasive *Streptococcus pneumoniae* infection in Quebec, Canada, from 1984 to 1986: serotype distribution, antimicrobial susceptibility, and clinical characteristics. *J Clin Microbiol* 1989; 27: 1–5.

28. Low DE, de Azavedo J, Weiss CA, *et al.* Antimicrobial resistance among clinical isolates of *Streptococcus pneumoniae* in Canada during 2000. *Antimicrob Agents Chemother* 2002; 46: 1295–301.

29. Baquero F, Garcia-Rodriguez JA, Garcia de Lomas J, Aguilar L. Antimicrobial resistance of 1,113 *Streptococcus pneumoniae* isolates from patients with respiratory tract infections in Spain: results of a 1-year (1996–1997) multicenter surveillance study. The Spanish Surveillance Group for Respiratory Pathogens. *Antimicrob Agents Chemother* 1999; 43: 357–359.

30. Marchese A, Tonoli E, Debbia EA, Schito GC. Macrolide resistance mechanisms and expression of phenotypes among *Streptococcus pneumoniae* circulating in Italy. *J Antimircob Chemother* 1999; 44: 461–464.

31. Descheemaeker PR, Chapelle S, Devriese LA, Butaye P, Vandamme P, Goossens H. Macrolide resistance and erythromycin resistance determinants among Belgian *Streptococcus pyogenes* and *Streptococcus pneumoniae* isolates. *J Antimircob Chemother* 2000; 45: 167–173.

32. Simor AE, Louie M, Low DE. Canadian national survey of prevalence of antimicrobial resistance among clinical isolates of *Streptococcus pneumoniae*. Canadian Bacterial Surveillance Network. *Antimicrob Agents Chemother* 1996; 40: 2190–2193.

33. Khan W, Ross S, Rodriguez W, *et al. Haemophilus influenzae* type B resistant to ampicillin. A report of two cases. *J American Med Ass* 1974; 229: 299–301.

34. Tomeh MO, Starr SE, McGowan JE Jr, Terry PM, Nahmias AJ. Ampicillin-resistant *Haemophilus influenzae* type B infection. *J American Med Ass* 1974; 229: 295–297.

35. Daum RS, Murphey-Corb M, Shapira E, Dipp S. Epidemiology of ROB β-lactamase among ampicillin-resistant *Haemophilus influenzae* isolates the United States. *J Infect Dis* 1988; 157: 450–455.

36. Sykes RB, Matthew M, O'Callaghan CH. R-factor mediated β-lactamase production by *Haemophilus influenzae* type B infection. *J Medical Microb* 1975; 8: 437–441.

37. Hoban D. and Felmingham D. The PROTEK surveillance study: antimicrobial susceptibility of *Haemophilus* and *Moraxella catarrhalis* from community-acquired respiratory tract infections. *J Antimicrob Chemother* 2002; 50: Suppl. S1, 49–59.

38. Marchese A, Schito GC. Italian Epidemiological Observatory for monitoring resistance to antimicrobials in community-acquired respiratory pathogens (1997–99) [Osservatorio Epidemiologico Italiano per il Monitoraggio delle Resistenze agli Antibiotici nei Patogeni Respiratori Comunitari 1997–1999: Significato per la Pratica Clinica]. *GIMMOC* 2000; IV: 51–58.

39. Thornsberry C, Sahm DF, Kelly LJ, *et al.* Regional trends in antimicrobial resistance among clinical Isolates of *Streptococcus pneumoniae*, *Haemophilus influenzae*, and *Moraxella catarrhalis* in the United States: results from the TRUST surveillance preogram, 1999–2000. *Clin Infect Dis* 2002; 34: Suppl. 1, 4–16.

40. Bootsma HJ, van Dijk H, Vauterin P, Verhoef J, Mooi FR. Genesis of BRO beta-lactamase-producing *Moraxella catarrhalis*: evidence for transformation-mediated horizontal transfer. *Mol Microbiol* 2000; 36: 93–104.

41. Bradley JS, Kaplan SL, Klugman KP, Leggiadro RJ. Consensus: Management of infections in children caused by *Streptococcus pneumoniae* with decreased susceptibility to penicillin. *Pediatr Infect Dis J* 1995; 14: 1037–1041.

42. Friedland IR, McCraken GH Jr. Management of infections caused by antibiotic-resistant *Streptococcus pneumoniae*. *N Engl J Med* 1994; 331: 377–382.

43. Friedland IR, Shelton S, Paris M, *et al.* Dilemmas in diagnosis and management of cephalosporin-resistant *Streptococcus pneumoniae* meningitis. *Pediatr Infect Dis J* 1993; 12: 196–200.

44. Paris MM, Ramilo O, McCraken GH Jr. Management of meningitis caused by penicillin-resistant *Streptococcus pneumoniae*. *Antimicrob Agents Chemother* 1995; 39: 2171–2175.

45. Dagan R. Clinical significance of resistant organisms in otitis media. *Pediatr Infect Dis J* 2000; 19: 378–382.

46. Dagan R, Piglansky L, Fliss DM, *et al.* Bacteriologic efficacies of oral azithromycin and cefaclor treatment of acute otitis media in infants and young children. *Antimicrob Agents Chemother* 2000; 44: 2590–25922.

47. Pallares R, Gudiol F, Linares J, *et al.* Risk factors and response to antibiotic therapy in adults with bacteremic pneumonia caused by penicillin-resistant penumococci. *N Engl J Med* 1997; 317: 18–22.

48. Pallares R, Linares J, Vadillo M, *et al.* Resistance to penicillin and cephalosporin and mortality from severe pneumococcal pneumonia in Barcelona, Spain. *N Engl J Med* 1995; 333: 474–480.

49. Friedland IR. Comparison of the response to antimicrobial therapy of penicillin-resistant and penicillin-susceptible pneumococcal disease. *Pediatr Infect Dis* 1995; 14: 885–890.

50. Choi EH, Lee HJ. Clinical outcome of invasive infections by penicillin-resistant *Streptococcus pneumoniae* in Korean children. *Clin Infect Dis* 1998; 26: 1346–1354.

51. Winston LG, Perlman JL, Rose DA, Gerberding JL. Penicillin-nonsusceptible *Streptococcus pneumoniae* at San Francisco General Hospital. *Clin Infect Dis* 1999; 29: 580–585.

52. Deeks LS, Palacio R, Ruvinsky R, *et al.* Risk factors and course of illness among children with invasive penicillin-resistant *Streptococcus pneumoniae*. The *Streptococcus pneumoniae* Working Group. *Pediatrics* 1999; 103: 409–413.

53. Ewig S, Ruiz M, Torres A, *et al.* Pneumonia acquired in the community through drug-resistant *Streptococcus pneumoniae*. *Am J Respir Crit Care Med* 1999; 159: 1835–1842.

54. Turett GS, Blum S, Fazal BA, Justman JE, Telzak EE. Penicillin resistance and other predictors of

mortality in pneumococcal bacteremia in a population with high human immunodeficiency virus seroprevalence. *Clin Infect Dis* 1999; 29: 321–327.

55. Metlay JP, Hofmann J, Cetron MS, *et al.* Impact of penicillin susceptibility on medical outcomes for adult patients with bacteremic pneumococcal pneumonia. *Clin Infect Dis* 2000; 30: 520–528.

56. Feikin DR, Schuchat A, Kolczak M, *et al.* Mortality from invasive pneumococcal pneumonia in the era of antibiotic resistance, 1995–97. *Am J Public Health* 2000; 90: 223–229.

57. Metlay JP, Singer DE. Outcomes in lower respiratory tract infections and the impact of antimicrobial drug resistance. *Clin Infect Dis* 2002; 8: Suppl. 2, 1–12.

58. Heffelfinger JD, Dowell SF, Jorgensen JH, *et al.* Management of community-acquired pneumonia in the era of pneumococcal resistance: a report from the Drug-Resistant *Streptococcus pneumoniae* Therapeutic Working Group. *Arch Intern Med* 2000; 160: 1399–1408.

59. Feldman C, Kallenbach JM, Miller SD, Thornburn JR, koornhoof HJ. Community-acquired pneumonia due to penicillin-resistant pneumococci. *N Engl J Med* 1985; 313: 615–617.

60. Sacho H, Klugman KP, Koornhof HJ. Ruff P. Community-acquired pneumonia in an adult due to a multiply-resistant pneumococcus. *J Infect* 1987; 14: 188–189.

61. Austrian R, Gold J. Pneumococcal bacteremia with special reference to bacteremic pneumococcal pneumonia. *Ann Inter Med* 1964; 60: 759–776.

62. Kelley MA, Weber DJ, Gillingan P, Cohen MS. Breakthrough pneumococcal bacteraemia in patients being treated with azithromycin and clarithromycin. *Clin Infect Dis* 2000; 31: 1008–1011.

63. British Thoracic Society Standards of Care Committee. BTS guidelines for the management of community-acquired pneumonia in adults. *Thorax* 2001; 56: Suppl. 4, 1–64.

64. Dagan R, Klugman KP, Craig WA, Baquero F. Evidence to support the rationale that bacterial eradication in respiratory tract infection is an important aim of antimicrobial therapy. *J Antimicrob Chemother* 2001; 47: 129–140.

65. Bartlett JG, Dowell SF, Mandell LA, File Jr TM, Musher DM, Fine MJ. Practice guidelines for the management of community-acquired pneumonia in adults. *Clin Infect Dis 200* 31: 347–382.

66. Amsden GW. Pneumococcal macrolide resistance-myth or reality? *J Antimicrob Chemother* 1999; 44: 1–6.

67. Doern GV, Bruggemann AB, Huynh H, Wingert E. Antimicrobial resistance with *Streptococcus pneumoniae* in the United States, 1997–98. *Emerg Infect Dis* 1999; 5: 757–765.

68. Fogarty C, Goldschimidt R, Bush K. Bacteremic pneumonia due to multidrug-resistant pneumococci in 3 patients treated unsuccessfully with azithromycin and successfully with levofloxacin. *Clin Infect Dis* 2000; 31: 613–615.

69. Lonks JR, Garau J, Gomez L, *et al.* Failure of macrolide treatment of erythromycin-resistant *Streptococcus pneumoniae*. *Clin Infect Dis* 2002; 35: 556–564.

70. Chen DK, McGreer A, De Azavedo JC, Lowe DE. Decreased susceptibility of *Streptococcus pneumoniae* to fluoroquinolones in *Canada*. *N Engl J Med* 1999; 341: 233–239.

71. Weiss K, Restieri C, Gauthier R, *et al.* A nosocomial outbreak of fluoroquinolone-resistant *Streptococcus pneumoniae*. *Clin Infect Dis* 2001; 33: 517–522.

72. Ho PL, Que TL, Tsang DN, Ng TK, Chow KH, Seto WH. Emergence of fluoroquinolone resistant among multiply resistant strains of *Streptococcus pneumoniae* in Hong Kong. *Antimicrob Agents Chemother* 1999; 43: 1310–1313.

73. Ho PL, Yam WC, Que TL, *et al.* Target site modification and efflux phenotype in clinical isolates of *Streptococcus pneumoniae* from Hong Kong with reduced susceptibility to fluoroquinolones. *J Antimicrob Chemother* 2001; 47: 655–658.

74. Ho PL, Tse WS, Tsang KW, *et al.* Risk factors for acquisition of levofloxacin-resistant *Streptococcus pneumoniae*: a case-control study. *Clin Infect Dis* 2001; 32: 701–707.

75. Davidson RJ, De Azavedo J, Bast D, *et al.* Resistance to levofloxacin and failure of treatment of pneumococcal pneumonia. *N Engl J M* 2002; 346: 747–750.

76. Bach PB, Brown C, Gelfand SE. McCrory DC, American College of Physicians-American Society of Internal Medicine, Ameican College of Chest Physicians. Management of acute exacerbations

of chronic obstructive pulmonary disease: a summary and appraisal of published evidence. *Ann Intern Med* 2001; 134: 600–620.

77.   Saint B, Bent S, Vittinghoff E. Antibiotics in chronic obstructive pulmonary disease exacerbations. A meta-analysis. *JAMA* 1995; 273: 957–960.

78.   Howard DH, Scott II RD, Packard R, Jones D. The global impact of drug resistance. *Clin Infect Dis* 2003; 36: Suppl. 1, S4–10.

79.   Wood MJ, Moellering RC. Microbial resistance: bacteria and more. *Clin Infect Dis* 2003; 36: Suppl. 1, S2–3.

CHAPTER 9

Lower respiratory tract infections: when are antibiotics mandatory?

L.A. Mandell

Henderson Hospital, Ontario, Canada.

Correspondence: L.A. Mandell, Henderson Hospital, 5th Floor 40 Wing, 711 Concession Street, Hamilton Ontario, L8VIC3, Canada.

Antibiotics were one of the most significant discoveries in the 20th century and are ranked amongst the most important medical advances in history. They have had an enormous impact upon patient morbidity and mortality and have helped to vanquish many of the infections that plagued man. Unfortunately due to their general widespread misuse and abuse, antimicrobial resistance now threatens, returning us to to a pre-antibiotic era.

The purpose of this article, ostensibly, is to discuss when antibiotics are mandatory for treatment of lower respiratory tract infections (LRTIs). In doing so both sides of the antibiotic question needs to be discussed *i.e.* when antibiotics are deemed mandatory and when they should not be used. Each of these in turn is associated with a number of issues *e.g.* if/when used are there advantages to particular classes, are there times when their use is indicated initially but then they must be streamlined or discontinued?

Situations requiring antibiotic use

As it is not possible to discuss all the various situations requiring antibiotic, this chapter will concentrate on community-acquired pneumonia (CAP), hospital-acquired or nosocomial pneumonia (HAP) and acute exacerbations of chronic bronchitis (AECB).

Community-acquired pneumonia

Introduction. Unlike the old adage pneumonia CAP is not the "old man's friend". It is estimated that ~4,000,000 cases of CAP occur annually in the US resulting in ~600,000 hospitalisations, 64,000 deaths and 64,000,000 days of restricted activity [1, 2]. The economic impact of the disease is vast with an estimated $4 billion is spent annually on the care of CAP patients [2]. Another important point for consideration, from the perspective of treatment decisions, is that the costs associated with inpatient therapy are in the order of 20-fold higher than those associated with outpatient care [2]. Within the total population of CAP sufferers ~80% are appropriately treated as outpatients whereas 20% require admission to hospital. The mortality rates in these two groups differ substantially with the rate in the former group being <1% and in the latter group ~20% [3]. The major problem in the management of CAP is the inability to determine the aetiological pathogen. Even in tertiary care university hospitals in which aggressive interventional diagnostic steps such as bronchoscopy or thoracentesis are more likely to be performed the etiological agent may remain undiscovered. This is compounded by the fact that more

Eur Respir Mon, 2004, 28, 146–164. Printed in UK - all rights reserved. Copyright ERS Journals Ltd 2004; European Respiratory Monograph; ISSN 1025-4408X. ISBN 1-904097-32-4.

than one pathogen may be responsible for the infection in any given patient. The concept of microbial synergy has been recognised for a long time in other infections *e.g.* as peritonitis, an intra-abdominal abscess, synergistic gangrene *etc.* One pathogen may inhibit the interaction of the host defenses with other pathogens, it may provide essential nutrients, or it could alter the local microenvironment so that the other pathogen(s) can thrive [4]. It has been shown that in nosocomial pneumonia more than one pathogen is present in more than one half of the cases presented [5]. The association of *Staphylococcus aureus* with *Haemophilus influenzae* infection in the same patient may be explained by the fact that the staphylococci produce nicotinomide dinucleotide which is necessary for the *H. influenzae* to grow [6].

In CAP, copathogens may also be found [1, 7, 8]. The type of pathogen is determined by the nature of the host (smoker *versus* nonsmoker, young *versus* old), the site of acquisition of the infection and the severity of illness. Regardless of these considerations however, the single most important pathogen is *Streptococcus pneumoniae*. A meta-analysis of studies spanning 30 yrs showed that of 7,000 pneumonia patients in whom an aetiological agent was found, *S. pneumoniae* was identified in 66% patients. It was also responsible for two out of three deaths from pneumonia [3].

The usual pathogens are listed in table 1. For outpatients, these include atypical examples *e.g. Mycoplasma pneumoniae* and *Chlamydia pneumoniae*, pneumococcus and *H. influenzae*. *H. influenzae* is more likely to occur in smokers or those with chronic bronchitis (CB).

As shown in table 1, although the pneumococcus must be considered in all cases, Gram-negative rods may also be important. Although Gram-negative bacilli do not occur with the same frequency as *S. pneumoniae* or *M. pneumoniae*, they are important because of the high mortality rate associated with them which is in the order of 33% [9].

The treatment of any infectious disease can be either "directed" or "empirical". The former assumes that the physician knows the specific pathogen causing the infection whereas the latter approach is essentially an educated guess. There are several advantages associated with directed therapy *e.g.* a reduction in polypharmacy, reduced costs, fewer adverse drug reactions and less antibiotic selection pressure. Unfortunately however, empirical therapy is used in the vast majority of cases. Its clear though that there are sufficiently compelling reasons to institute empirical therapy in patients with CAP, these include: 1) the impact of the disease; 2) the number of possible pathogens; 3) the presence of co-pathogens; and 4) the limitations of diagnostic testing. Unfortunately there are insufficient rapid, sensitive and specific tests to enable the rapid identification of the aetiological pathogen. The fact that the present diagnostic tests may not always be helpful underscores the fact that empirical treatment must be appropriate, particularly in severely ill patients. Therefore, it is necessary to carefully consider the various risk factors and epidemiological circumstances and initiate treatment with antibiotics able to effectively treat the most likely pathogens causing the infection.

One of the most important treatment decisions is the initial site of care *i.e.* will the patients be managed in the hospital setting (medical ward or intensive care unit: ICU) or will

Table 1. – Usual pathogens in community-acquired pnuemonia and nursing home-acquired pneumonia

Outpatients	Inpatients	Nursing Home
Streptococcus pneumoniae	*S. pneumoniae*	*S. pneumoniae*
Atypicals (2)	Atypicals (3)	Atypicals [3]
Haemophilus influenzae	*H. influenzae*	*Staphlococcus, aureus*
	GNR	GNR

GNR: Gram-negative rods.

the patient be treated in the home? A couple of recent articles suggest that the initial site of treatment should be selected in a systematic three-step process [10, 11]. Step one involves the assessment of any pre-existing conditions that could compromise treatment in the home setting. These include the presence of coexisting conditions which require hospitalisation, the presence of haemodynamic instability, acute hypoxaemia or severe social or psychiatric problems and the inability to take oral medicines. Step two involves the determination of the pneumonia port severity index, and step three involves the use of clinical judgment to determine the overall health of the patient and suitability for home care.

Treatment. Currently in the US and Canada there are three sets of CAP guidelines. One from the Infectious Diseases Society of America (IDSA), one from the American Thoracic Society (ATS) and one that is a joint statement from the Canadian Infectious Disease Society (CIDS) and the Canadian Thoracic Society [12–14]. The IDSA guidelines seem to regard outpatients almost as a single entity but with modifying factors such as suspected penicillin-resistant *S. pneumoniae* (PRSP) infection, suspected aspiration or infection in the young adult [12]. The ATS approach however, is to divide the group into those who are younger and without comorbidity and those who are older or with comorbidity [13]. The Canadian document goes to some lengths to categorise the patients into those without modifying factors, those with chronic obstructive lung disease (COPD) and patients who

Table 2. – Empirical antimicrobial selection for adult patients with community-acquired pneumonia

Type of patient and factor(s) involved	Treatment	
	First choice	Second choice
Outpatient with no modifying factors	Macrolide[#]	Doxycycline
Outpatient with modifying factors		
COLD no recent antibiotics or PO steroids within 3 months	Newer macrolide[¶]	Doxycycline
COLD recent antibiotics or PO steroids within 3 months; *Haemophilus influenzae* and enteric Gram-positive rods implicated	"Respiratory" fluoroquinolone[+]	Amoxicillin/clavulanate+macrolide or 2G cephalosporin+macrolide Respiratory fluoroquinolone (*e.g.* levofloxacin)+clindamycin or
Suspected macroaspiration: oral anaerobes	Amoxicillin/clavulanate± macrolide	metronidazole
Nursing home resident		
Streptococcus pneumoniae, enteric Gram-negative rods, *H. influenzae* implicated	"Respiratory" fluorquinolone alone or amoxicillin/ clavulanate and macrolide	2G cephalosporin+macrolide
Hospitalised	Identical to treatment for other hospitalised patients	
Hospitalised patient on medical ward		
S. pneumoniae, *Legionella pneumophila*, *Clamydia pneumoniae* implicated	"Respiratory" fluoroquinolone	2G, 3G, or 4G cephalosporin+ macrolide
Hospitalised patient in ICU		IV macrolide+cefotaxime, ceftriaxone
Pseudomonas aeruginosa not suspected; *S. pneumoniae*, *L. pneumophila*, *C. pneumoniae* Gram stain justifies Gram-negative rods implicated *P. aeruginosa* suspected	IV respiratory fluoroquinolone+ cefotaxime, ceftriaxone, or β-lactam/β-lactamase inhibitor Antipseudomonal fluoroquinolone *e.g.* ciprofloxacin+ antipseudomonal β-lactam	or β-lactam/β-lactamase inhibitor Triple therapy with antipseudomonal β-lactam (*e.g.* ceftazidime, aminoglycoside piperacillin-tazobactam imipenem, or meropenem)+aminoglycoside (*e.g.* gentamicin, tobramycin or amikacin)+macrolide

COLD: chronic obstructive lung disease; PO: oral; 2G: second generation; 3G: third generation; 4G: fourth generation; ICU: intensive care unit; IV: intravenous; [#]: erythromycin, azithromycin, or clarithromycin; [¶]: azithromycin or clarithromycin; [+]: levofloxacin, gatifloxacin, or moxifloxacin; trovafloxacin restricted because of potential severe hepatotoxicity.

may have aspirated (table 2) [14]. To date, no data exists that can definitively demonstrate that any one approach to treatment of CAP patients is superior to another. Given the low mortality rate associated with outpatients however, it is unlikely that any differences will be demonstrated in the future unless other outcome measures are used. The main concern most physicians have is that the overuse of any one class of antibiotics will result in an increased antimicrobial resistance, whether it involves the macrolides, the fluoroquinolones or the β-lactams. A reasonable approach is to continue to assess risk factors such as comorbid illness and risk factors for infection with PRSP and design therapeutic regimens accordingly.

Risk factors that have been identified for infection with PRSP include the use of beta β-lactams within the previous 3 months, immunosuppression, <5 yrs of age, hospitalisation within 6 months and nosocomial acquisition [15]. Others have argued that PRSP is so widespread now that it is no longer worth considering its risk factors in individual patients.

For those without risk factors for PRSP or without comorbid illness a fluoroquinolone is unnecessary and a macrolide or doxycycline should suffice. For patients with reduced pulmonary reserve who also are at risk of infection with PRSP or Gram-negative rods, a fluoroquinolone would be more appropriate.

Recently there has also been some concern about macrolide resistance. There are two types of macrolide resistances depending upon the mechanism involved. A change in target is mediated by the *erm* gene and results in the macrolide-lincosamide streptogramin b (MLSb) phenotype which is associated with high level resistance while efflux is mediated by the *mef* gene and results in the M phenotype which is associated with low level resistance [16]. In the US ~1–2% of pneumococcal isolates have both genes while in another 1–2% of mutants resistance may be based on other alterations in the macrolide binding site *e.g.* at ribosomal proteins L4 and L22 [17–19].

There have been a number of reports recently of clinical failures or breakthrough bacteremias with *S. pneumoniae* associated with macrolide usage [20–23]. However the current feeling is that macrolides still have a role to play and may be used as monotherapy in those with milder outpatient infections or in combination with β-lactams for those who are more seriously ill. In such cases a β-lactams *e.g.* cefotaxime or ceftriaxone would be virtually certain to cover the pneumococcus while the macrolide could be used for the atypical pathogens.

Resistance to fluoroquinolones has also become a concern but the overall level in the US regarding pneumococcal quinolone resistance is currently ~1–2%. However, a recent report on the failures to treat pneumococcal pneumonia associated with levofloxacin use did indicate that a mutation resulting in resistance and clinical failure may occur within a few days [23].

The currently available "respiratory" fluoroquinolone agents used for CAP include moxifloxacin, gatifloxacin and levofloxacin.

For those treated in hospital, all three of the North American guidelines differentiate between patients admitted to a medical ward and those requiring treatment in an ICU. For those treated in a ward all three guidelines recommend a β-lactam plus a macrolide or monotherapy with one of the respiratory fluoroquinolones.

Those treated in an ICU setting require broad spectrum therapy. In the absence of any risk factors for *Pseudomonas aeruginosa* such as severe structural lung disease, a non pseudomonal beta lactam plus a macrolide or respiratory fluoroquinolone may be used.

Initially the recommendation that combination therapy be used in such situations was based upon the fact that there were no randomised control trials using monotherapy with a fluoroquinolone for patients with severe pneumonia. Three retrospective studies have suggested that combination therapy which included a macrolide resulted in reduced mortality of bacteremic pneumococcal pneumonia [24–26].

If Pseudomonas is a concern then the regimen given in table 2 should be used. Data have shown that inappropriate antibiotic therapy in those with severe CAP results in increased mortality rates [27]. Based upon a review of >13,000 Medicare hospitalised patients who had not received antibiotics prior to their admission, suggested that administration of initial therapy within 4 h of arrival at hospital was associated with reduced mortality in the hospital [28].

There are no data based upon properly conducted randomised control trials to inform on how long patients must be treated. By conversion they are usually treated for 1–2 weeks based upon their initial presentation and subsequent response to therapy.

Hospital-acquired pneumonia

Introduction. HAP is a serious disease which is associated with considerable morbidity and mortality. By definition it is pneumonia occurring 48 h or more following admission to hospital. It is the second most common nosocomial infection but the one most likely to result in a fatal outcome. It also has a significant economic and sociological impact as it increases the length of stay by 8 days on average [29].

Ventilator-associated pneumonia (VAP) is a subset of HAP that develops in patients receiving mechanical ventilation. While it's estimated that the annual incidence of HAP is 5–10 cases per 1,000 admissions, in those undergoing mechanical ventilation this figure may increase to 20 fold [30, 31].

The usual pathogens encountered in nosocomial pneumonia are Gram-negative rods and certain Gram-positive cocci. The former include Enterobacteriaceae, *H. influenzae* and on occasions *P. aeruginosa* and *Acinetobacter spp.* while the latter includes *S. aureus* and *S. pneumoniae* [32]. The Enterobacteriaceae of concern include *Escherichia coli*, *Klebsiella sp.*, *Enterobacter sp.*, *Proteus sp.* [32]. A study by BARTLETT *et al* [5] showed conclusively that in over half of the HAP cases more than one pathogen could be found. In an attempt to simplify matters the CIDS and the ATS suggested that a "core" group of pathogens should be used when dealing with cases of HAP [29, 33]. The idea was to have a number of bacteria that clinicians would recognise as being potential causes of HAP and that represent an irreducible group of etiological agents that must be treated when antibiotic therapy is started. The pathogens that can cause mild–to–moderate HAP or early VAP and severe HAP or late VAP are listed in table 3.

One of the main challenges in the management of HAP is to overcome the resistance issues which have become so important and common over the past several years. Bacteria can become resistant either by mutating or by acquiring new genetic information. This in turn can result in the production of enzymes which could inactivate the antibiotic, reduce accessibility of the antibiotic to the target sites, provide a change in the target site itself, cause an efflux of the antibiotic or enable the inhibited pathways of the pathogen to be bypassed.

Bacteria are capable of producing a number of enzymes which can inactivate

Table 3. – Commonly encountered pathogens in hospital-acquired pneumonia (HAP) and ventilator-associated pneumonia (VAP)

Mild-to-moderate/early (core)	Severe/late
Enterobacteriaceae Haemophilus influenzae Staphylococcus aureus Streptococcus pneumoniae	Core+Pseudomonas aeruginosa, Acinonacter sp.

Table modified from [32].

antibiotics as diverse as β-lactams, aminoglycocides and chloramphenical and one of the most common mechanisms of bacterial resistance is β-lactamase production which can be mediated either by a plasmid or a chromosome. There are currently >75 plasmid mediated β-lactamases and the most clinically relevant, at present, are the extended spectrum β-lactamases (ESBLs). These are usually found in *K. pneumoniae* and are less frequent in other Enterobacteriaceae and can confer resistance to many of the broad spectrum cephalosporins such as ceftriaxone, cefotaxime and ceftazidime and the monobactam aztreonam [34, 35]. Drugs which remain active against pathogens producing ESBLs are the carbapenems *e.g.* imipenem and meropenem, β-lactam/β-lactamase inhibitors such as piperacillin-tazobactam and the fluoroquinolones [34, 36].

The chromosomal β-lactamases are also important. A clinically relevant example is the spontaneous mutation occurring in the bacterial genome of *Enterobacter sp.* in patients who are being treated with third generation cephalosporins. This mutation may result in the production of a stably derepressed mutant which is a hyper producer of β-lactamase [47, 38]. The only β-lactams which are effective against chromosomal β-lactamases are cefipime and the carbapenems. In general the fluoroquinolones and aminoglycosides are always useful.

Access of the drug to the target site may be changed by alterations in the porin proteins which make up the diffusion channels through which the drug normally crosses the bacterial outer membrane. Examples of such mechanisms of resistance include *P. aeruginosa* and *E. aerogenes* to imipenem and *Serratia marcescens* and *P. aeruginosa* to fluoroquinolones [39–41]. Active efflux or pumping out of the antibiotic has been described as a resistance mechanism with tetracyclines and fluoroquinolones [42, 43].

It is of some concern that certain antimicrobials which are unaffected by more common resistance mechanisms such as inactivating enzymes, are precisely those agents whose use appears to select out multidrug resistant mutants which over produce multidrug efflux pumps. In *E. coli*, over production of the main multi drug pump occurs as a result of the increased production of a global regulator (Mar A) which is produced in response to the presence of antibiotics in the environment [44].

If the antibiotic does reach the target and has not been inactivated by enzymes, resistance may still occur as a result of a change in the target site itself. While there are three ways of achieving this, the most common is due to a change in the target enzyme. This is important for resistance to both β-lactams and fluoroquinolones.

The penicillin binding proteins are bacterial enzymes involved in the synthesis of peptidoglycan and also serve as the target sites of action for β-lactam antibiotics. Changes in these sites result in resistance to β-lactam antibiotics with the most relevant examples being *S. pneumoniae* resistance to penicillin and in selected instances to second and third generation cephalosporins and *S. aureus* having resistance to β-lactams *i.e.* methicillin-resitant *S. aureus* (MRSA) [45, 46].

Deoxyriboenucleic acid (DNA) gyrase and topoisomerase IV are enzymes necessary for super coiling and decatination respectively of bacterial DNA and also serve as target sites of action for fluoroquinolones. Mutations in the genes regulating these enzymes (*gyr A, gyr B, par C* and *par E*) respectively may result in changes in these enzymes with resultant resistance to fluoroquinolones [47, 48]. Changes in more than one site can result in very substantial increases in minimal inhibitory concentrations (MICs) to the various fluoroquinolones.

Changes in cell wall precursor targets and in ribosomal binding sites have been implicated in resistance of enterococci to vancomycin and of Gram-positive cocci to macrolides, lincosamides and in some cases tetracyclines.

As a general rule resistance is more likely to be encountered when dealing with VAP cases than HAP cases on the medical wards. VAP cases are more likely to have been exposed to prior antibiotics and generally have spent more time in hospital than the average HAP case.

S. aureus is the predominant Gram positive pathogen in HAP and VAP. Coma is the primary risk factor for VAP caused by methacillin sensitive *S. aureus* and risk factors for VAP caused by MRSA include corticosteroid therapy, mechanical ventilation longer than 6 days, >25 yrs of age, prior diagnosis of COPD, and previous use of antibiotics [49].

Many of the diagnostic issues discussed earlier relating to CAP also pertain to HAP. Often empirical therapy is required although when dealing with VAP patients the physician is more likely to obtain deep suction aspirates which may help with initial treatment and if not, may help once culture data becomes available. When dealing with HAP either a clinical approach; or a clinical plus an invasive/quantitative approach can be undertaken. The former relies upon information gathered from a carefully taken history, physical examination and selected laboratory tests and procedures such as a chest roentgenogram and cultures of blood and sputum. The latter method relies upon more sophisticated testing techniques such as bronchoscopy with protected specimen brush (PSB) or bronchoalveolar lavage (BAL). Occasionally other methods *e.g.* transthoracic needle aspiration or lung biopsy may be used.

One study that compared noninvasive and invasive strategies for the management of suspected VAP randomised patients to each of these methods for making a diagnosis. The noninvasive method utilised the clinical approach plus nonquantitative cultures of endotracheal aspirate. The invasive approach relied upon PSB or BAL with quantitative cultures. The primary outcome measures were as follows: mortality at 14 days; the presence of multiple organ dysfunction at 7 days; and antibiotic free days at 14 days. In all cases the invasive approach yielded data that were statistically significantly better than the noninvasive approach [50].

Treatment. There are a number of challenges facing the physician who must initiate treatment of HAP or VAP. The following issues must be born in mind with each case: 1) the disease itself may be associated with significant morbidity and mortality; 2) data suggests that inappropriate initial therapy or delayed appropriate therapy is associated with increased mortality [51–53]; 3) the currently available diagnostic tests are of limited utility; 4) resistance may be an issue; and 5) co-pathogens may be present in more than half of the number of cases presented.

This means that the physician is often put in the position of having to initiate empirical therapy using reasonably broad spectrum agents which will cover the likely pathogens. The approach used by the ATS and CIDS is based upon the following variables: 1) risk factors; 2) severity of illness; and 3) time of onset [29, 33]. Patients with VAP are divided into those with early infection (<5 days) or late infection (≥5 days).

Both guidelines have divided patients into three groups based upon the variables referred to earlier. These are: 1) patients with mild-to-moderate nosocomial pneumonia with no unusual risk factors, onset anytime, or patients with severe HAP with early onset; 2) patients with mild to moderate HAP with risk factors, onset anytime; 3) patients with severe HAP with risk factors, early onset or patients with severe HAP late onset.

When selecting any antibiotic regimen the first step is to choose an agent to which the pathogen is known or likely to be susceptible. Other factors that need to be considered include pharmacokinetic and pharmacodynamic properties, toxicity, drug interactions and cost. Pharmacokinetics refers to the absorption, distribution and elimination of drugs while pharmacodynamics is the relationship between the concentration of the drug in serum and its pharmacological and toxicological effects. Depending upon the class of antibiotic being used, different pharmacokinetic/pharmacodynamic parameters correlate approximately with clinical or therapeutic efficacy. For β-lactam drugs, macrolides and clindamycin, the time during which the antibiotic concentration at the site of action in the tissues is greater that the MIC of the organism correlates best with efficacy [54]. For aminoglycosides, fluoroquinolones and vancomycin the area under the curve after 24 h (AUC$_{24}$)/MIC ratio correlates best [54]. Higher ratios of peak serum concentrations to MIC have been shown to prevent the emergence of resistance during treatment with fluoroquinolones and aminoglycosides.

As a general rule, doses sufficient to achieve levels above the MIC of a particular pathogen at the site of infection should be administered. In immunocompetent patients however, even subinhibitory concentrations of an antibiotic may at times be effective. Although the drug may not be able to kill or even inhibit the pathogen it may alter it sufficiently so that it is more readily disposed of by host defenses such as the obsinons and phagocytes.

The treatment of mild-to-moderate HAP or early onset VAP involves the use of a single agent such as a β-lactam/β-lactamase inhibitor or a nonpseudomonal β-lactam *e.g.* cefotaxime or ceftriaxone or a fluoroquinolone will suffice. Combination therapy is generally used to extend antimicrobial coverage, provide synergy or prevent the emergence of resistance. The issue of broader coverage was of greater concern years ago before the introduction of such broad spectrum agents as the carbapenems or various β-lactam/β-lactamase inhibitors. Now drugs *e.g.* piperacillin-tazobactam or *imipenem etc.* provide coverage for most of the aerobic and anaerobic pathogens of concern. The issue of synergistic or additive activity is being re-evaluated. Historically combination therapy seemed to be of benefit for treatment of *P. aeruginosa*, enterococcal infections and *S. aureus* bacteremia. Patients with bacteremic pneumococcal pneumonia may also benefit from combination therapy as discussed in the section on CAP treatment.

It should be noted that *Enterobacter sp.* are the most common of the Enterobacteriaceae implicated as causes of HAP. One of the major concerns with infection caused by such organisms is that in the presence of a third generation cephalosporin a mutation in the bacterial genome may occur resulting in a pathogen that becomes a hyper producer of β-lactamases and is thus resistant to selected penicillins and cephalosporins [38].

For HAP patients who are severely ill or late onset VAP patients, aggressive combination therapy should be instituted initially. If the patient was not receiving prior antibiotics and deep suction aspirates or bronchoscopy fail to yield *P. aeruginosa* or other often resistant pathogens such as *Acinetobacter spp.* treatment may be modified to a single drug regimen [29, 32].

The same issues pertaining to the length of treatment applied to CAP also apply to HAP and VAP. Therapy is typically given for 10–14 days depending upon the initial severity of illness and the clinical and radiological response. However there is increasing interest in shorter courses of therapy and data suggests that even in selected VAP cases the pathogens are eradicated and the parameters which are used to suggest infection were resolved within a week [55, 56]

Acute exacerbations of chronic bronchitis

Introduction. In order to understand AECB and its management and treatment the disease pool from which this entity arises must first be understood. COPD is a slow progressive pulmonary condition whose major characteristic is chronic airflow limitation. The disease progresses over years and is largely irreversible. Most definitions of COPD define it as a spectrum of respiratory disease which includes entities as CB, emphysema and small airways disease with some mixture of chronic cough, increased sputum production, dyspnoea, airflow limitation and impaired gas exchange. CB is usually defined clinically as a disorder with expectoration of sputum on most days during at least three consecutive months for more than two successive years, with other causes of cough and sputum having been excluded [57]. CB accounts for ~85% of COPD and often coexists with emphysema and small airways disease. While many people refer to the acute flare ups as AECB some use the term exacerbations of COPD, there is obviously considerable overlap.

One of the difficulties has been in defining exactly what is meant by AECB. Like the disease itself chronic bronchitis, exacerbations are defined clinically and the most commonly used system to assess severity of an acute exacerbation is that developed by ANTHONISEN et al. [58]. In this system patients with type I (severe) exacerbations have all three of the main clinical findings which typically include increased cough and volume of sputum, increased purulence of sputum and increased dyspnoea. Those with type II (moderate) exacerbations have two of the three findings and those with type III (mild) exacerbations have at least one of the clinical findings. SEEMUNGAL et al. [59] have proposed major and minor criteria which can be used to define an exacerbation. The major criteria are the three mentioned prevoiously while minor criteria include wheeze, sore throat, cough and symptoms of the common cold such as nasal congestion or discharge. They defined an exacerbation as the presence of at least two major symptoms or one major and one minor symptom for at least two consecutive days. Unfortunately at present there are no rating systems for severity of exacerbation that have been validated.

The impact of airway disease is substantial. In the US, COPD afflicts 20% of the population and is the fourth leading cause of death [60, 61]. Acute bronchitis (AB) and AECB together account for ~14 million visits to the physician per year and in the UK it's estimated that bronchitis is associated with 28 million lost working days and 5% of deaths per year [62, 63]. Unfortunately most physicians do not differentiate among various entities that comprise LRTIs including AB, AECB, and CAP.

AECBs may result in hospitalisation which is associated with a 4% short term mortality rate for patients with mild-to-moderate disease but can be as high as 24% for patients requiring care in an ICU [64–68]. Patients with severe disease have been reported to have 1 yr mortality rates as high as 46% and unfortunately many patients requiring hospitalisation for management of an episode of AECB will require subsequent readmissions because of persistent symptoms [65–69].

Exacerbations have been reported following exposure to allergens, environmental pollutants or infection. Even with infection it's clear that viruses may play a role in a considerable number of cases [70]. There is however a growing body of evidence suggesting that bacterial infection plays an important role. In patients experiencing an exacerbation, investigators have demonstrated an increase in the numbers of bacteria, neutrophils and inflammatory mediators in purulent sputum as well as an acute antibody response in serum to various bacterial pathogens [71–73]. A recent paper in the *New England Journal of Medicine* further supported the role of bacterial infection as a cause of AECB by demonstrating that the acquisition of a new strain of pathogenic bacterial species by a patient with COPD but with no pre-existing immunity to the strain can lead to an exacerbation [74].

The bacterial aetiology of AECB is not straightforward. While pathogens such as *H. influenzae*, *S. pneumoniae* and *Moraxella catarrhalis* are commonly seen in mild-to-moderate cases it has been observed that with a decline in pulmonary function there is an increase in the prevalence of pathogens such as enteric Gram-negative bacilli and *P. aeruginosa* [78].

A process termed the "vicious circle hypothesis" has been invoked to explain the pathogenesis of bacterial damage and subsequent exacerbations [76]. Initiating factors such as smoking or childhood respiratory disease may lead to airway damage with impaired mucociliary clearance. This in turn may result in bacterial colonisation of the airways which results in release of various bacterial products and induces the host's inflammatory response. The resultant damage to the airways makes it easier for further colonisation to occur and the process is repeated. Progressive airway damage is a result of the bacterial products themselves as well as the various cytokines and enzymes which represent the patient's response to the microbial pathogens.

The diagnosis of AECB is typically a clinical one. There are no characteristic physical findings and the lack of a clear definition has interfered with proper investigation of this entity. There is a lack of a reproducible rating system to determine severity and the differences in the definitions for ABs and the lack of standard outcome measures, have made it exceedingly difficult to evaluate studies dealing with its management. Over the past 40 yrs >11,000 patients have been enrolled in randomised placebo control trials of antibiotic treatment of AECB but none have been of identical design and the patient populations have not been uniform. It is clear that there is a great deal of work to be done in this area.

For now the diagnosis is based upon the presence or absence of the cardinal symptoms of AECB which were described earlier as part of the ANTHONISEN et al [58] criteria i.e. increased sputum production, increased sputum purulence and increased dyspnoea. The presence of any one, two or three of these in someone with a diagnosis of CB suggests a diagnosis of an AECB.

Treatment. Despite a growing body of evidence supporting the role of antibiotics there continues to be questions regarding the use of these agents. A landmark study by ANTHONISEN et al. [58] was among the first to demonstrate a benefit for antibiotics in the management of such patients. It was shown that patients with type I (severe) or type II (moderate) exacerbation had a demonstrable benefit from antimicrobial therapy while those with a type III (mild) exacerbation did not benefit. A recent meta-analysis involving nine randomised placebo control trials concluded that there was a benefit associated with antibacterial therapy in the management of AECB [77]. However, concerns have been raised about many of these studies including the fact that the ANTHONISEN et al. [58] classification only had a 50% sensitivity and 60% specificity in predicting a bacterial exacerbation [78].

If it is accepted that antibiotics play a role in the treatment of AECB the immediate question becomes "are certain antibiotics better than others?" A retrospective study looked at three outcome measures these were: failure rates; time to relapse (in weeks); and the percentage of patients hospitalized, these were correlated with the types of antibiotics used [79]. First line antibiotics were amoxicillin, cotrimoxazole, tetracycline and erythromycin, second line antibiotics were cefuroxime, cefaclor and cefprozil and third line antibiotics were amoxicillin-clavulanic acid, azithromycin and ciprofloxacin. There was a strong correlation between potency and spectrum of antibiotics and improved response rates. Other investigators have examined the role of fluoroquinolones in the management of AECB and found significant benefit associated with their use. The GLOBE study looked at gemifloxacin versus clarithromycin and found a significant improvement in the prevention of relapse rates with the use of a fluoroquinolone agent. In a prospective health economical study, ciprofloxacin was compared with any nonquinolone based therapy in the management of AECB [80, 81]. Although overall there was no benefit associated with either regimen it was noted that those who used ciprofloxacin with patients that had risk factors it resulted in an improved clinical outcome, a higher quality of life and at a lower cost [81].

It is clear that even routine antimicrobial therapy results in failure in 13–25% of treated exacerbations [82, 83]. Such failure results in increased cost of care as a result of additional physician visits, additional tests and possibly repeated treatment with antibiotics. Secondary costs resulting from loss work days are incurred and in some cases failure may result in hospitalisation. A number of factors have been reported as predictive of failure of initial antimicrobial therapy including coexistent cardio-pulmonary disease, a number of prior exacerbations and the advanced age of the patient [84]. Those at particularly high risk are patients with >4 exacerbations in the previous year requiring systemic corticosteroid medications, and those with significant impairment function of lung [82–84]. For those requiring admission to hospital the risk factors for increased mortality included >65 yrs of age, comorbid organ dysfunction and length of stay in hospital prior to ICU admission [85].

It was hoped that by stratifying patients into various risk categories the physician may be able to select those at greatest risk and use more potent antimicrobials in their management. A number of schema have been developed which essentially categorise patients according to severity of their underlying disease and risk of failure with antibacterial therapy [86–88]. Table 4 shows the patient stratification scheme proposed by BALTER et al. [86] and is included in the Canadian Guidelines for the management of AECB. Group I refers to acute exacerbation which is a separate entity from CB and will be discussed in detail in a subsequent section. It was purposely included in the AECB guidelines in order to draw attention to this problem and the fact that it is all too often over treated. Group II deals with patients with simple CB and can be managed with an amino penicillin. Group III refers to those with moderate-to-severe CB and it is clear that such patients require somewhat broader and more potent agents. Group IV is similar to Group III but with the presence of significant comorbid illness. The suggested treatment regimens are similar but this author would not use trimethoprim sulpha because of increasing resistance problems and concerns relating to increased reports of adverse drug reactions with sulphas in the elderly. Group V refers to those with advanced structural lung disease such as bronchiectasis. These patients may frequently be colonised with pathogens e.g. P. aeruginosa and require treatment aimed at this organism.

Streamlining, de-escalating and shortening therapy

By necessity initial antibiotic therapy is usually empirical rather than directed and may at times be somewhat broader in spectrum than is required. One study suggested that location-specific antibiotic regimens which were tailored to the susceptibility patterns of the local microbial flora, were most likely to be effective [89]. However it is also recognised that these initial regimens may often be streamlined or de-escalated thereby narrowing the spectrum of activity and reducing antibiotic selection pressure but without compromising patient care. In addition to narrowing coverage, the duration of antimicrobial treatment may be shortened and ideally limited to the shortest, yet effective, course of treatment.

Use of antibiotic practice guidelines, various critical pathways and protocols have proven to be helpful in maximising the utility of therapeutic regimens. Automated and partially nonautomated approaches have been utilised and both have proven to be successful. An example of the former is the computerised system in place at LDS Hospital in Salt Lake City, Utah [90, 91]. This system has been shown to significantly improve the prescribing of antibiotics and to reduce costs. Similar results have been seen with non or partially automated systems including reductions in unnecessary antibiotics and antibiotic related costs [92, 93].

The use of shorter courses of antibiotic treatments is also under investigation and is

Table 4. – Risk classification and suggested antimicrobial therapy

Group	Basic clinical state	Symptoms and risk factors	Probable pathogens	First choice	Alternatives for treatment failures
0	Acute trachobronchitis	Cough and sputum without previous pulmonary diseas	Usually viral	None unless symptoms persist for >7–10 days	Macrolide or tetracycline
I	CB without risk factors (simple)	Increased cough and sputum, sputum purulence and increased dyspnoea	*Haemophilus influenzae* *Haemophilus* spp. *Moraxella catarrhalis,* *Streptococcus pneumoniae*	2G macrolide, 2G/3G cephalosporin, amoxicillin, doxycycline trimethoprim/ sulphamethoxazole	Fluoroquinolone, β-lactam/ β-lactamase inhibitor
II	CB with risk factors (complicated)	As in class I plus one or more of: FEV1<50% predicted ≥4 exacerbations per yr ≥ Age >65 yrs Significant co-morbidity (especially heart disease) Use of home oxygen Chronic oral steroid use Antibiotic use in the past 3 months			
III	Chronic suppurative bronchitis	As in class II with constant purulent Some have bronchiectasis FEV1, usually <35% pred sputum Multiple risk factors (*e.g*) frequent exacerbations and FEV1 <50%	As in class II plus *Pseudomonas aeuroginosa* and mulitresistant	Ambulatory patients: tailor treatment to airway pathogen *P. aeuroginosa* common (ciprofloxacin) Hospitalised patients: parenteral therapy usually required	

Table taken from BALTET *et al.* [86]. 2G: second generation; 3G: third generation; FEV1: forced expiratory volume in one second.

likely to become the general practice in a number of situations. The advantages of shorter courses are obvious and include reduced costs, reduced adverse drug reactions and antibiotic selection pressure. For CAP, two studies with garenoxacen for five days *versus* a control agent from another class for 10 days have been completed and apparently show the five day regimen to be as effective (personal communication D. Webb). Studies in VAP patients have shown that if an appropriate antibiotic regimen is used the markers of infection and host response to infection, such as elevated leukocyte count and temperature and $Pa,O_2/FI,O_2$ ratios have normalised by day six and most cultures obtained by endotracheal aspirate have cleared [55, 56].

The GLOBE trial which compared a 5-day gemifloxacin course with a 7-day clarithromycin cours for AECB showed similar efficacy for the two agents but the fluoro-quinolone was superior in preventing further exacerbations and hospitalisations [80].

Situations which do not require antibiotic use

It is clear that the majority of LRTIs require antibiotic therapy, however, there are at least two situations that may not demand the same treatment. One is type three

AECB and the other is acute bronchitis (AB). The former is a mild form of exacerbation and refers to a patient with only one of the cardinal symptoms of exacerbation; there are no specific studies that have addressed this subset exclusively. Instead, patients with all gradations of severity were included in two studies and the various sub-groups separated [68, 94]. The studies by ANTHONISEN et al. [58] and ALLEGRA et al. [95] failed to show any benefit for antibiotics over placebo for patients with mild flare ups of CB. This supports the argument that antibiotics are not necessary for all cases of AECB and that viruses play an important role in the etiology of this entity as reports have indicated.

AB is one of the most common illnesses seen in primary care. It is an acute illness in otherwise healthy individuals lasting 1–2 weeks and is frequently caused by respiratory viruses. It is characterised by cough with or without sputum, fever and/or substernal discomfort without any radiographical infiltrates.

The Cochrane database reviewed nine randomised placebo controlled trials involving >750 patients including smokers and nonsmokers [96]. Overall, antibiotics appeared to have a modest beneficial effect in patients with AB but the magnitude of this benefit was similar to that of the detriment from potential adverse effects.

There are, however, two reviews of AB that do not support antibiotics for the treatment of this disease [97, 98]. The paper by GONZALEZES [97] concluded that available data from randomised placebo controlled trials do not support routine antibiotic treatment of uncomplicated AB and the McKAY [98] paper comes to the same conclusion but also reported that albuteral had an advantage over erythromycin.

It is clear that antibiotics have a definite role to play in many LRTIs but in a few they do not. However, it is also clear that physicians often misuse these drugs and by doing so threaten to render them useless. It is therefore of great importance that the use of these agents to treat patients is carried out in both a careful and an appropriate manner so that they are preserved and consequently can be used for generations to come.

Summary

This chapter deals with community-acquired pneumonia (CAP), hospital-acquired pneumonia (HAP), and acute exacerbations of chronic bronchitis (AECB). It first considers those situations which require the use of antibiotics before briefly discussing the various issues surrounding the streamlining, de-escalation and shortening of treatment as well as situations that do not require the use of antibiotics. Situations that require antibiotics the need for streamlining, de-escalation and shortening of treatment as well as situations that do not require antibiotic use will be discussed in different degrees of details.

CAP can be treated either with directed therapy or using empirical therapy. The former involves use of a narrow spectrum antibiotic directed against a known pathogen whereas the latter essentially is an educated guess involving broader spectrum agents directed against a variety of pathogens in the hope that the correct one will be eradicated. While there is no question that the former is more desirable the latter is almost always the one used.

Various treatment guidelines are currently available including those from the Infectious Diseases Society of America (IDSA), the American Thoracic Society (ATS) and the Canadian Infectious Disease Society/Canadian Thoracic Society (CIDS/CTS). The Canadian Guidelines are presented in tabular format.

Antimicrobial resistance has become a legitimate concern over the past 1–2 decades and this issue is discussed in some detail. Hospital-acquired pneumonia (HAP) is the second most common nosocomial infection and ventilator-associated pneumonia (VAP) represents a subset of HAP. Here too, a large number of potential pathogens may be encountered but a "core group" are felt to be the most likely pathogen in most cases.

Just as with CAP, empirical therapy is often caused in HAP as well. The reasons for this are that HAP/VAP may be associated with significant morbidity and mortality and there are good data to show that inappropriate initial therapy or delayed appropriate therapy are associated with increased mortality. The treatment recommendations for HAP and VAP represent slight modification of the original CIDS and ATS recommendations.

Again various resistance issues are discussed particularly as they relate to Gram-negative pathogens. For AECB the definition and classification is discussed and major and minor criteria are proposed. The major criteria are: 1) increased cough and volume of sputum; 2) increased purulence of sputum; and 3) increased dyspnoea while the minor criteria include: wheeze, sore throat, cough and symptoms such as nasal congestion or discharge. The presence of two major symptoms or one major and one minor for at least 2 consecutive days define an acute exacerbation. A variety of pathogens may be responsible for flare ups but it has become fairly clear that the aetiological agent will vary depending upon pulmonary function.

A number of treatment schemes have stratified patients according to severity of underlying disease and risk of failure with antibacterial therapy. British, German and Canadian Guidelines have been proposed based upon such a stratification scheme. The Canadian Guidelines are presented in one of the papers.

Initial regimens are often, by necessity, more broad spectrum than may be required. They may be streamlined or de-escalated allowing a narrowing of the spectrum of activity thereby reducing antibiotic selection pressure and hopefully minimizing resistance without compromising patient care. A variety of approaches including antibiotic practice guidelines, critical pathways and protocols have been helpful. Also automated and partially nonautomated approaches have also been of use.

The use of shorter course treatment is being looked at very carefully in CAP, HAP and AECB and data already exists showing that treatment may be shortened in all three of these disease entities.

Finally some situations which do not require antibiotic use were also considered. These include Type III AECB and acute bronchitis. The former consists of only one of the cardinal manifestations and the latter is typically of viral aetiology.

Keywords: Acute exacerbations of chronic bronchitis, community-acquired pneumonia, guidelines, hospital-acquired pneumonia, resistance.

References

1. Dixon RE. Economic costs of respiratory tract infections in the United States. *Am J Med* 1985; 78: 45.
2. National Center for Health Statistics: National hospital discharge survey; Annual summary 1990. *Vital Health Stat* 1992; 13: 1–225.
3. Fine MJ, Smith MA, Carson CA, *et al.* Prognosis and outcomes of patients with community-acquired pneumonia. *JAMA* 1996; 275: 134–141.
4. Rotstein OD, Pruett TL, Simmons RL. Mechanisms of microbial synergy in polymicrobial surgical infections. *Rev Infect Dis* 1985; 7: 151–170.

5.   Bartlett JG, O'Keefe P, Talley F, *et al.* Bacteriology of hospital-acquired pneumonia. *Arch Intern Med* 1986; 145: 868–871.

6.   Mandell LA, Loeb M. Microbiology of hospital-acquired pneumonia. *Semin Respir Crit Care Med* 1997; 18: 111–120.

7.   Marston BJ, Plouffe JF, File TM, *et al.* Incidence of community-acquired pneumonia requiring hospitalizations: Results of a population-based active surveillance study in Ohio. *Arch Intern Med* 157: 1709–1718.

8.   Mundy LM, Auwaerter PG, Oldach D, *et al.* Community-acquired pneumonia: Impact of immune status. *Am J Respir Crit Care Med* 1995; 152: 1309–1315.

9.   Gilbert K, Fine MJ. Assessing prognosis and predicting patient outcomes in community-acquired pneumonia. *Semin Respir Infect* 1994; 9: 140–152.

10.   Halm E. Management of community-acquired pneumonia. *New Engl J Med* 2002; 347: 2039–2045.

11.   Fine MJ. A prediction rule to identify low risk patients with community-acquired pneumonia. *New Engl J Med* 1997; 336: 243–250.

12.   Bartlett JG, Dowell SF, Mandell LA, *et al.* Practice guidelines for the management of community-acquired pneumonia in adults. *Clin Infect Dis* 2000; 31: 347–382.

13.   American Thoracic Society. Guidelines for the management of adults with community-acquired pneumonia. Diagnosis, assessment of severity, antimicrobial therapy, and prevention. *Am J Respir Crit Care Med* 2001; 163: 1730–1754.

14.   Mandell LA, Marrie TJ, Grossman RF, *et al.* Canadian guidelines for the initial management of community-acquired pneumonia: an evidence-based update by the Canadian Infectious Diseases Society and the Canadian Thoracic Society. *Clin Infect Dis* 2000; 31: 383–421.

15.   Nava JM, Bella F, Garau J, *et al.* Predictive factors for invasive disease due to penicillin-resistant *Staphylococcus pneumoniae*. A population-based study. *Clin Infect Dis* 1994; 19: 884–890.

16.   Shortridge V, Doern G, Brueggeman A, *et al.* Prevalence of macrolide resistance mechanisms in Streptococcus pneumoniae isolates from a multicenter antibiotic resistance surveillance study conducted in the United States in 1994–1994. *Clin Infect Dis* 1999; 29: 1186–1188.

17.   Depardieu F, Courvalin P. Mutation in 23SrRNA responsible for resistance to 16-member macrolides and streptogramins in *Streptococcus pneumoniae*. *Antimicrob Agents Chemother* 2001; 45: 319–323.

18.   Tait-Kamradt A, Davies T, Cronan M, *et al.* Mutations in 23 SrRNA and ribosomal protein L4 account for resistance in pneumococcal strains selected in vitro by macrolide passage. *Antimicrob Agents Chemother* 2000; 44: 2118–2125.

19.   Tait-Kamradt A, Davies T, Appelbaum PC, *et al.* Two new mechanisms of macrolide resistance in clinical strains of *Streptococcus pneumoniae* from Eastern Europe and North America. *Antimicrob Agents Chemother* 2000; 44: 3395–3401.

20.   Fogarty C, Goldschmidt R, Bush K. Bacteremic pneumonia due to multidrug resistant pneumococci in 3 patients treated unsuccessfully with azithromycin and successfully with levofloxacin. *Clin Infect Dis* 2000; 31: 613–615.

21.   Kelley MA, Weber DJ, Gilligan P, *et al.* Breakthrough pneumococcal bacteremia in patients on azithromycin/clarithromycin therapy. *Clin Infect Dis* 2000; 31: 1008–1011.

22.   Lonks JR, Garau J, Gomez L, *et al.* Failure of macrolide antibiotic treatment in patients with bacteremia due to erythromycin-resistant *Streptococcus pneumoniae*. *Clin Infect Dis* 2002; 35: 556–564.

23.   Davidson R, *et al.* Resistance to levofloxacin and failure of treatment of pneumococcal pneumonia. *New Engl J Med* 2002; 346: 747–750.

24.   Martinez JA, Horcajada JP, Almela M, *et al.* Addition of a macrolide to a β-lactam-based empirical antibiotic regimen is associated with lower in-hospital mortality for patients with bacteremic pneumococcal pneumonia. *Clin Infect Dis* 2003; 36: 389–395.

25.   Waterer G. Monotherapy may be suboptimal for severe bacteremic pneumococcal pneumonia. *Arch Intern Med* 2001; 161: 1837–1842.

26. Mufson MA, Stanek RJ. Bacteremic penumococcal pneumonia in one American city: a 20-year longitudinal study. *Am J Med* 1999; 107: 34S–43S.

27. Leroy O, Santre C, Beuscart C. A 5-year study of severe community-acquired pneumonia with emphasis on prognosis in patients admitted to an ICU. *Intensive Care Med* 1995; 21: 24–31.

28. Houck PM, Bratzler DW, Nsa W, *et al.* Timing of antibiotic administration and outcomes for Medicare patients hospitalized with pneumonia. In review at Archives of Internal Medicine.

29. Campbell GD, Niederman MS, Broughton DE, *et al.* Hospital-acquired pneumonia in adults: diagnosis, assessment of severity, initial antimicrobial therapy, and preventative strategies. A consensus statement of the American Thoracic Society. *Am J Respir Crit Care Med* 1996; 153: 1711–1725.

30. Celis RA, Torres A, Gatell JM, *et al.* Nosocomial pneumonia: A mutivariate analysis of risk and prognosis. *Chest* 1988; 93: 318–324.

31. Torres A, Aznar R, Gatell JM, *et al.* Incidence, risk and prognosis factors of nosocomial pneumonia in mechanically ventilated patients. *Am Rev Respir* 1990; 152: 523–528.

32. CDC NNIS System. National Nosocomial Infections Surveillance Report. *Am J Infect Control* 1966; 24: 380–388.

33. Mandell LA, Marrie TJ, Niederman MS. Canadian Hospital Acquired Pneumonia Consensus Conference Group (1993). Initial antimicrobial treatment of hospital-acquired pneumonia in adults: a conference report. *Can J Infect Dis* 1993; 4: 317–321.

34. Livermore DM. β-lactamases in laboratory and clinical resistance. *Clin Microbiol Rev* 1995; 8: 557–584.

35. Philippon A, Labia R, Jacoby GA. Extended spectrum β-lactamases. *Antimicrob Agents Chemother* 1989; 33: 1131–1136.

36. Jacoby GA, Carreras I. Activities of β-lactam antibiotics against *Escherichia coli* strains producing extended-spectrum β-lactamases. *Antimicrob Agents Chemother* 1990; 34: 858–862.

37. Sanders CC, Sanders WE. Clinical importance of inducible β-lactamases in gram-negative bacteria. *Eur J Clin Microbiol* 1987; 6: 435–438.

38. Chow JW, Fine MJ, Shlaes DM, *et al.* Enterobacter bacteremia - clinical features and emergence of antibiotic resistance during therapy. *Ann Int Med* 1991; 115: 585–590.

39. Trias J, Nikaido H. Outer membrane protein D2 catalyzes facilitated diffusion of carbapenems and penems through the outer membrane of *Pseudomonas aeruginosa*. *Antimicrob Agents Chemother* 1990; 34: 52–57.

40. Hopkins JM, Towner KJ. Enhanced resistance to cefotaxime and imipenem associated with outer membrane protein alterations in *Enterobacter aerogenes*. *J Antimicrob Chemother* 1990; 225: 49–55.

41. Sanders CC, Sanders WE Jr, Goering RV, Werner V. Selection of multiple antibiotic resistance by quinolones, beta-lactams, and aminoglycosides with special reference to cross-resistance between unrelated drug classes. *Antimicrob Agents Chemother* 1984; 26: 797–801.

42. McMurray L, Petrucci RE, Levy SB. Active efflux of tetracycline encoded by four genetically different tetracycline resistance determinants in *Escherichia coli*. *Proceedings of the National Academy of Sciences USA* 1980; 70: 3974–3977.

43. Cohen SP, Hooper DC, Wolfson JS, *et al.* Endogenous active efflux of norfloxacin in susceptible Escherichia coli. *Antimicrob Agents Chemother* 1988; 32: 1187–1190.

44. Nikaido H. The role of outer membrane and efflux pumps and the resistance of Gram negative bacteria. Can we improve drug access? *Drug Resistance Updates* 1998; 1: 93–98.

45. Austrian R. Confronting drug-resistant pneumococci. *Ann Int Med* 1994; 121: 807–809.

46. Jacoby GA, Archer GL. New mechanisms of bacterial resistance to antimicrobial agents. *New Eng J Med* 1991; 324: 601–612.

47. Nakamura S, Nakamura M, Kojima T, Yoshida H. gyrA and gyrB mutations in quinolone-resistant strains of Escherichia coli. *Antimicrob Agents Chemother* 1989; 33: 128–130.

48. Wolfson JS, Hooper DC. The fluoroquinolones: structures, mechanisms of action resistance, and spectra of activity *in vitro*. *Antimicrob Agents Chemother* 1985; 28: 581–586.

49. Rello J, Torres A, Ricart M, *et al.* Ventilator-associated pneumonia by Staphylococcus aureus: Comparison of methicillin-resistant and methicillin-sensitive episodes. *Am J Respir Crit Care Med* 1994; 150: 1545–1549.

50. Fagon J, *et al.* Invasive and noninvasive strategies for management of suspected VAP. *Ann Int Med* 2000; 132: 621–630.

51. Celis R, Torres A, Gatell JM, *et al.* Nosocomial pneumonia: A multivariate analysis of risk and prognosis. *Chest* 1988; 93: 318–324.

52. Torres A, Aznar R, Gatell JM, *et al.* Incidence, risks and prognosis factors of nosocomial pneumonia in mechanically ventilated patients. *Am Rev Resp Dis* 1990; 142: 523–528.

53. Luna C, Vujacich P, Niederman MS, *et al.* Impact of BAL data on the therapy and outcome of ventilator-associated pneumonia. *Chest* 1997; 111: 676–685.

54. Craig WA. Pharmacokinetic pharmcodynamic parameters: Rationale for antibacterial dosing of mice and men. *Clin Infect Dis* 1998; 26: 1–12.

55. Denneson P. Resolution of infectious parameters after antimicrobial therapy in patients with VAP. *Am J Resp Crit Care Med* 2001; 163: 1371.

56. Luna CM. Resolution of VAP: prospective evaluation of the clinical pulmonary infection score as an early clinical prediction of outcome. *Crit Care Med* 2003; 31: 1.

57. Definition and classification of chronic bronchitis for clinical and epidemiological purposes. A report to the Medical Research Council by their Committee on the Aetiology of Chronic Bronchitis. *Lancet* 1965; 1: 775–779.

58. Anthonisen NR, Manfreda J, Warren CP, Hershfield ES, Harding GK, Nelson NA. Antibiotic therapy in exacerbations of chronic obstructive pulmonary disease. *Ann Intern Med* 1987; 106: 196–204.

59. Seemungal TA, Donaldson GC, Bhowmik A, Jeffries DJ, Wedzicha JA. Time course and recovery of exacerbations in patients with chronic obstructive pulmonary disease. *Am J Respir Crit Care Med* 2000; 161: 1608–1613.

60. US Bureau of the census: statistical abstract of the United States, Edn 14. Washington, US Bureau of the Census, 1994: pp. 95.

61. Woolcock AJ. Epidemiology of chronic airways disease. *Chest* 1989; 96: Suppl. 3, 302–306.

62. Verheij TJM, Kaptein AA, Mulder JD. Acute bronchitis: etiology, symptoms and treatment. *J Fam Pract* 1989; 6: 66–69.

63. Turner-Warwick M, Hodson ME, Corrin B, *et al.* Clinical atlas of respiratory diseases. London, Gower Medical Publishing, 1990.

64. Mushlin AI, Black ER, Connolly CA, Buonaccorso KM, Eberly SW. The necessary length of hospital stay for chronic pulmonary disease. *JAMA* 1991; 266: 80–83.

65. Connors AF, Dawson NV, Thomas C, *et al.* Outcomes following acute exacerbation of severe chronic obstructive lung disease. The SUPPORT investigators (Study to Understand Prognoses and Preferences for Outcomes and Risks of Treatments). *Am J Respir Crit Care Med* 1996; 154: 959–967.

66. Burk RH, George RB. Acute respiratory failure in chronic obstructive pulmonary disease. Immediate and long-term prognosis. *Arch Intern Med* 1973; 132: 865–868.

67. Seneff MG, Wagner DP, Wagner RP, *et al.* Hospital and 1-year survival of patients admitted to intensive care units with acute exacerbation of chronic obstructive pulmonary disease. *JAMA* 1995; 274: 1852–1857.

68. Cydulka RK, McFadden ER Jr, Emerman CL, *et al.* Patterns of hospitalization in elderly patients with asthma and chronic obstructive pulmonary disease. *Am J Resp Crit Care Med* 1997; 156: 1807–1812.

69. Osman IM, Godden DJ, Friend JA, *et al.* Quality of life and hospital readmission in patients with chronic obstructive pulmonary disease. *Thorax* 1997; 52: 67–71.

70. Seemungal T, Harper-Owen R, Bhowmik A, *et al.* Respiratory viruses, symptoms, and inflammatory markers in acute exacerbations and stable chronic obstructive pulmonary disease. *Am J Respir Crit Care Med* 2001; 164: 1618–1623.

71. Fisher M, Akhtar AJ, Calder MA, *et al.* Pilot study of factors associated with exacerbations of chronic bronchitis. *Br Med J* 1969; 4: 187–192.

72. Medici TC, Chodosh S. The reticuloendothelial system in chronic bronchitis. *Am Rev Respir Dis* 1972; 105: 792–804.

73. Stockley RA, Burnett D. Serum derived protease inhibitors and leucocyte elastase in sputum and the effect of infections. *Bull Eur Physiolpathol Respir* 1980; 16: 261–271.

74. Sethi S, Evans N, Brydon JB, *et al.* New strains of bacteria and exacerbations of chronic obstructive pulmonary disease. *New Engl J Med* 2002; 347: 465–471.

75. Eller J, Ede J, Rossdeutscher W, *et al.* Sputum bacteriology of acute infective exacerbation: Chronic obstructive pulmonary disease *versus* bronchiestasis. *Eur Respir J* 1996; 9: Suppl, 23 107.

76. Cole P, Wilson R. Host-microbial interrelationships in respiratory infection. *Chest* 1989; 95: Suppl. 217–221.

77. Saint S, Bent S, Vittinghoff E, *et al.* Antibiotics in chronic obstructive pulmonary disease exacerbations. A meta-analysis. *JAMA* 1995; 273: 957–960.

78. Sethi S, Paluri R, Grant E, *et al.* Prediction models for the etiology of acute exacerbations of COPD. *Am J Resp Crit Care Med* 1999; 159: A819.

79. Destache C, *et al.* Clinical and economic considerations in acute exacerbations of chronic bronchitis. *J Antimicrob Chemother* 1999; 43: Suppl. A, 107–113.

80. Wilson R, *et al.* A comparison of gemifloxacin and clarithromycin in acute exacerbations of chronic bronchitis and long term clinical outcomes. *Clin Ther* 2002; 24: 639–652.

81. Grossman RF, Mukerjee J, Vaughan D, *et al.* A one-year community based health economic study of ciprofloxacin vs. usual antibiotic treatment in acute exacerbations of chronic bronchitis. *Chest* 1998; 113: 131–141.

82. Ball P, Harris JM, Lowson D, *et al.* Acute infective exacerbation of chronic bronchitis. *Q J Med* 1995; 88: 61–68.

83. MacFarlane JT, Colville A, Guion A, *et al.* Prospective study of aetiology and outcome of adult lower-respiratory tract infections in the community. *Lancet* 1993; 341: 511–514.

84. Niroumand M, Grossman RF. Airway infection. *In*: Moellering RC Jr, ed. Infectious Disease Clinics of North America, Lower Respiratory Tract Infections. Philadelphia, WB Saunders Company, 1998: pp. 671–688.

85. Seneff MG, Wagner DP, Wagner RP, *et al.* Hospital and 1-year survival of patients admitted to intensive care units with acute exacerbation of chronic obstructive lung disease. *JAMA* 1995; 274: 1852–1857.

86. Balter MS, La Forge J, Low DE, Mandell L. Canadian guidelines for the management of acute exacerbations of chronic bronchitis. *Can Resp J* 2003; Suppl. 3B, 3B–32B.

87. Lode H. Respiratory tract infections: when is antibiotic therapy indicated? *Clin Ther* 1991; 13: 149–156.

88. Wilson R. Outcome predictors in bronchitis. *Chest* 1995; 108: Suppl. 53–57.

89. Trouillet JL, Chastre J, Vuagnat A, *et al.* Ventilator-associated pneumonia caused by potentially drug-resistant bacteria. *Am J Respir Crit Care Med* 1998; 157: 531–539.

90. Evans RS, Classen DC, Pestotnik SL, *et al.* Improving empiric antibiotic selection using computer decision support. *Arch Intern Med* 1994; 154: 878–884.

91. Evans RS, Pestotnik SL, Classen DC, *et al.* A computer-assisted management program for antibiotics and other anti-infective agents. *N Engl J Med* 1998; 338: 232–238.

92. Bailey TC, Ritchie DJ, McMullin ST, *et al.* A randomized, prospective evaluation of an interventional program to discontinue intravenous antibiotics at two tertiary care teaching institutions. *Pharmacotherapy* 1997; 17: 277–281.

93. Leibovici L, Gitelman V, Yehezkelli Y, *et al.* Improving empirical antibiotic treatment: prospective, nonintervention testing of a decision support system. *J Intern Med* 1997; 242: 395–400.

94. Allegra L, Grasi E, Pozzi E. Puolo degli antibiotici nel trattamento delle riacutizza della bronchite cronica. *Ital J Chest Dis* 1991; 45: 138–148.

95. Greenberg SB. Respiratory consequences of rhinovirus infection. *Arch Intern Med* 2003; 163: 278–284.

96. Smucny J, Fahey T, Becker L, *et al.* Cochrane database of systematic reviews.

97. Gonzales R. Uncomplicated acute bronchitis. *Ann Intern Med* 2000; 133: 981–991.

98. McKay DM. Treatment of acute bronchitis in adults without underlying lung disease. *J Gen Intern Med* 1996; 11: 557–562.

CHAPTER 10

Epidemiological impact of antibiotic use/misuse in the community

T. Welte

Dept of Pneumology and Intensive Care Medicine, University of Magdeburg, Magdeburg, Germany.

Correspondence: T. Welte, Dept of Pneumology and Intensive Care Medicine, University of Magdeburg, Leipziger 44 Street, 39120 Magdeburg, Germany.

Resistance of bacterial pathogens against modern antimicrobial agents has been a problem since the late 1950s. In the 1970s there existed an uncritical optimism that challenges of antibiotic resistance could be solved with the development of new drugs. Today, however, the opposite has been revealed to be true. The release of new substances became slower, while the development of resistance by various bacterial pathogens became faster [1]. Resistance by bacteria was scarce at the beginning of the 1980s, but a number of worldwide surveillance programs, like the Alexander Project [2], revealed resistances against all substances in use today (*Streptococcus pneumoniae* resistance against penicillin is 18.2%, against macrolides is 24.6%, and against fluorchinolones is 1.1%; β-lactamase producing *Haemophilus influenzae* in 16.9 %, *Moxarella. catarrhalis* in 92.1%). Three major reasons for these findings are under discussion: 1) the widespread application of antibiotics in animals; 2) the growing use of antibiotics in all developed countries; and 3) the fast spreading of resistances due to travelling and globalisation. However, resistance patterns vary greatly from continent to continent, and from country to country. Even in different regions of the same country different resistance patterns had been found. No valid explanation can be given for this phaenomenon until today.

Nowadays it is unclear, whether or not the growing rates of resistances have an impact on the prognosis of respiratory infections in shorter or longer terms, there may be major differences between pathogens. Therefore the question is open as to which measures might be helpful for the prevention of further development of resistances.

Use of antibiotics in animals

Antibiotics are used in animal farms for two reasons: 1) to treat and prevent diseases; and 2) to improve the efficacy of nutrition and growth (table 1).

The individual treatment of a diseased animal would be possible, but often it is easier to treat the whole group of animals which are kept in the same place. In some species (chicken or fish) this is the only way of treatment. Large doses of antibiotics are used to treat a small number of diseased animals and to prevent the rest of the cohort (so called metaphylaxis). Prophylactic antibiotic treatment is allowed by most authorities for animals in high risk situations *e.g.* long haul transportation. The correlation of prophylactic antibiotic treatment and improvement of growth is less well documented than the benefit of curing diseased animals. Nevertheless a number of substances can be legally applied in subtherapeutic doses.

Eur Respir Mon, 2004, 28, 165–174. Printed in UK - all rights reserved. Copyright ERS Journals Ltd 2004; European Respiratory Monograph; ISSN 1025-448x. ISBN 1-904097-32-4.

Table 1. – Reasons for the use of antimicrobials in food animals

Type of antimicrobial use	Purpose	Route or vehicle of administration	Administration to individuals or groups[#]	Diseased animals
Therapeutic	Therapy	Injection, feed, water	Individual or group	Diseased individuals; in groups, may include some animals that are not diseased or are subclinical
Metaphylactic	Disease prohylaxis, therapy	Injection (feedlot calves), feed, water	Group	
Prophylactic	Disease prevention	Feed	Group	None evident, although some animals may be subclinical
Subtherapetic	Growth promotion Feed efficiency	Feed	Group	None
		Feed	Group	None
	Disease prohylaxis	Feed	Group	None

[#]: food animals are usually grouped by pen, flock, pond, barn, or other. Adapted from McEwen *et al.* [3].

Animal production grew enormously since the end of World War II although the number of farms became continuously reducing, the total amount of produced meat (cattle, chicken, fish) has increased.

The increase in animal production has been associated with a fast growing production of antibiotics. Data from Denmark during 1994 in a report by Aarestrup *et al.* [4] revealed that this small country has a consumption of 260,000 kg of antimicrobials in the farming industry. Several systematic reviews revealed a close association between the use of antibiotics and the rate of resistance in pathogens [3]. The major problem is the development of resistances in enteric commensals (enterococci and most of the *Escherichi coli* strains) and pathogens (Salmonella, Campylobacter, Yersinia, *E.coli*), since these bacteria can be easily transferred to humans. Resistance genes in commensal microorganisms were probably transferred to the enteropathogens [3].

Theoretically it would be possible that resistances spread to other bacterial species (*e.g.* from enterococci to staphylococci), and this would aggravate the situation in humans tremendously [5]. The huge increase of resistant enteropathogens in humans and the increase of deaths from polyresistent salmonella, resulted in most countries in more restrictive laws concerning the use of antibiotics in animals. The sole use of antibiotics to improve growth in livestock is forbidden. This resulted in an increase in infectious diseases, in animals, however this stance did improve measures of hygiene and the introduction of aseptic products (*e.g.* zink oxide in piglets) counterbalanced the problem [6]. The total consumption of antibiotics was estimated to have been reduced by 60%. This was accompanied by a reduction of resistant microbial pathogens in farm animals, but a complete elimination of resistant strains was not possible. This might be due to a persistence of resistant microbial organisms in the wild animals, and repeated re-infections might be possible *via* direct contact or compounds of nutrition.

The ban of antimicrobials in subtherapeutic doses was associated with a reduction in meat production and the economic damage was huge. In the US, this was estimated to be in the range of $1.2–2.5 billion, which means $5–10 *per capita* [3]. The damage was lowest in chicken livestock and it was the highest in cattle livestock.

In conclusion, the application of antibiotics in animals resulted in a high resistance of animal pathogens and to a lesser extent, in resistance of human pathogens. The invention of restrictive laws had been successful. Table 2 shows a list of the antimicrobials approved for use in livestock in the US. The economical consequences in animal

Table 2. – Antimicrobials approved for use in food animals in the US

Purpose	Cattle	Swine	Poultry	Fish
Treatment of various infections	Amoxicllin Cephapirin Erythromycin Fluoroquinolone Gentamicin Novobiocin Penicillin Sulphonamides Tilicosin Tylosin	Amoxicllin Ampicillin Chlortetracycline Gentamici Linomycin Sulfamehtazine Tiamulin Tylosin	Erythromycin Fluoroquinolone Gentamicin Neomycin Penicillin Spectinomycin Tetracyclines Tylosin Virginiamycin	Ormetoprim Sulphonamide Oxytetracycline
Growth and feed efficiency	Bacitracin Chlortetracycline Lasalocid Monensin Oxytetracycline	Asanilic acid Bacitracin Bambermycin Chlortetracycline Erythromycin Penicillin Tiamulin Tylosin Virginiamycin	Bambermycin Bacitracin Chlortetracycline Penicillin Tylosin Virginiamycin	

Table adapted from McEwen *et al.* [3].

production might not been neutralised by government financial support, therefore close microbiological surveillance is necessary to prevent further illegal use of antibiotics.

Growing use of antibiotics worldwide

A correlation between antibiotic use and bacterial resistance has been demonstrated repeatedly. In the case of *S. pneumoniae*, links between antibiotic use and resistance have been consistently found at every etiological level these have included: 1) patients [7]; 2) small, human communities [8]; 3) different geographical areas of the same country [9]; and 4) nationally and internationally [10]. The best way to demonstrate the link between spreading of resistant clones and the selection pressure of antibiotics is the simultaneous proof of resistance from different bacterial species. In Spain, a 1-yr prevalance survey revealed a parallel increase of resistance in *S. pneumoniae* and *Streptococcus pyogenes*, depending on the consumption of macrolides [11]. Theoretically, the above mentioned gene transfer could be responsible for this observation, but varying determinants of resistances render this inprobable.

The correlation between resistances and consumption of antibiotics is not linear and is shown in figure 1.

The current view on antibiotic resistance assumes that a certain minimum consumption is necessary to create resistance. The amount of this consumption, whether it is the same for different antibiotics, and whether it is the same for different countries, is not clear yet [12]. If resistance is present, the high consumption seems to promote further resistance [13]. Sepala *et al.* [14] could demonstrate the course and the pattern of resistance in A streptococci in a multicentre study in Finland, resulting from a guideline recommendation for macrolides as a first-line treatment option. After recognition of this problem, and restrictions on the use of macrolides had been implemented, a marked reduction of resistance had been observed in the following years, but without complete remission. Nasrin *et al.* [15] could demonstrate similar results after the reduction of β-lactam consumption, concerning the resistances of *S. pneumoniae*.

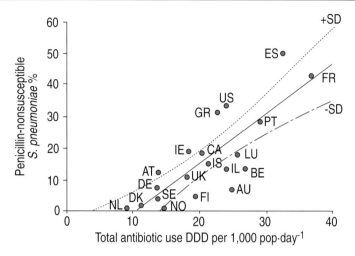

Fig. 1. – Correlation between antibiotic consumption and penicillin resistance by *Streptococcus pneumoniae*. DDD: Defined daily dose; POP: population; AT: Austria; AU: Australia; BE: Belgium; CA: Canada; DE: Germany; DK; Denmark; ES: Spain; FI: Finland; FR: France; GR: Greece; IE: Ireland; IS: Iceland; IT: Italy; LU: Luxemburg; NL: The Netherlands; NO: Norway; PT: Portugal; SE: Sweden; UK: United Kingdom; US: United States of America; ········· +SD; ·—·—·: -SD. Reproduced with kind permission from S. Harbarth (personnel communication; University of Geneva Hospitals, Geneva, Switzerland).

The risk of selection-resistant pathogens is not the same for all antibiotics. This is highly dependent on the pharmacocinetics and pharmacodynamics of the substances. The eradication rate for microbial pathagens colonising the oropharynx varies widely between certain antibiotics, depending on bactericidal properties, the mechanism of action, the peak and trough concentrations and the way the substance is metabolised. Underdosing increases the risk on resistance as well as prolonged and repeated application [16]. NASRIN *et al.* [15] demonstrated in a study with β-lactam treatment in children, that the risk of antibiotic resistance grows by approximately 4% per day. High-dose short-term treatment goes along with a reduced selection of resistances, at least in S. pneumoniae [17]. The same phaenomenon could be found in early nosocomial pneumonia, which is typically caused by the same pathogens [18].

In the future, much more attention needs to be spent on the pharmadynamical aspects to obtain treatment regimens specially adapted for certain groups of patients and antibiotics. The major problem of the previous pharmacokinteic studies was that the observation had been obtained from young individuals in an experimental setting (nonsmokers, no excessive fluid intake), and the transfer of these findings onto elderly and polymorbid patients is problematic.

The increasing workload in the Western World and the risk of workers losing their employment was one of the reasons for the early use of antibiotics in uncomplicated diseases, instead of waiting spontaneous remission. More than 50% of patients with uncomplicated infections of the upper airways are reportedly treated with antibiotics in present day society [19]. The acute bronchitis (AB) is responsible for >70% of all disorders in the upper airways [20]. Nearly in all cases viral infections are the underlying reason, and superinfection with bacteria can be found in a small number of patients only. Purulent secretions are frequently misinterpreted as a sign of bacterial infection. Large meta-analyses revealed that there is no advantage of antibiotic therapy in terms of duration of the disease, number of days off work, and the level of activity of the patients [21–23]. All the studies concluded that there is no evidence for the use of antibiotics as a routine measure in AB. One intervention study showed that teaching programmes for

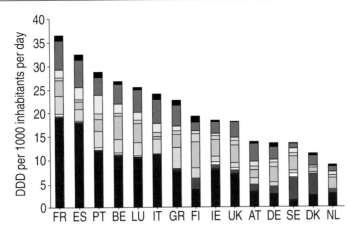

Fig. 2. – Use of antibiotics in Europe adapted from [30]. DDD: defined daily dose; for country codes refer to fig. 1; ●: others; ● macrolides and lincosamides J01F; ●: quinalones J01M; ●: trimethprim J01EA; ●: tetracyclins J01D; ●: cephalosporins J01CF; ○ penicillinase-resistant penicillins J01CF; ●: narrowspectrum penicillins J01CE; ● Broad spectrum penicillins J01CA.

primary physicians and for patients resulted in a significant reduction of prescriptions [24]. However, >60 % of such patients are treated with antibiotics. The situation is nearly the same in acute rhinosinusitis, which is also caused in the majority of cases by viral infection. Bacterial infection can be assumed if symptoms persist for >7 days [25]. One meta-analysis suggests a slightly better effect by antibiotics compared with the placebo, however, this is not evidence for the routine application of antibiotics [26]. If antibiotics had been used, there was no convincing advantage of modern broad-spectrum substances compared with amoxicillin [27]. The situation is different in patients with exacerbated chronic obstructive pulmonary disease (COPD). In these cases, depending on the severity of the disease, early antibiotic treatment of exacerbations had been shown to improve the course of the disease [28]. Nevertheless, many more patients with COPD are treated with antibiotics as would be necessary according to the current guidelines.

The number of prescribed antibiotics for outpatients has been growing in the last few years at a continuous rate. The differences in sociological and epidemiological factors, in healthcare systems, in marketing strategies of pharmaceutical companies, and differences in the traditions of treatment may be the reason for the varying growth rates of antibiotic consumption in different countries [29, 30]. Children are the most frequent carriers of *S. pneumoniae* (50–60 % of infants aged 1–2 yrs), a high proportion of children within the community correlates with higher rates of resistance [31]. The transmission of pathogens is enhanced by daycare centres. In countries with high proportion of these centres, higher rates of resistance can be found [32]. Children may transfer resistant pathogens to parents and grandparents. WHITNEY *et al.* [33] could prove, that vaccination of children against pneumococci reduced the incidence of invasive pneumococcal disease not only in children, but also in elderly people (>65 yrs). The currently used vaccines against pneumococci infections are less than ideal. They prevent invasive infections only, local infections are not covered, and they are not effective against all serotypes. However, a recently developed 9-valent vaccine could accomplish a reduction in the rate of pneumonia. This vaccine was also efficient in HIV positive patients, in whom no positive effects had been expected yet [34].

The consumption of antibiotics is closely related to the epidemiology of viral respiratory tract infections and other diseases. In France and Spain, correlation to the appearance of flue-like illness and the consumption of β-lactams and macrolides could be demonstrated [12]. In Scandinavia and in The Netherlands, which belong to a group of countries with high prevalence of vaccination against influenza, no increase was found for the same time, in which no epidemic had been present. It can be understood that antibiotics are misused in patients with viral infections, especially in elderly people. It can be assumed, even in the absence of valid data, that similar mechanisms produced resistance in respiratory pathogens, by the treatment of Helicobacter associated ulcer wtih macrolides or the treatment of urinary tract infections with fluoroquinolones.

The situation is the worst in south European countries, where drugs need no prescription but can be independently bought at each pharmacy (fig. 2). Telephone interviewers found a higher storage of antibiotics in households in southern Europe, and that these substances are frequently applied without consultation of a physician [35]. However, increasing use of antibiotics is closely associated with bacterial resistances. Pathogens, which are exposed to selection pressure by antibiotic treatment, quickly develop mechanisms to survive under the applied anti-infective agent.

Influence of antibiotic resistance for the outcome of community-acquired infections

Large investigations in patients with nosocomial infections revealed that resistant pathogens negatively impact on the morbidity and mortality of patients. This was shown for metacillin resistant *Staphlococcus aureus* [36], as well as for *Enterobacteriacae sp.* [37]. However, these findings cannot be transferred to the community-acquired pathogens, especially *S. pneumoniae*. In a multicentre study, which involved 844 patients with invasive pneumococci infection, YU *et al.* [38] could not demonstrate a relationship between mortality and resistance. This confirms other findings from patients with meningitis, caused by pneumococci [39]. Also in cephalosporines, no direct impact of resistance on the outcome of patients could be proven [40].

In opposition to these studies, 5 % of patients with severe community-acquired pneumonia (CAP) did not respond to treatment due to resistance [41]. This contradiction could possibly be explained by the fact that in many cases of pneumococcal resistance, it is a low level resistance (MIC ≤ 2 μg·m^{-1}). Adequate dosing of β-lactams is indeed effective in these cases. In Spain high level resistance could be detected, which was associated with treatment failure of β-lactam antibiotics. The situation seems to be different in macrolides. Low level (*mef* mediated), as well as high level (*erm* mediated) resistance result in a high rate of treatment failure [42]. Even if no elevated mortality was documented, a higher mortality must be assumed [43]. According to case reports, resistance against chinolones is also related to more severe courses of pneumonia [44].

The assumption of high prevalence of atypical pneumonia resulted in recommendations of international scientific societies, that macrolides should be applied as first line therapy in atypical pneumonia an example of this is given by NIEDERMAN *et al.* [45]. The growing resistance against macrolides resulted in a switch to the use fluorochinolons. This could be documented by the Community Acquires Pneumonia Network for several regions in Germany. Further studies on the impact of resistance on the outcome of community-acquired infections seem to be urgently necessary for a more appropriate treatment and an adaptation of the guidelines in the future.

Spread of resistance

The continuous globalisation of the modern societies is associated with frequent and long distance travelling. Completely new dimensions for the spread of infectious diseases have now been opened, as was observed with the severe acute respiratory syndrome (SARS) outbreak at the beginning of 2003 [46]. The spread of resistance is enhanced by the same mechanisms. An example is the appearance of the Spanish Clone, the *S. pneumoniae* serotype 23F, in Germany, which was largely responsible for the resistance against penicillin by this organism [47]. *S. pneumoniae* with resistance against macrolides represents the Scandinavian serotype. Untypical resistances, which are not known from other countries, can rarely been found [48].

Larger surveillance networks as the Alexander or the Protect Project reconstructed the mechanisms and ways of resistance worldwide.

Conclusion

Resistance against common antibiotics is a fast growing problem for all bacterial pathogens causing community-acquired infections. There are various reasons for this problem, however the increasing consumption of antibiotics within many countries is thought to play a major role. In countries with high level antibiotic treatment strategies and attachment to the actual guidelines resistance was not a major problem in the past. Due to the progressive globilisation and the associated transfer of resistance there is an increasing risk of reduced antibiotic efficiency for these countries, too.

Worldwide teaching programs about the management of community-acquired infections, based on current guidelines, would be a cornerstone for improvement of the resistance problems. These concepts must be developed and must be established worldwide. Presently Programmes of the European Union are under way. Since respiratory tract infections have a huge medical and economical impact, pulmonologists should play a central role in the development of such programmes.

Summary

Respiratory infections are among the most frequent reasons for prescribing antibiotics. Despite the widely accepted consensus that antibiotic therapy is not appropriate for the treatment of most cases of acute bronchitis, sinusitis and pharyngitis, ~50 % of patients diagnosed with upper respiratory tract infections are treated with these drugs. Several studies strongly support the hypothesis that the excessive use of antibiotics in such patients has contributed to the emergence and spreading of antibiotic resistance. Countries with the highest per capita antibiotic consumption have the highest frequency and patterns of resistance. The emergence of penicillin-resistant *Streptococcus pneumoniae* is related to the consumption of penicillin, cephalosporinines and macrolides. Macrolid prescription correlates significantly with the level of macrolid resistance of group A streptococci. Oral cephalosporin use might be associated with the increase of β-lactamase producing strains of *Moxarella catarrhalis* and *Haemophilus influenzae*. This resulted in progressive use of fluorchinolones in outpatients, which is associated with resistance in *S. pneumoniae*, *Escherichia. coli* and other Gram-negative bacteria. Paediatric bacterial isolates are more often resistant to various antimicrobial agents than isolates from adult patients. This might be due to more frequent use of antibiotics in children and extensive child-to-child transmission.

The three major reasons for the rise in microbial resistance rates which include: 1) the widespread application of antibiotics in animals; 2) the growing use of antibiotics in all developed countries; and 3) the fast spread of resistances due to travelling and globalisation, are discussed in this chapter. The increasing use of antibiotics reflects a shift in the attitude of the communities towards disorders and diseases. Prevention programs have to be multimodal and integrative. Infections of the respiratory tract play an important role for further developments, since they have an enormous medical and economical impact. Therefore pulmonologists should be integrated in the further conception of such programmes.

Keywords: Antibiotics, antibiotic resistance, community-acquired infection, epidemiology.

References

1.   Guillemot D. Antibiotic use in humans and bacterial resistance. *Curr Opin Microbiol* 1999; 2: 494–498.

2.   Jacobs MR, Felingham D, Appelbaum PC, Gruneberg RN. The Alexander Project 1998–2000: susceptibility of pathogens isolated from community-acquired respiratory tract infections commonly used antimicrobial agents. *J Antimicrob Chemother* 2003; 52: 229–246.

3.   McEwen SA, Fedorka-Cray PJ. Antimicrobial use and resistance in animals. *Clin Infect Dis* 2002; 34: Suppl. 3, S93–106.

4.   Aarestrup FM, Seyfarth AM, Emborg HD. Effect of abolishment of the use of antimicrobial agents for growth promotion on occurrence of antimicrobial resistance in fecal enterococci from food animals in Denmark. *Antimicrob Agents Chemother* 2001; 45: 2054–2059.

5.   Filutowicz M, Rakowski SA. Regulatory implications of protein assemblies at the gamma origin plasmid R6K – a review. *Gene* 1998; 223: 195–204.

6.   Grecko C. Sweden and the European Union: what is happening in relation to antibiotics in feed? *In*: Annual Conference Proceedings of Australian Veterinarians in Industry and Australian Veterinarians in Public Health, Perth, Australian Veterinary Association Annual Conference, 2000: 18–22.

7.   del Castillo F, Baquero–Artigao F, Garcia-Perea A. Influence of recent antibiotic therapy on antimicrobial resistance of *Streptococcus pneumoniae* in children with acute otitis media in Spain. *Pediatr Infect Dis J* 1998; 17: 94–97.

8.   Garcia-Rey C, Aguilar L, Baquero F, Casal J, Dal-Re R. Importance of local variations in antibiotic consumption and geographical differences of erythromycin and penicillin resistance in *Streptococcus pneumoniae*. *J Clin Microbiol* 2002 Jan; 40: 159–164.

9.   Granizo JJ, Aguilar L, Casal J, Dal-Re R, Baquero F. Streptococcus pyogenes resistance to erythromycin in relation to macrolide consumption in Spain (1986–1997). *J Antimicrob Chemother.* 2000 Dec; 46: 959–964.

10.   Baquero F, Barrett JF, Courvalin P, Morrissey I, Piddock L, Novick WJ. Epidemiology and mechanisms of resistance among respiratory tract pathogens. *Clin Microbiol Infect* 1998; 4: Suppl. 2, S19–S26.

11.   Perez-Trallero E, Fernandez-Mazarrasa C, Garcia-Rey C, *et al.* Spanish Surveillance Group for Respiratory Pathogens. Antimicrobial susceptibilities of 1,684 *Streptococcus pneumoniae* and 2,039 *Streptococcus pyogenes* isolates and their ecological relationships: results of a 1-year (1998–1999) multicenter surveillance study in Spain. *Antimicrob Agents Chemother* 2001; 45: 3334–3340.

12.   Baquero F, Baquero-Artigao G, Canton R, Garcia-Rey C. Antibiotic consumption and resistance selection in *Streptococcus pneumoniae*. *J Antimicrob Chemother.* 2002; 50: Suppl. S2, 27–37.

13.   Austin DJ, Bonten MJ, Weinstein RA, Slaughter S, Anderson RM. Vancomycin-resistant enterococci in intensive-care hospital settings: transmission dynamics, persistence, and the impact of infection control programs. *Proc Natl Acad Sci U S A.* 1999; 96: 6908–6913.

14.   Seppala H, Klaukka T, Vuopio-Varkila J, *et al.* The effect of changes in the consumption of macrolide antibiotics on erythromycin resistance in group A streptococci in Finland. Finnish Study Group for Antimicrobial Resistance. *N Engl J Med* 1997; 337: 441–446.

15.   Nasrin D, Collignon PJ, Roberts L, Wilson EJ, Pilotto LS, Douglas RM. Effect of beta lactam antibiotic use in children on pneumococcal resistance to penicillin: prospective cohort study. *BMJ* 2002; 324: 28–30.

16.   Guillemot D, Carbon C, Balkau B, *et al.* Low dosage and long treatment duration of beta-lactam: risk factors for carriage of penicillin-resistant Streptococcus pneumoniae. *JAMA* 1998; 279: 365–370.

17.   Schrag SJ, Pena C, Fernandez J, *et al.* Effect of short-course, high-dose amoxicillin therapy on resistant pneumococcal carriage: a randomized trial. *JAMA* 2001; 286: 49–56.

18.   Singh N, Rogers P, Atwood CW, Wagener MM, Yu VL. Short-course empiric antibiotic therapy for patients with pulmonary infiltrates in the intensive care unit. *Am J Respir Crit Care Med* 2000; 162: 505–511.

19.   Gonzales R, Steiner JF, Sande MA. Antibiotic prescribing for adults with cold, upper respiratory tract infection, and bronchitis by ambulatory care physicans. *JAMA* 1997; 278: 901–904.

20.   Gonzales R, Bartlett JG, Besser RE. Principles of appropriate antibiotic use for treatment of uncomplicated acute bronchitis. *Background Ann Intern Med* 2001; 134: 521–529.

21.   Bent S, Saint S, Vittinghoff E. Antibiotics in acute bronchitis: a meta-analysis. *Am J Med* 1999; 102: 62–67.

22.   Fahey T, Stocks N, Thomas T. Quantitative systemic review of randomized controlled trials comparing antibiotic with placebo for acute cough in adults. *BMJ* 1998; 316: 906–106.

23.   Smuczny JJ, Becker LA, Glazier RH. Are antibiotics effective treatment for acute bronchitis? A meta-analysis. *J Fam Pract* 1998; 47: 453–460.

24.   Gonzales R, Steiner JF, Lum A. Decreasing antibioic use in ambulatory practice: impact of multidimensional intervention on treatment of uncomplicated acute bronchitis in adults. *JAMA* 1999; 281: 1512–1519.

25.   Hickner JM, Bartlett JG, Besser RE. Principles of approbriate antibiotic use for acute sinusitis in adults. Background. *Ann Intern Med* 2001; 134: 498–505.

26.   Williams JW Jr, Aguilar C, Makela M. Antibiotic therapy for acute sinusitis: a systematic literature review. The Cochrane Library. Oxford: update Software 1997.

27.   Snow V, Mottur-Pilson C, Gonzales R. Principles of approbriate use for acute sinusitis in adults. *Ann Intern Med* 2001; 134: 495–497.

28.   Global Strategy for the Diagnosis, Managment, and Prevention of Chronic Obstructive Pulmonary Disease (2003). www.Goldcopd.com: 98–107. Updated 2003.

29.   Carrie AG, Zhanel GG. Antibacterial use in community practice: assessing quantity, indications and appropriateness, and relationship to the development of antibacterial resistance. *Drugs* 1999; 57: 871–881.

30.   Cars O, Molstad S, Melander A. Variation in antibiotic use in the European Union. *Lancet* 2001; 9: 357: 1851–1853.

31.   Clavo-Sanchez AJ, Giron-Gonzalez JA, Lopez-Prieto D, *et al.* Multivariate analysis of risk factors for infection due to penicillin-resistant and multidrug-resistant Streptococcus pneumoniae: a multicenter study. *Clin Infect Dis* 1997; Jun 24: 1052–1059.

32.   Sa-Leao R, Tomasz A, Sanches IS, *et al.* Carriage of internationally spread clones of *Streptococcus pneumoniae* with unusual drug resistance patterns in children attending day care centers in Lisbon, Portugal. *J Infect Dis* 2000; 182: 1153–1160.

33.   Whitney CG, Farley MM, Hadler J, *et al.* Decline in invasive pneumococcal disease after the introduction of protein-polysaccharide conjugate vaccine. *N Engl J Med* 2003; 348: 1737–1746.

34.   Klugman KP, Madhi SA, Huebner RE, Kohberger R, Mbelle N, Pierce N, Vaccine Trialists Group. A trial of a 9-valent pneumococcal conjugate vaccine in children with and those without HIV infection. *N Engl J Med* 2003; 349: 1341–1348.

35. Orero A, Gonzalez J, Prieto J. Antibiotics in Spanish households. Medical and socioeconomical implications. URANO Study Group. *Medicina Clinica* 1997; 109: 782–785.

36. Cosgrove SE, Cosgrove SE, Sakoulas G, *et al.* Comparison of mortality associated with methicillin-resistant and methicillin-susceptible *Staphylococcus aureus* bacteremia: a meta-analysis. *Clin Infect Dis* 2003; 36: 53–59.

37. Cosgrove SE, Kaye KS, Eliopoulous GM, Carmeli Y. Health and economic outcomes of the emergence of third-generation cephalosporin resistance in *Enterobacter species*. *Arch Intern Med* 2002; 162: 185–190.

38. Yu VL, Chiou CC, Feldman C, *et al.* An international prospective study of pneumococcal bacteremia: correlation with *in vitro* resistance, antibiotics administered, and clinical outcome. *Clin Infect Dis* 2003 Jul 15; 37: 230–270.

39. Auburtin M, Porcher R, Bruneel F. Pneumococcal meningitis in the intensive care unit: prognostic factors of clinical outcome in a series of 80 cases. *Am J Respir Crit Care Med* 2002; 165: 713–717.

40. Pallares R, Capdevila O, Linares J, *et al.* The effect of cephalosporin resistance on mortality in adult patients with nonmeningeal systemic pneumococcal infections. *Am J Med* 2002; 113: 120–126.

41. Rello J, Badi M, Mariscal D, *et al.* Microbiological testing and outcome of pts. with severe CAP. *Chest* 2003; 123: 174–180.

42. Lonks JR, Garau J, Gomez L, *et al.* Failure of macrolide antibiotic treatment in patients with bacteremia due to erythromycin-resistant *Streptococcus pneumoniae*. *Clin Infect Dis* 2002; 35: 556–564.

43. Jacobs MR. *In vivo* veritas: in vitro macrolide resistance in systemic *Streptococcus pneumoniae* infections does result in clinical failure. *Clin Infect Dis* 2002: 1; 35: 565–569.

44. Davidson R, Cavalcanti R, Brunton JL, *et al.* Resistance to levofloxacin and failure of treatment of pneumococcal pneumonia. *N Engl J Med* 2002; 346: 747–50.

45. Niederman MS, Mandell LA, Anzueto A, *et al.* Guidelines for the management of adults with community-acquired pneumonia. Diagnosis, assessment of severity, antimicrobial therapy, and prevention. *Am J Respir Crit Care Med* 2001; 163: 1730–1754.

46. Groneberg DA, Zhang L, Welte T, Zabel P, Chung KF. Severe acute respiratory syndrome: global initiatives for disease diagnosis. *QJM* 2003; 96: 845–852.

47. Reinert RR, Muckel S, Al-Lahham A, *et al.* Characterization of German penicillin non-susceptible serotype 23F pneumococci using multilocus sequence typing. *J Med Microbiol* 2003; 52: 981–987.

48. Reinert RR, Wild A, Appelbaum P, Lutticken R, Cil MY, Al-Lahham A. Ribosomal mutations conferring resistance to macrolides in Streptococcus pneumoniae clinical strains isolated in Germany. *Antimicrob Agents Chemother* 2003; 47: 2319–2322.

CHAPTER 11

Antibiotics and new guidelines for the treatment of lower respiratory tract infections

G. Di Maria, L. Spicuzza, R. Polosa

Dept Medicina Interna e Medicina Specialistica, Sezione Malattie Respiratorie, University of Catania, Italy.

Correspondence: G. DiMaria, Dept di Medicina Interna e Medicina Specialistica, Sezione Malattie Respiratorie, University of Catania, Italy.

At the turn of the 21st century lower respiratory tract infections (LRTIs), including community-acquired pneumonia (CAP) and chronic bronchitis (CB), are still amongst the most common infectious diseases of humans, representing a major cause of morbidity and mortality worldwide [1–4]. It is now widely recognised that LRTIs are important determinants of disability-adjusted life-years [5], and comprise of a large percentage of disease entities treated by primary care physicians. In addition, LRTIs due to the cost of hospitalisation and antibiotic therapy in particular the newer agents, represent a relevant economic burden for most of the healthcare systems [6].

As a consequence of such high prevalence the subsequent usage rates of antimicrobials in the treatment of LRTIs have increased substantially during the past few decades and important progress in controlling LRTIs has been made. This progress is mostly explained by the introduction of a variety of classes of powerful antibiotics with improved pharmacokinetic and broad-spectrum activity against many common microbial pathogens [3, 4].

The key pathogens associated with community-acquired LRTIs, include *Streptococcus pneumoniae*, and other significant pathogens, such as *Haemophilus influenzae*, *Staphylococcus aureus* and *Pseudomonas aeruginosa*. In current clinical practice, etiological pathogens are seldom identified either before or after initiation of therapy, and objective criteria decreasing the level of uncertainty in choosing effective antimicrobial agents are lacking. It is also important to take into account that the relationship between the pathogenic microorganisms and the susceptible host is highly complex and shaped by conflicting forces. After the discovery and use of antibiotics for therapeutic purposes, pathogens have developed strategies that enable them to use metabolic processes to resist the antibiotic's actions. As a consequence, the spread of microbial resistance towards multiple antibiotics has further complicated this already complex arena. However the key factor appears to be whether or not microbial resistance is able to affect the clinical outcomes of antibiotic treatment. Most importantly, a variety of characteristics including aetiology and individual risk factors appear to be associated with mortality and other medical outcomes of LRTIs. Taken together, these problems have raised concern both in clinicians and patients. This concern is mainly reflected by the aptitude of many physicians to prescribe simultaneously two different classes of antibiotics in order to widen the spectrum of pathogens potentially involved and to increase the rate of successful treatment.

Physicians may often have a limited appreciation of bacterial sensitivity or resistance, therefore the prescribing of initial antibiotic therapy for community-acquired LRTIs is

Eur Respir Mon, 2004, 28, 175–188. Printed in UK - all rights reserved. Copyright ERS Journals Ltd 2004; European Respiratory Monograph; ISSN 1025-448x. ISBN 1-904097-32-4.

primarily empiric. For different and obvious reasons these facts have prompted the development and validation of guidelines aiming to reduce variability and help physicians to establish a more rational approach to the diagnosis and treatment of LRTIs. In the last decade, a number of guidelines for the management of CAP put forth by the American Thoracic Society (ATS) and other reputed scientific societies have recommended choices in therapeutic regimens based on the presence of risk factors and severity of illness [7–13]. These guidelines have been subsequently implemented and used in many countries around the world as a basis for management protocols in general practice [14, 15]. However despite the progress during the above mentioned 10-yr span, many new recommendations covering the assessment and management of pneumonia do not sufficiently cover the much larger group of nonpneumonic LRTIs which include exacerbations of chronic obstructive pulmonary disease (COPD), nor do they deal with respiratory infections of patients with predisposing illnesses such as cancer or acquired immunodeficency syndrome, and are based on the lowest grades of evidence. Under these circumstances many decisions largely depend upon personal experience and clinical judgement, which remains in the domain of the "art of medicine".

In current guidelines for the management of adults with CAP, the selection of initial antimicrobial treatment and/or the triaging decision about hospitalisation or intensive care unit (ICU) admission are largely based on the assessment of pneumonia severity [10–13]. Some of the proposed severity criteria are mainly derived from studies determining predictors of adverse outcome [16–21]. Based on a number of predictors, which include age, male sex, comorbidity, acute respiratory failure, sepsis or septic shock, radiographic extension of lung infiltrates, and bacteraemia, the calculation of a pneumonia severity index (PSI) has been proposed [16]. In order to achieve a more rational therapeutic approach, some of the most recent guidelines have endorsed the use of PSI [10, 11]. Furthermore, several guidelines recommend the use of decision pathways to assist clinical judgement and subsequent choice of antibiotic treatment. In this article the antibiotic classes that are most frequently used for the treatment of LRTIs are reviewed along with the criteria by which the new guidelines help clinicians in choosing the most suitable therapeutic approach.

Microbial patterns in the aetiology of lower respiratory tract infections

The knowledge of predominant microbial patterns in CAP and other LRTIs, although not sufficient, represent the basis for any initial decisions about empirical antimicrobial treatments [7, 10–13]. A wide variety of pathogens are implicated in the aetiology of respiratory infections, and the patterns of aetiology for CAP and acute exacerbations of CB (AECB), have been the subject of extensive investigation in several local settings during the last 20 yrs [2, 16, 22–25]. Although, the occurrence of the five most common pathogens reported by several previous series is similar, these patterns have differed considerably depending on the geographic area and studied population, as well as the methods used for the microbiologic analysis. *S. pneumoniae* has been unanimously found to be the leading pathogen in both CAP and AECB, whereas *H. influenzae* has been reported to account for 4–11% of CAP episodes [22]. In other series, *C. pneumoniae* accounted for 3–18%, influenza viruses A and B for 3–8%, and *Legionella spp.* for 2–16% [26]. More recently, a rate of viral aetiology up-to 21% (including 13 of 39 (33%) cases of mixed viral/bacterial infections) and a relatively high percentage (6%) of Gram-negative enteric bacilli (GNEB) have been reported among 395 hospitalised patients with CAP [19]. Therefore, the importance of viral and other nonpneumococcal agents in the aetiology of CAP should not be underestimated.

One main difficulty in attempting to determine the different etiologic agents is that the causative microorganism is not detected in up to 60% of patients, and in 5% to 10% of cases copathogens are identified [12, 13, 24]. In addition, studies have occasionally reported unusually high frequencies of viral infections [19]. This can contribute to increase the variability of the clinical response to antibiotics or even low the rate of successful treatment in patients with CAP. Similar considerations apply to patients with exacerbated COPD [28–30]. The lack of etiological diagnosis in a relevant proportion of cases and the possibility that patients with chronic bronchitis or COPD develop exacerbations due to causes other than infections are widely recognised. Thus the role of infection and the efficacy of antibiotics in AECB remains debatable and yet incompletely understood. It must be stressed, however, that although the causative role of infections is questioned, their importance is greatly increased by the application of newer and more sensitive investigative techniques [28, 29]. Under these circumstances it is likely that up-to 70–80% of AECB are caused by infections with 40–50% due to bacteria [28].

Antibiotic management of lower respiratory tract infections

Guidelines are an important means by which professional associations and governments have sought to improve the quality and costeffectiveness of disease management for infectious respiratory diseases. Problems in the management of CAP arise mainly from the causal pathogens remaining unknown, thus preventing the choice of optimal treatment for individual patients. Other unresolved problems related to CAP management consist in the emergence of new pathogens, in the changed susceptibility to antibiotics among traditional pathogens and in the increasing number of elderly and immunocompromised patients who are likely to develop severe pneumonia or have the disease complicated by other pathological events. In combination these factors, along with a general trend towards an evidence-based approach, have provided a strong input for the major scientific respiratory societies to develop new guidelines for a more effective management of this disease. This should determine an improvement in the clinical outcomes and a reduction in the costs. The optimisation of the antibiotic regimens should also minimise the occurrence of bacterial resistance to antibiotics, which is constantly increasing. In the last decades a number of guidelines have been published in North America, in some European (namely UK, France, Spain, and Italy) as well as in some Asiatic countries. Many guidelines recommend diagnostic strategies as well as antibiotic alternatives specific for patients' categories and provide a mean to standardise the clinical management of these patients. Although developed in different countries and with different approaches, all these guidelines, particularly the European ones, have a number of common themes and exhibit a substantial agreement on the empirical antibiotic therapy [9]. Despite consistency among guidelines, in the clinical practice several factors including local experience, antibiotics availability and commercial strategies may influence the physicians' aptitude and the strategies they adopt against LRTIs. These factors rather than evidence-based guidelines might explain the major differences in antibiotic use that have been reported in different countries or even in different regions within the same country.

Choice of therapy: basis for empirical approach

One of the major problems in managing patients with CAP is that in 25–60% of the cases, the pathogen cannot be isolated and identified [33]. Despite the introduction of new technologies there is no easy and rapid diagnostic test available. Serology only allows pathogens to be identified retrospectively. In many patients sputum is difficult to obtain and contamination of the sample with pathogens colonising the upper airways is difficult to exclude. It is also important to note that only 1 day of antibiotic treatment will affect results of the sputum culture. For these reasons the guidelines published by the ATS in 1993 clearly stated that searching the pathogen in the sputum of patients with CAP is not necessary [7] and this concept was also supported by other guidelines [13]. The guidelines published by the ATS in 2001 further stress this aspect outlining limitation of sputum's Gram staining, *e.g.* the difficulty in obtaining an adequate sample, observers independent interpretations and the inability to detect atypical pathogens [12]. Direct staining of sputum, with non-Gram stain methods may be a useful diagnostic tool for some pulmonary infections *e.g.* those due to *Mycobacterium sp.*, *Legionella sp.* and *Pneumocytis carinii.* These new guidelines once again also underline the poor sensitivity and specificity of bacterial cultures of the sputum, although recovery of organisms that are not usually part of the normal flora may be meaningful. Microbiological investigations are not recommended routinely by the British Thoracic Society (BTS) to manage patients in the community, while examination of the sputum should be considered for patients who do not respond to empirical antibiotic treatment. In view of these considerations there is a general agreement that the initial pharmacological management of CAP, especially when managed in the community, has to be empirical. In the hospitalised patients the aetiology may be determined in order to modify the initial empirical treatment. Antibiotic drug overuse and inappropriate antibiotic drug selection have been pointed out as a possible determinant of increased drug resistance among respiratory pathogens (most notably, *S. pneumoniae*), possible progression to chronic disease, and increased treatment costs. Therefore, physicians should be aware of clinical manifestations that help differentiate viral from bacterial infections in that the appropriate use of antimicrobial agents for respiratory infections could be associated with a potential reduction of the emergence of antibiotic resistance. Concentrated, sustained efforts are needed to secure physicians' use of guidelines. The information should be put into a simple format available at the point of prescribing and supported by other behavioural change techniques.

Factors determining the choice of antibiotics

A number of factors should be taken into consideration when choosing an antibiotic therapy. These factors include epidemiological data, risk factors (*e.g.* age of the patient, the status of his/her immune system, and the presence of comorbidities), the severity of respiratory infection, and the antibiotic susceptibility and/or resistance in each specific geographic area. However it should be taken into account that evidence has been provided for the importance of the initiation of early empiric antimicrobial treatment for a favourable outcome of CAP. Variations of microbial patterns are only in part due to different epidemiological settings. Therefore, initial empiric antimicrobial treatment will also have to take into account local trends of microbial patterns.

The spectrum of pathogens causing CAP is narrow and no major differences exist among different geographic areas. Epidemiological studies indicate that *S. pneumoniae* accounts for ~80% of community-acquired infections, followed by *Mycoplasma pneumoniae*, *Legionella sp.*, *H. influenzae* and *S. aureus* [1]. Gram-negative bacilli such as *Escherichia coli*, *Klebsiella pneumuniae* and *P. aeruginosa*, usually associated with nosocomial pneumonia, may have a role also in CAP in the presence of comorbidities and in the elderly and the ATS and Canadian guidelines [11], but not the BTS guidelines

[13], recommend antibiotic coverage against these pathogens in those patients included in the risk category. The attribution of a clinical feature to specific microbial agents is common in the clinical practice. Thus a syndromic approach based on clinical and radiological presentation of CAP has been proposed to distinguish between "typical" and "atypical" or nonpneumococcal pneumonia in order to better support the empirical choice of antibiotics in the absence of laboratory data. However, evidence has been provided that clinical and radiographic features of "typical" pneumonia were neither sensitive nor specific for the differentiation of pneumococcal and nonpneumococcal aetiologies. Yet a significant correlation has been found between aetiologies and a number of factors including age and comorbidity [19, 31, 32]. This evidence supports a management approach based on the associations between aetiology and age, comorbidity, and severity, instead of the traditional syndromic approach to CAP.

One problem when dealing with this aspect is that clinical features are not always determined by the infecting pathogens and a number of studies have shown that there is no correlation between clinical features and aetiological agents [33–34]. In addition, no typical radiological patterns are generally associated to specific pathogens [35]. Therefore, particularly in children, in the elderly and in severe conditions classic clinical signs to fit the patient in one of the two groups may lack. The recent ATS guidelines have stressed the concept that it is not possible to rely on clinical features including history, physical examination, routine laboratory and radiological evaluation, for an aetiological diagnosis of pneumonias [12]. More importantly, clinical features may have some relevance in the assessment of the severity of the diseases which is an important determinant in the choice of the antibiotic treatment as pointed out by the guidelines. The empirical treatment of pneumonia should be largely based on criteria such as the age of the patients, the presence of comorbidities and the severity of the condition. One study on a large number of patients has shown that patients aged <60 yrs were at significant risk of atypical bacterial aetiology and the presence of comorbidities as well as current cigarette smoking and alcohol abuse were associated to distinct aetiological patterns. In contrast, clinical and radiographical features of typical pneumonia were neither sensitive nor specific for the differentiation of pneumococcal and nonpneumococcal aetiologies [19]. The BTS has recently proposed to abandon the term "atypical" as this incorrectly implies that there is a characteristic clinical presentation.

In choosing the antibiotic regimen it should be considered the problem of the increased incidence of resistance to antibiotics among respiratory pathogens, particularly *S. pneumoniae*, reported by multiple studies during the 1990s. According to the ATS guidelines more than 40% of all pneumococci are resistant according to the *in vitro* definition of resistance [36]. When implicated in cases of pneumonia, *S. pneumoniae* should be considered susceptible if penicillin minimum inhibitory concentration (MIC) ≤ 1 $\mu g \cdot mL^{-1}$, of intermediate susceptibility if MIC is 2 $\mu g \cdot mL^{-1}$, and resistant if MIC is ≥ 4 $\mu g \cdot mL^{-1}$. In addition, for penicillin-resistant pneumococci *in vitro* resistance has been also reported for cephalosporins and macrolides [37]. However the relevance of drug-resistant *S. pneumoniae* (DRSP) in clinical practice is still controversial as outlined by both the ATS and BTS. The current definition of resistance includes an "intermediate-level" of resistance (MIC≥ 2 $\mu g \cdot mL^{-1}$) and most of the studies have shown that this intermediate resistance does not significantly increase the mortality as compared to patients infected with sensitive microorganisms [11–13]. An MIC value ≥ 4 $\mu g \cdot mL^{-1}$ is associated with increased risk of mortality [37] and when documented, the guidelines recommend to consider alternative agents to penicillin. The newer antipneumococcal fluoroquinolones, ketolides and vancomicyn are active against drug-resistant pneumo-cocci according to the ATS, although few reports on the resistance to fluoroquinolones are beginning to appear in the literature. Factors associated to DRSP include age >65 yrs, multiple comorbidities and previous β-lactam therapies [12]. The impact of penicillin resistance on medical outcomes of CAP has been investigated. One recent study reported that the incidence of drug-resistant pneumococci was high, with risk factors for resistance including patient advanced age and comorbidity, but concluded that the outcome was not significantly affected by drug resistance [32]. Conflicting with this observation are the results of a retrospective cohort study investigating drug susceptibility of pneumococci isolated from adult patients with bacteremic pneumococcal pneumonia [38]. Of the 192 study patients, 44 (23%) were infected with pneumococcal strains that demonstrated some degree of penicillin nonsusceptibility. Compared with patients infected with penicillin-susceptible pneumococcal strains, patients whose isolates were nonsusceptible had a significantly greater risk of in-hospital death due to pneumonia, although only risk of suppurative complications remained statistically significant after adjustment for baseline differences in severity of illness.

Both bacterial and individual host factors that could help achieve the most appropriate use of antimicrobial agents should be carefully evaluated in order to foster the objective of optimal treatment of respiratory tract infections.

Patients stratification and antibiotic treatments

Although the assessment of illness severity of patients with LRTIs might be helpful in improving the treatment and outcomes of the disease, there is no agreement on what constitutes the best approach to this. This is reflected by the considerable variability in rates of hospitalisation of patients with CAP, in part because of physicians' uncertainty in assessing the severity of illness at presentation. This uncertainty might also influence the choice of antibiotic(s). In order to choose the empirical antibiotic therapy the BTS classifies patients according to the severity of the condition and to the setting of treatment (home or hospital). A more articulate classification is provided by the recent ATS guidelines which distinguish four group of patients: outpatients with or without cardiopulmonary diseases or other modifying factors, hospitalised patients (with or without cardiopulmonary diseases or modifying factors) and ICU-admitted patients (with or without risk of *P. aeruginosa*). Specific pathogens associated to each group are indicated in the guidelines. As the empirical treatment is primarily directed towards *S. pneumoniae*, oral aminopenicillins namely amoxicillin are the antibiotic of choice for the treatment of nonsevere outpatients with CAP according to the BTS and other guidelines issued in Europe, whereas macrolides, erythromycin or clarithromycin, represent an alternative for patients intolerant to amoxicillin. The recommendation of amoxicillin as a first choice antibiotic by the new BTS guidelines rely on the observation that highly resistant strains of pneumococci in the UK are uncommon and that the clinical relevance of pneumococci with low or intermediate degree of resistance is uncertain. However, the new BTS guidelines state that the dosage of amoxicillin should be higher than previously recommended [13]. Considered that *M. pneumoniae* occurs periodically every four to five times it seems inappropriate to cover this pathogen with the initial empiric therapy. Oral amoxicillin (or ampicillin if IV injection is needed) plus a macrolide is recommended for nonsevere patients admitted in the hospital while third generation cephalosporin in combination with a macrolide should be used in severe hospitalised patients. According to the BTS the view that the presence of comorbidites is associated to specific pathogens is not supported by data in the literature for these reason no alternative regimens are recommended for patients with associated comorbidities. Similarly to the BTS the European Respiratory Society (ERS) do not recommend coverage of atypical pathogens in outpatients [9]. Differently from the BTS, the ATS recommend advanced generation macrolides (azithromycin and clarithromycin) or doxycycline as the first choice therapy for outpatients [12]. Coverage of atypical organisms in outpatients with CAP is recommended also by the Infectious Disease Society of America (IDSA) and (Canadian Infectious Disease Society/Canadian Thoracic Society (CIDS/CTS) guidelines [10, 11]. In the presence of cardiopulmonary diseases and/or other modifying factors, β-lactam (oral cephalosporins, high dose amoxicillin, amocixicillin/clavulanate or parental ceftriaxone) associated to macrolides or doxycycline or an antipneumococcal fluoroquinolone should be used. Modifying factors include the risk for DRSP, Gram-negative enterobacters and *P. aeruginous*, in this group of patients the presence of DRSP as well as the risk of Gram-negative infection is more likely. Intravenous β-lactam plus a macrolide or IV fluoroquinolones exhibiting antipneumococcal activity alone should be used in hospitalised (non- ICU) patients in the presence of cardiopulmonary diseases and/or other modifying factors whereas IV azithromycin alone or IV antipneumococcal fluoroquinolone alone can be used in the absence of cardiopulmonary diseases and modifying factors. It should be considered that some studies have shown a polymicrobial aetiology in 10–40% of patients admitted with CAP [39]. The effectiveness of the association between β-lactam and macrolide in reducing mortality in hospitalised patients is supported by recent studies [12]. Generally a narrow spectrum approach is recommended in mild case while a broad-spectrum regimen is recommended in severe cases and in presence of risk factors.

Specific recommendation for CAP on the basis of penicillin MIC have also been recently issued by the DRS Therapeutic Working Group (DRSPTWG) [37]. These includes the use of macrolide, doxycicline, oral β-lactam as a first choice therapy in outpatients with penicillin MIC ≤ 0.06. Fuoroquinolones are not indicated as a first choice therapy for concerns about emerging resistance, however with increasing levels of penicillin MIC fluoroquinolones become the antibiotic of choice in both outpatients and hospitalised (non-ICU) patients.

Newer antibiotics

A number of fluoroquinolones with antipneumococcal activity, including levofloxacin, sparfloxacin, gatifloxacin and moxifloxacin have been developed in recent years. The advantage of these new fluoroquinolones consist in their wider spectrum, covering Gram-positive, Gram-negative and atypical pathogens. In addition quinolones penetrate well into the lung (high levels can be detected in lung tissues), are highly bioavailable and the serum concentrations obtained with oral therapy are similar to those achieved by the IV route. For this reason they might be useful to treat outpatients with oral therapy or to switch more rapidly from IV treatment in hospitalised patients [12]. Some concerns have been expressed on the emerging resistance to fluoroquinolones. Although the MIC values of these agents for *S. pneumoniae*, ranging from 0.12–2 mg·DL^{-1}, are similar for penicillin-sensitive and penicillin-resistant pneumococci, high level of penicillin resistance can be associated with resistance to quinolones [40, 12]. Indeed a number of studies have shown the efficacy of fluoroquinolones in the treatment of CAP [41, 42] and currently fluoroquinolones are included by the most recent guidelines, although the BTS guidelines underline that these are expensive antibiotics and so far have not been shown to be more efficacious than standard therapy. For this reason, and for some concern on the side effect profile, these are considered as an alternative regimen for those patients who are intolerant to penicillins or macrolides [12, 13].

New antibiotics will continue to have a role in disease management. Rapid, costeffective diagnostic techniques are also required and.

Route of administration and duration of therapy

The recent BTS guidelines underline how parenteral treatment is often unnecessarily used in the management of hospitalised patients and that only 30–50% of the patients admitted with CAP will require parenteral antibiotics [13]. Other than in community-managed patients, oral antibiotics can be used in non severe hospital managed patients in absence of contraindications such as inability to swallow or inadequate absorption [13].

The optimal duration of antibiotic therapy is still debated and differences exist among the guidelines. The presence of comorbidities, bacteremia and the severity of the condition should generally determine the duration of the therapy. For patients with *S. pneumoniae* the duration of the therapy ranges from 7 (in mild cases) to 10 days in more severe cases. Atypical pneumonia should be treated for 10–14 days according to both ATS and BTS guidelines, while for *Legionella sp.* infections a 10–14 day treatment is recommend. The treatment should be prolonged (14–21 days) also in case of Gram-negative pathogens or *S. aureus* infections. The choice to switch from parenteral to oral therapy is based on clinical assessment. Both the ATS and the BTS recommend clinical criteria, including resolution of fever, dyspnoea and cough [12, 13]. If the clinical response is generally favourable the switch to oral therapy can be made even if the patient is not completely afebrile [12]. However the decision should be strongly individualised for each patient.

Antibiotic treatment of drug-resistant *Staphylococcus pneumoniae*

Identification of the causal microorganisms in AECB is often difficult. Two major studies have shown that *H. influenzae*, *S. pneumoniae* and *M. catarrhalis* are the most common pathogens isolated in patients with COPD exacerbations [43, 44]. *S. aureus* and GNEB have been also identified cause of exacerbation in a small number of subjects. In particular infection by *P. aeruginosa* is more likely to occur in patients with severe obstruction, hypoxaemia, malnutrition and more frequent hospitalisation [45]. Virus can also be a cause of exacerbation and serum viral antibody titres increase in approximately one third of these patients. The role of atypical pathogens such as *M. pneumoniae* and *Chlamydia pneumoniae* in AECB is still debated. Most of the studies suggest that these pathogens are an uncommon cause of AECB accounting for <10% of the cases, as suggested by serological tests. However it has to be considered that not all exacerbations of COPD are of bacterial origin and therefore an antibiotic treatment is not always required. Bacterial pathogens can be cultured from lower airways in 50% of exacerbations. Alternatively positive cultures have been reported in 22% of the patients with chronic bronchitis without clinical signs of exacerbation, and *H. influenzae* has been detected in the secretions of patients in stable conditions [46]. In light of these considerations the value of antibiotic treatment in COPD exacerbation has been object of intense debate.

The hypothesis of the "vicious circle" proposes that airway damage from chronic infection can occur in patients with CB when bacteria determine the release of inflammatory mediators in the airways. After airway damage has occurred the repair process is associated to the production of some surface molecules promoting the binding of pathogens such as *H. influenzae*. This can somehow account for the positive correlation between repeated infections and decline in lung function [47]. Viral infections can also induce damage of the bronchial mucosa leading to bacterial colonisation, and in many patients, although the initial insult causing cough and sputum is viral, exacerbations can be complicated by bacterial infections.

The usefulness of antibiotics in the treatment of AECB is supported by many studies. Antibiotics were shown to be useful in the treatment of >80% of patients in the presence of at least two of the following symptoms: increased dyspnoea, increased sputum volume and increase sputum purulence (Anthonisen criteria) [48]. The study, also known as the Winnipeg study, showed that the greater the number of symptoms present, the better the response to the antibiotic treatment as compared to placebo. A recent meta-analysis has shown that patients with severe lung function impairment are those who will benefit more from the antibiotic treatment [49]. Another meta-analysis has shown some clinical benefits of antibiotic treatment in patients with AECB, particularly in those with low baseline flow rates [50]. According to the ERS the antibiotic treatment is always recommended in severe exacerbations or in nonsevere exacerbations in the presence of Anthonisen criteria [51].

In light of previous consideration, as for CAP, the antibiotic strategy for AECB should be empirical. In addition it has to be noted that there is no single antibiotic which can cover the pathogens potentially involved in the exacerbation process. Aminopenicillin (amoxicillin and ampicillin) are the most commonly used agents for COPD exacerbation in mild-moderate cases. In particular high doses of aminopenicillins in combination with a β-lactam inhibitor have been shown effective against *H. influenzae* and *M. catarrhalis*, and represent a better choice for the initial treatment of AECB as compared to aminopenicillins alone or cephalosporins [52]. The high incidence of β-lactamase has to be considered producing strains associated to AECB. New fluoroquinolones, with wider spectrum activity, have been shown to be highly effective in the management of AECB as compared to β-lactams. In fact although some concern about their antipneumococcical activity it has to be considered that they are highly potent against *H. influenzae* and *M. catarrhalis* and that their penetration into bronchial tissues is superior as compared to other traditional agents. The increasing resistance of pathogens to β-lactams is another factor which contribute to the elevation of fluoroquinolones to potential first choice antibiotics for the future treatment of AECB.

Although erythromycin has poor activity against *H. influenzae*, other macrolides such as clarythromicyn and the azalide azythromicin exhibit a higher activity against this pathogen as well as a good penetration into the lung tissue. In addition, an anti inflammatory activity of these agents has been recently identified. In more severe cases, however, a better activity against *H. influenzae* and *M. catharralis* is maintained by IV cephalosporins.

The BTS consider aminopenicillins as a first choice therapy, unless previously proven to be ineffective. In this case second-line alternatives are broad spectrum cephalosporins or new macrolides [51]. Broad spectrum agents such as tetracyclines, erythromicine, amoxicillin and cefaclor are recommended by the ATS, with broad spectrum cephalosporins as a second choice [53]. European guidelines suggest amoxicillin plus a β-lactamase inhibitor as a first choice agent and cephalosporins, new macrolides and fluoroquinolones as second choice antibiotics [9]. Recent publicationd recommend antibiotic treatment on the basis of risk stratification [52]. This approach, based on the severity of the condition (from class I–IV) allows an appropriate, patient-focused treatment which reduce the risk of treatment failure. According to this scheme acute tracheobronchitis should not receive antibiotic treatment, while the antibiotic regimen recommended for more severe conditions, class II–IV, takes into account spectrum of activity, resistance to inactivation by B-lactam penetration into sputum and bronchial tissues, and MIC values. In patients not responding to traditional treatment infection by *P. aeruginosa* or *S. aureus* must be considered. The possibility that *M. pneumoniae* or

C. pneumoniae might also be the cause of infections refractory to traditional treatment should be taken into account.

Conclusion

Respiratory tract infections represent the most common reason of consultation in primary care medicine. Their treatment is associated with the prescription of ~200 million courses of antibiotics each year in Europe. Despite the development of novel antibiotic agents and the proliferation of practice guidelines and treatment recommendations, the management of bacterial LRTIs still represents a difficult task and an important challenge for physicians. This is partly due to the heterogeneity of this condition on both the aetiological and clinical site. Microbiology is therefore extremely important for accurate bacterial identification and testing of microbial susceptibility to antibiotics in that microbiologically documented data may provide a more reliable basis for making appropriate therapeutic decisions. All the procedures involved in pathogen identification and susceptibility testing imply an unavoidable delay, which constitutes a limitation to the early onset of treatment and imposes the initiation of an empiric antibiotic therapy. For any microbiological examination to be helpful, the results should be immediately available at the time that therapeutic decision is made. Despite these limitations, direct microscopical examination of Gram-stained sputum or bronchial aspirate and rough identification based on morphology and Grams stain is recommended. In addition, most patients with LRTIs are treated as outpatients and choice of therapy is empirical because the etiological agent remains unknown. As a consequence, therapy with antibiotics should include coverage for both typical and atypical organisms. Recommendations by three major evidence-based guidelines support the use of a regimen that possesses activity against both typical and atypical microorganisms. Thus an integral role for macrolides and fluoroquinolones in the management of these conditions has been recently emphasised.

When implicated in cases of pneumonia, *S. pneumoniae* should have its susceptibility carefully tested. Among adults with bacteremic pneumococcal pneumonia, infection with penicillin-nonsusceptible pneumococci is associated with an increased risk of adverse outcome. For outpatient treatment of CAP, suitable empirical oral antimicrobial agents include a macrolide (*e.g.* erythromycin, clarithromycin, azithromycin), doxycycline (or tetracycline) for children aged ≥8 yrs or an oral β-lactam with good activity against pneumococci (*e.g.* cefuroxime axetil, amoxicillin, or a combination of amoxicillin and potassium clavulanate). Suitable empirical antimicrobial regimens for inpatient pneumonia include an intravenous β-lactam such as cefuroxime, ceftriaxone sodium, cefotaxime sodium, or a combination of ampicillin sodium and sulbactam sodium plus a macrolide. New fluoroquinolones with improved activity against *S. pneumoniae* can also be used to treat adults with CAP. To limit the emergence of fluoroquinolone-resistant strains, the new fluoroquinolones should be limited to adults [1] for whom one of the above regimens has already failed, [2] who are allergic to alternative agents, or [3] who have a documented infection with highly drug-resistant pneumococci (*e.g.* penicillin MIC ≥4 µg·mL^{-1}). Vancomycin hydrochloride is not routinely indicated for the treatment of CAP or pneumonia caused by DRSP.

As not all the acute exacerbations of CB and COPD are due to bacterial infections, antibiotics might not always be required. Unfortunately objective criteria to distinguish between bacterial and nonbacterial AECB are not available and therefore the decision to treat the individual patient with antibiotics should be based upon the presence of all the clinical characteristics (*i.e.* increased sputum volume and purulence, and increased dyspnoea) that are currently used as general criteria for the definition of exacerbation. In addition, all severe exacerbations, due to their high mortality risk, should be treated with antibiotics. Among adults with bacteremic pneumococcal pneumonia, infections with penicillin-nonsusceptible pneumococci are associated with an increased risk of adverse outcome [38].

Several observations suggest that current practice of LRTIs is inadequate. In particular, the selection and use of antibiotics are not sufficient. Problems are mainly due to the lack of objective criteria to evaluate the severity of CAP and whether or not bacterial infection is responsible of AECB. Illness severity might usefully guide a number of management decisions in the care pathway of a patient with CAP. Whether a referral to hospital by the primary care physician, whether to admit by the hospital junior doctor, what investigations to perform, what antibiotic(s) to give, and whether or not patients should be admitted to the intensive care unit are just some examples. Of course, the association between antibiotic use and bacterial resistance requires physicians to evaluate regularly what constitutes best practice for antibiotic therapy for CAP and AECB, and this evaluation should be consciously integrated in strategies to control the emergence of antibiotic-resistant respiratory tract pathogens in order to optimise the management and outcomes of LRTIs.

Summary

Lower respiratory tract infections (LRTIs), including community-acquired pneumonia and acute exacerbation of chronic bronchitis are common infectious diseases of human beings and represent a major cause of morbidity and mortality worldwide. Key pathogens associated with community-acquired LRTIs, include *Streptococcus pneumoniae* and other significant pathogens, such as *Hemophilus influenzae*, *Staphylococcus aureus* and *Pseudomonas aeruginosa*. Rates of antimicrobial use for the treatment of LRTIs have increased substantially during the past few decades and important progress in controlling LRTIs has been made. This progress is mostly explained by the introduction of a variety of classes of powerful antibiotics with improved pharmacokinetic and broad-spectrum activity against many common microbial pathogens.

However, despite the development of novel antibiotic agents and the proliferation of guidelines and treatment recommendations, the management of bacterial LRTIs still represents a difficult task and an important challenge in clinical practice. This is partly due to the heterogeneity of this condition on both the etiological and clinical site. Major issues in the choice of antibiotic regimens for LRTIs include the identification of the pathogen, the occurrence of antibiotic resistance, the presence of specific risk factors and the severity of the condition.

Keywords: Acute exacerbations of chronic bronchitis, antibiotics, community-acquired pneumonia, *Streptococcus pneumoniae*.

References

1. Almirall J, Bolibar I, Vidal J, *et al.* Epidemiology of community-acquired pneumonia in adults: a population-based study. *Eur Respir J* 2000; 15: 757–763.

2. Woodhead M. Community-acquired pneumonia in Europe: causative pathogens and resistance patterns. *Eur Respir J* 2002; 20: Suppl. 36, 20s–27s.

3. Gin AS. Community-acquired pneumonia – What is the state of the Art? *J Inform Pharmacother* 2000; 3: 336–344.

4. Legnani D. Role of oral antibiotics in treatment of community-acquired lower respiratory tract infection. *Diagn Microbiol Infect Dis* 1997; 27: 41–47.

5. Murray CJL, Lopez AD. Evidence-based health policy-lessons from the Global Burden of Disease Study. *Science* 1996; 274: 740–743.

6. Niederman MS, McCombs JI, Unger AN, *et al.* The cost of treating community-acquired pneumonia. *Clin Ther* 1998; 20: 820–837.

7. Niederman MS, Bass JB Jr, Campbell GD, Kumar A, Popovian R. Guidelines for the initial management of adults with community-acquired pneumonia: diagnosis, assessment of severity, and initial antimicrobial therapy. American Thoracic Society. Medical Section of the American Lung Association. *Am Rev Respir Dis* 1993; 148: 1418–1426.

8. Gialdroni Grassi G, Bianchi L. Guidelines for the management of community-acquired pneumonia in adults. *Monaldi Arch Chest Dis* 1996; 30: 1 21–27.

9. Huchon G, Woodhead M, Gialdroni-Grassi G, P, *et al.* Guidelines for the management of adult community-acquired lower respiratory tract infections. *Eur Respir J* 1998; 11: 986–991.

10. Bartlett JG, Dowell SF, Mandell LA, File Jr TM, Musher DM, Fine MJ. Practice guidelines for the management of community-acquired pneumonia in adults. Infectious Diseases Society of America. *Clin Infect Dis* 2000; 31: 347–382.

11. Mandell LA, Marrie TJ, Grossman RF, *et al.* Canadian guidelines for the initial management of community acquired pneumonia: an evidence-based update by the Canadian Infectious Diseases Society and the Canadian Thoracic Society. The Canadian Community-Acquired Pneumonia Working Group. *Clin Infect Dis* 2000; 31: 383–421.

12. Niederman MS, Mandell LA, Anzueto A, *et al.* Guidelines for the management of adults with community-acquired pneumonia. Diagnosis, assessment of severity, antimicrobial therapy, and prevention. *Am J Respir Crit Care Med* 2001; 163: 1730–1754.

13. British Thoracic Society. BTS guidelines for the management of community acquired pneumonia in adults. *Thorax* 2001; 56: Suppl. IV, 1–64.

14. Suchyta MR, Nathan DO, Dean C, Narus S. Hadlock CJ. Effects of a practice guideline for community-acquired pneumonia in an outpatient setting. *Am J Med* 2001; 110: 306–309.

15. Cazzola M, Blasi F, Allegra L. Critical evaluation of guidelines for the treatment of lower respiratory tract bacterial infections. *Respir Med* 2001; 95: 95–108.

16. Neill AM, Martin IR, Weir R, *et al.* Community-acquired pneumonia: aetiology and usefulness of severity criteria on admission. *Thorax* 1996; 51: 1010–1016.

17. Fine MJ, Auble TE, Yealy DM, *et al.* A prediction rule to identify low-risk patients with community-acquired pneumonia. *N Engl J Med* 1997; 336: 243–250.

18. Ewig S, Ruiz M, Mensa J, *et al.* Severe community-acquired pneumonia. Assessment of severity criteria. *Am J Respir Crit Care Med* 1998; 158: 1102–1108.

19. Ruiz M, Ewig S, Marcos MA, *et al.* Etiology of community-acquired pneumonia: impact of age, comorbidity, and severity. *Am J Respir Crit Care Med* 1999; 160: 397–405.

20. Ewig S, Schafer H, Torres A. Severity assessment in community-acquired pneumonia. *Eur Respir J* 2000; 16: 1193–1201.

21. Lim WS, van der Eerden MM, Laing R, *et al.* Defining community-acquired pneumonia severity on presentation to hospital: an international derivation and validation study. *Thorax* 2002; 58: 377–382.

22. British Thoracic Society and the Public Health Laboratory Service. Community-acquired pneumonia in adults in British hospitals in 1982–1983: a survey of aetiology, mortality, prognostic factors and outcome. *Q J Med* 1987; 239: 195–220.

23. Örtquist AJ, Hedlund L, Grillner E, *et al.* Aetiology, outcome and prognostic factors in patients with community acquired pneumonia requiring hospitalisation. *Eur Respir J* 1990; 3: 1105–1113.

24. Fang G-D, Fine M, Orloff J, *et al.* New and emerging etiologies for community-acquired pneumonia with implications for therapy: a prospective multicenter study of 359 cases. *Medicine* 1990; 69: 307–316.

25. Lieberman D, Schlaeffer F, Boldur I, *et al.* Multiple pathogens in adult patients admitted with community-acquired pneumonia: a one year prospective study of 346 consecutive patients. *Thorax* 1996; 51: 179–184.

26. Mundy LM, Auwaerter PG, Oldach D, *et al.* Community-acquired pneumonia. Impact of immune status. *Am J Respir Crit Care Med* 1995; 152: 1309–1315.

27. Woodhead MA, McFarlane JT, McCracken JS, Rose DH, Finch RG. Prospective study of the aetiology and outcome of pneumonia in the community. *Lancet* 1987; 1: 671–674.

28. Miravitlles M. Exacerbations of chronic obstructive pulmonary disease: when are bacteria important? *Eur Respir J* 2002; 20: Suppl. 36, 9s–19s.

29. Akalin HE. The place of antibiotic therapy in the management of chronic acute exacerbations of chronic bronchitis. *Int J Antimicrob Agents* 2001; 18: Suppl. 1, 49–55.

30. Arancibia F, Ewig S, Martinez JM, *et al.* Antimicrobial Treatment Failures in Patients with Community-acquired Pneumonia. Causes and Prognostic Implications. *Am J Respir Crit Care Med* 2000; 162: 154–160.

31. Hoffken G. Epidemiology of respiratory tract infections. *Eur Respir Rev* 2000; 10: 149–155.

32. Ewig S, Ruiz M, Torres A, *et al.* Pneumonia acquired in the community through drug-resistant *Streptococcus pneumoniae*. *Am J Respir Crit Care Med* 1999; 159: 1835–1842.

33. Mckean MC. Evidence based medicine: Review of BTS guidelines for the management of community-acquired pneumonia in adults. *J Infect* 2002; 45: 213–218.

34. Niederman MS. Empirical therapy of community-acquired pneumonia. *Semin Respir Infect* 1994; 9: 192–198.

35. MacFarlane JT, Miller AC, Roderick Smith WH, Morris AH, Rose DH. Comparative radiographic features of community-acquired Legionnaires disease, pneumococcal pneumonia, mycoplasma pneumonia, and psittacosis. *Thorax* 1984; 39: 28–33.

36. Doern GV, Pfaller MA, Kugler K, Freeman J, Jones RN. Prevalence of antimicrobial resistance among respiratory tract isolates of *Streptococcus pneumoniae* in North America: 1997 results from the SENTRY antimicrobial Surveillance Program. *Clin Infect Dis* 1998; 27: 764–770.

37. Heffelfinger JD, Dowell SF, Jorgensen JH, *et al.* Management of community-acquired pneumonia in the era of pneumococcal resistance: a report from the drug-resistant *Streptococcus pneumoniae* Therapeutic Working Group. *Arch Intern Med* 2000; 160: 1399–1408.

38. Metlay JP, Hofmann J, Cetron MS, *et al.* Impact of penicillin susceptibility on medical outcomes for adult patients with bacteremic pneumococcal pneumonia. *Clin Infect Dis* 2000; 30: 520–528.

39. Fine MJ, Smith MA, Carson CA. Prognosis and outcomes of patients with community-acquired pneumonia: a meta-analysis. *JAMA* 1996; 275: 134–141.

40. Chen DK, McGeer A, De Azavedo JC, Low DE. Decreased susceptibility of *Streptococcus pneumoniae* to fluoroquinolones in Canada. *N Engl J Med* 1999; 341: 233–239.

41. Niederman MS, Traub S, Ellison W, Williams D. A double-blind, randomized, multicenter, global study in hospitalized community-acquired pneumonia (CAP) comparing trovafloxacin with ceftriaxone+erythromycin. Toronto, Canada 37th Interscience Conference on Antimicrobial Agents and Chemotherapy, 1997; ALM–72.

42. Sullivan JG, McElroy AD, Honsinger RW, McAdoo M, Garrison BJ, Plouffe JF, *et al.* Treating community-acquired pneumonia with once-daily gatifloxacin *vs* once-daily levofloxacin. *J Respir Dis* 1999; 20: S49–S59.

43. Monsò E, Ruiz J, Rossell A, *et al.* Bacterial infections in chronic pulmonary disease: a study of stable and exacerbated outpatiuents using the protected specimen brush. *Am J Respir Crit Care Med* 1995; 152: 1316–1320.

44. Fagon JY, Chastre J, Trouillet, *et al.* Characterization of distal bronchial microflora during acute exacerbation of chronic bronchitis: use of protected specimen brush technique in 54 mechanically ventilated patients. *Am Rev Respir Dis* 1990; 142: 1004–1008.

45. Eller J, Ede A, Schaberg T, Niederman MS, Mauch H, Lode H. Infective exacerbations of chronic bronchitis: relation between bacteriologic etiology and lung function. *Chest* 1998; 113: 1542–1548.

46. Sethi S. Infectious exacerbations of chronic bronchitis: diagnosis and management. *J Antimicrob Chemothr* 1999; 43: Suppl. A, 97–105.

47. Murphy TF, Sethi S. Bacterial infection in chronic obstructive pulmonary disease. *Am Rev Respir Dis* 1992; 146: 1067–1083.

48. Anthonisen NR, Manfreda J, Warren CPW, *et al.* Antibiotic therapy in exacerbation of chronic obstructive pulmonary disease. *Am Intern Med* 1987; 106: 196–204.

49. Taylor DC, Clancy RL, Cropps AW, *et al.* An alteration in the host-parasite relationship in subjects with chronic bronchitis prone to recurrent episodes of acute bronchitis. *Immunol Cell Biol* 1994; 72: 143–151.

50. Saint S, Bent S, Vittinghoff E, *et al.* Antibiotics in chronic obstructive pulmonary disease exacerbations. A meta-analysis. *J Am Med Assoc* 1995; 273: 957–960.

51. The COPD Guidelines Group of The Standards Care Committee of the BTS. BTS guidelines for the management of chronic obstructive pulmonary disease (COPD). *Eur Respir J* 1995; 8: 1398–1420.

52. Ball P, Wilson R. Causes epidemiology, and treatment of bronchial infections. *Infect Med* 2000; 17: 186–198.

53. American Thoracic Society. Standards for the diagnosis and care of patients with chronic obstructive pulmonary disease. *Am J Respir Crit Care Med* 1995; 152: S72–S120.

CHAPTER 12

Are antibiotics useful in acute exacerbations of chronic bronchitis?

F. Blasi, L. Allegra

Institute of Respiratory Diseases, University of Milan, IRCCS Ospedale Maggiore Milan, Milan, Italy.

Correspondence: F. Blasi, Institute of Respiratory Diseases, University of Milan, IRCCS Ospedale Maggiore Milan, Milan, Italy.

In the US chronic obstructive pulmonary disease (COPD) is present in 20% of the population [1]. Exacerbations of chronic bronchitis are a common occurrence in clinical practice, and are a leading cause for the prescription of antibiotics regarding respiratory infections. The causes that trigger an acute exacerbation of chronic bronchitis (AECB) are generally multifactorial and commonly include a combination of smoking habits, environmental irritants and infections [2]. It is perceived that up to 70% of respiratory infections are caused by bacteria, with the remaining 30% being attributed to "atypical" pathogens *e.g.* viruses, *Mycoplasma pneumoniae*, and *Chlamydia pneumoniae* [3]. However, the role of bacterial infections in AECB is still controversial. Findings commonly associated with bacterial infections, for example fever and leukocytosis, are often absent and despite the use of bacterial culture techniques and antibody titres, an association between exacerbations and acute bacterial infections has not been clearly demonstrated [4, 5].

The three most consistently reported pathogens causing AECB are as follows: *Haemophilus influenzae*, *Streptococcus pneumoniae*, and *Moraxella catarrhalis* [3–7]. *H. influenzae* is the most common pathogen isolated from expectorated sputum and is held responsible for 35–50% of exacerbations, whereas recent clinical trials confirm that *S. pneumoniae* is responsible for ≤20% of exacerbations. Viruses and *M. pneumoniae* account for approximately one third of acute exacerbations and ∼5% of patients with chronic bronchitis exacerbations are caused by *C. pneumoniae* infections [8, 9].

Undoubtedly, every episode induces a temporary decrease in the function of the lung and therefore, may pose a threat of respiratory failure or death in the more severely obstructed patients. It is still uncertain whether each new exacerbation may deteriorate the natural history of chronic bronchitis. Two recent studies support the role of respiratory infections as disease modifiers [10, 11]. Data from the Lung Health Study on mild COPD patients [10] indicated that continuous smokers who reported lower respiratory tract infections during the year preceding testing, showed a larger fall in their forced expiratory volume in one second ($FEV1$) than those who did not. These data were consistent with lower respiratory tract infections being associated with a decrease in lung function. There was an additive effect of smoking and lower respiratory tract infections on the 1-yr change in $FEV1$. Over the 5-yr study period the data was consistent with an effect of a lower respiratory tract infection on the decline of $FEV1$ in continuing and intermittent smokers that was not seen in sustained quitters. In another study a cohort of 109 moderate-severe COPD patients was prospectively evaluated over 4 yrs [11]. Patients with frequent exacerbations had a significantly faster decline in both the $FEV1$ and peak

Eur Respir Mon, 2004, 28, 189–197. Printed in UK - all rights reserved. Copyright ERS Journals Ltd 2004; European Respiratory Monograph; ISSN 1025-448x. ISBN 1-904097-32-4.

expiratory flow (PEF) when compared with infrequent exacerbators, and were more frequently admitted to hospital.

Exacerbations are usually defined as an increase in cough, a change in the colour or quantity of sputum, or an increase in the severity of dyspnoea [12].

A recent study described the diagnostic role of sputum purulence and colour in the identifaction of bacterial exacerbations [13]. A positive culture was obtained from 84% of purulent sputa compared with 38% from mucoid sputa. The presence of green sputum was 94% sensitive and 77% specific for a high bacterial-load yield. Interestingly, resolution of sputum purulence was shown to relate to the resolution of symptoms [14]. All patients producing mucoid sputum improved without antibiotic therapy, and sputum characteristics remained the same even when the patients had returned to their stable clinical state.

Antibiotics and AECB

If the role of bacterial infections is still controversial, the efficacy of antimicrobial therapy in AECB is even more uncertain.

In order to evaluate the effect of antibiotics on AECB and chronic bronchitis' natural history two approaches have been used. The first is the prophylactic use of antibiotics that should lead to a decrease in the number and frequency of AECB. Many studies tried to address this issue, amongst these nine were placebo-controlled studies involving ≥ 25 patients (table 1) [15–23].

MURPHY and SETHI [24] analysed the trials that showed a benefit from antibiotic prophylaxis, and observed that patients who were more likely to experience beneficial effects of prophylaxis, were those with a more relevant clinical impairment (as determined by the number of past exacerbations). Patients who experienced many exacerbations ($\sim 4 \cdot yr^{-1}$) are most likely to benefit from antibiotic prophylaxis whereas this effect is less likely to occur in patients with one or two exacerbations per yr. Therefore, it is indicated from the available studies that antibiotic prophylaxis strategies should be limited to patients with more severe clinical impairment, which can be determined by the number of exacerbations the patient undertook in the in the previous years.

The other possible approach in evaluating the role of antibiotic treatment in exacerbations of chronic bronchitis, is to assess the efficacy of antibiotic therapy on the severity and course of a single exacerbation, after its onset.

Table 1. – Placebo-controlled clinical trials of chemoprophylaxis of acute exacerbations of chronic bronchitis

Trials	Benefit
The Working Party on Trials of Chemotherapy in Early Chronic Bronchitis of The Medical Research Council. [15]	No reduction in the frequency of exacerbations Reduced time loss from work in the antibiotic group
DAVIS et al. [16]	No reduction in the frequency of exacerbations
PRIEDIE et al. [17]	No reduction in the frequency of exacerbations
FRANCIS RS et al. [18]	No reduction in the frequency of exacerbations Reduced time loss from work in the antibiotic group
JOHNSTON et al. [19]	No reduction in the frequency of exacerbations.
DAVIS et al. [20]	Statistically significant reduction in the frequency of exacerbations
BUCHANAN et al. [21]	Statistically significant reduction in the frequency of exacerbations
PINES [22]	Statistically significant reduction in the frequency of exacerbations
JONHSTON et al. [23]	Statistically significant reduction in the frequency of exacerbations

At least 10 placebo-controlled studies have been performed to answer the question on the possible beneficial effects of an antibiotic treatment in patients with AECB (table 2) [25–34].

A meta-analysis of randomised, placebo-controlled trials of patients on antibiotic treatment with AECB demonstrated only a small, though statistically significant improvement, attributable to antimicrobial therapy [35]. Major difficulties in defining the true value of antibiotic treatment are the lack of unifying definitions of an exacerbation as well as the heterogeneity of chronic bronchitis patients in terms of severity of the underlying disease. It is important to bear in mind that both baseline severity and exacerbation severity may be associated with unusual bacterial aetiologies for example *Pseudomonas aeruginosa*. [36–38].

ALLEGRA *et al.* [34] analysed the data of a prospective study on chronic bronchitis patients with acute exacerbations treated with amoxicillin/clavulanic acid or matched placebo. The authors retrospectively reclustered patients on the basis of the severity of baseline lung function as follows: Cluster 1 (104 patients) mean screening FEV_1 32.67±6.83 (±SD); Cluster 2 (109 patients) mean screening FEV_1 54.12±5.56; Cluster 3 (122 patients) mean screening FEV_1 71.54±5.51. The success rate in the antibiotic group was significantly greater compared to the placebo group ($p<0.001$). When clinical improvement was analysed on the basis of patient re-clustering, 31.4% of Cluster 1 (severe COPD) patients treated with amoxicillin/clavulanate showed clinical improvement, however success was recorded in 58.8%. In contrast 13.2% of Cluster 1 patients receiving placebo improved and 17% successfully recovered ($p<0.001$). Mild and moderate COPD patients (Clusters 2 and 3) were grouped together. In these two combined groups, 31.2% and 53.6% of patients receiving antibiotic treatment showed improvement or recovery, respectively, compared to 29.2% improvements and 30.2% successful recoveries among placebo-treated patients ($p<0.001$). In placebo-treated patients the improvement/success *versus* failure rate was significantly different in Cluster 1 patients compared to the combined Cluster 2 and 3 subjects ($p<0.01$, Chi-square test). The difference in final FEV_1 values in the treatment group and placebo group were significantly different ($p<0.01$) in favour of the active treatment group. Among more severe patients (Cluster 1), the comparison between screening and follow up FEV_1 values showed an improvement following antibiotic treatment and a decline after placebo ($p<0.01$). In Clusters 2 and 3 the difference between screening and follow up FEV_1 values was not significant for both treatment groups. The data of this study suggest that patients with severe functional impairment and higher number of exacerbations per year are those who derive the greatest benefit from antibiotic treatment.

Another study on AECB patients requiring mechanical ventilation, analysed the effect of antibiotic treatment on the clinical outcome [39]. A total of 93 COPD patients admitted to the intensive care unit (ICU) were randomly assigned to receive either once daily oral ofloxacin or placebo. No patient received corticosteroids. The overall mortality was significantly lower in ofloxacin-treated patients when compared with the placebo group (4% *versus* 22%, respectively). The combined frequency of in-hospital death and need for additional antibiotics was also significantly lower in patients assigned to ofloxacin. The authors concluded that antibiotic treatment is beneficial for those patients with severe AECB requiring mechanical ventilation and suggest that bacterial infections play an important role in these patients AECB.

Antibiotic-associated improvement may, therefore, be particularly significant in those patients with greater baseline pulmonary dysfunction and severe exacerbations, although it is still unclear whether all COPD patients need antibiotic treatment.

Table 2. – Placebo-controlled clinical trials of antibiotic treatment in acute exacerbations of chronic bronchitis

Reference	Year of publication	Patients n (exacerbations)	Treatment	Outcome measured	Results
Elmes et al. [25]	1957	88 (113)	Oxytetracycline	Days of illness	The treated group lost an average of 5.2 fewer days from work per exacerbation compared with the placebo group.
Berry et al. [26]	1960	53 (53)	Oxytetracycline	Severity score	Treated patients recovered sooner and deteriorated less often than the controls. This advantage is statistically significant for patients with moderately severe attacks but not for those with mild attacks.
Fear and Edwards [27]	1962	62 (119)	Oxytetracycline	Duration of exacerbation Clinical response	The duration of the relapses in the treated patients was reduced by half.
Elmes et al. [28]	1965	56 (56)	Ampicillin	Mortality Length of hospital stay Relapses in hospital Relapses after discharge Change in PEFR	No conclusive evidence that ampicillin was beneficial. Higher (not significantly) mortality in the control group. In-hospital relapses occurred significantly more often in the control group. Higher (not significantly) increase in PEFR in the treated group
Petersen et al. [29]	1967	19 (19)	Chloramphenicol	Change in lung function tests	The lung function tests showed no significant different response to treatment.
Pines et al. [30]	1972	259 (259)	Tetracycline (89) or chloramphenicol (84)	Clinical score Change in PEFR	Clinically, antibiotic treatment was superior to the placebo. Patients treated with chloramphenicol benefited little more than those given tetracycline, except that chloramphenicol was much better tolerated. PEFR improved by a mean 10.7%, 12.6%, and 4.7% in tetracycline, chloramphenicol and placebo groups, respectively.
Nicotra et al. [31]	1982	40 (40)	Tetracycline	P_{a,O_2} Change in PEFR Clinical response	More pronounced improvement in oxygenation occurred in the tetracycline group. No difference in PEFR changes.
Anthonisen et al. [32]	1987	173 (362)	Trimethoprim-sulfamethoxazole or amoxicillin or doxycycline	Change in lung function tests	The success rate with placebo was 55% and with antibiotic 68%. The rate of failure with deterioration was 19% with placebo and 10% with antibiotic. There was a significant benefit associated with the antibiotic. PEFR recovered more rapidly with antibiotic treatment than with placebo.
Joergensen et al. [33]	1992	268	Amoxicillin	Clinical response Change in PEFR	Type 1 exacerbations (increased dyspnoea, sputum volume, and sputum purulence) showed a relatively large advantage for antibiotic therapy. No difference in terms of success rate and PEFR increase
Allegra et al. [34]	2001	335 (335)	Amoxicillin/clavulanic acid (7:1)	Clinical score Change in lung function tests	The failure rate with placebo was 49.7% and with the antibiotic 13.6%. FEV1 recovered more rapidly with antibiotic than with placebo.

PEFR: P_{a,O_2}: arterial oxygen tension; FEV1: forced expiratory volume in one second.

Which antibiotic

Studies of AECB therapy generally do not show clear superiority of one agent over another, as often they are designed to show equivalence between a new agent and an approved one.

The recommendations of the European Respiratory Society [40] can be roughly described as follows: The need for exacerbation severity and functional impairment assessment is beginning to break through. Antibiotic therapy is always recommended in severe exacerbations, but it is also recommended for nonsevere exacerbations if the increase in sputum purulence and volume are present, together with an increase in the severity of dyspnoea. Treatment should always last a minimum of 7 days.

The choice of the antibiotic employed depends on the habitual prescribing behaviour of the clinician and, when available, local pathogen epidemiological considerations, in addition to information on previous antibiotic failures. The impact on the cost of treatment differs widely according to the antibiotic employed, although drug expenses never account for >10–16% of the total costs. The rate of relapse following antibiotic treatment is a fundamental determinant of expenses, because patients with more relapses burn up more health resources. Alternatively slow remission of an exacerbation also expands total treatment expenses.

Comparing the time span between one exacerbation and the next after the use of a first choice (amoxicillin, tetracycline, erythromycin, or cotrimoxazole), second choice (oral cephalosporins), or third choice antibiotic (co-amoxiclav, ciprofloxacin and azithromycin) DESTACHE et al. [41] showed that first and second line antibiotics allowed exacerbation-free intervals of 18.3 and 23.7 weeks respectively, whereas third choice antibiotics gave an interval of 33 weeks.

Treatment for all patients should target the core organisms that include *H. influenzae, M. catarrhalis*, and *S. pneumoniae*. This applies for patients with uncomplicated AECB, with fewer than four exacerbations per year, no comorbid illness, and a FEV1 >50% of predicted. Patients aged >65 yrs who have greater than four exacerbations per year, serious comorbidities or FEV1 <50%, are at risk form the core organisms and are more likely to have drug-resistant pathogens (organisms that produce β-lactamase and resistant pneumoccus) and possibly enteric Gram-negative bacteria. Recommended treatment for this group of patients is based on fluoroquinolones with antipneumococcal activity or amoxicillin/clavulanate or, newer macrolides if only one risk factor is present. In patients with risk factors for *P. aeruginosa* infection, e.g. chronic bronchial sepsis, the need for corticosteroid therapy and frequent courses of antibiotics (>4·yr^{-1} instances), or a FEV1 <35%, the suggested treatment is an oral antipseudomonal fluoroquinolone for outpatients.

In addition to the probable spectrum of organisms involved, the choice of which antibiotic treatment to use should also be guided by pharmacokinetic and pharmacodynamic considerations.

The optimal duration of therapy treatment is as yet undefined, although many trials have shown efficacy with a 5–7-day courses in uncomplicated cases. In more severely ill patients with more complex diseases, the duration of treatment should follow the resolution of symptoms, and it might be reasonable to extend the duration to 10–14 days to avoid a relapse.

A patient's prior treatment with antibiotics has been shown in CAP cases as a risk factor, as there is an increased probability of acquiring infections by resistant organisms in [42], and antibioticrotation has been suggested. This hypothesis seems attractive, but whether this could apply to AECB remains to be verified.

The suggested empirical antibiotic treatment according to a patient's characteristics is

Table 3. – The stratification scheme for empirical antibiotic treatments according to patients characteristics

Condition	Treatment
Simple, uncomplicated AECB	Macrolide (clarithromycin azithromycin)
≤4 exacerbations	or
No comorbid illness	New cephalosporin (cefpodoxime, cefuroxime, cefprozil)
FEV1>50%	or
	Doxycycline
Complicated AECB	Fluoroquinolones
>64 yrs	or
>4 exacerbations/yr	Amoxicillin/clavulanate
Serious comorbid illness	
FEV1<50%	
Complicated AECB at risk of	Fluoroquinolone with antipseudomonal activity
Pseudomonas aeruiginosa	
Pts with chronic bronchial sepsis	
Need for chronic corticosteroid therapy	
and frequent (>4 yr^{-1}) courses of	
antibiotics	
FEV1<35% predicted	

AECB: acute exacerbations of chronic bronchitis; pts: patients; FEV1: forced expiratory volume in one second.

shown in table 3. This stratification scheme should be viewed as a hypothesis that needs testing with prospective studies evaluating whether patient outcome can be improved by adherence to the suggested protocol. Preliminary data do support the general approach proposed.

Conclusions

Exacerbations of chronic bronchitis are a common occurrence in clinical practice and are a leading cause of antibiotic prescription among respiratory infections. On the basis of recent studies it is now thought that each new exacerbation is involved in deteriorating the natural history of chronic bronchitis, although definitive proof is still lacking. Undoubtedly, every episode induces a temporary decline in lung function and may therefore pose a threat of respiratory failure or death in more severely obstructed patients.

The overall impression from the studies performed on antibiotic value in AECB is that antibiotic treatment induces an improvement of both clinical and functional parameters. These benefits are in some studies relatively small but may be clinically significant, especially in those patients with a more severe impairment of respiratory function.

In conclusion, the role of antibiotic treatment in chronic bronchitis exacerbations seems to be confirmed in terms of mid-term functional recovery, and to be relevant to patients with severe functional impairment and higher number of exacerbations per year in whom antibiotic treatment induces the greatest benefit.

Summary

Atypical pathogens are increasingly being implicated in the aetiology of lower respiratory tract infections (LRTIs) in both adults and children. The lack of simple, standardised diagnostic tests and the difficulty in differentiating infections due to atypical pathogens on clinical or radiological evidence alone, leads to under-recognition and potentially ineffective empirical treatment of these infections. A wide range of figures for the prevalence of *Chlamydia pneumoniae* and *Mycoplasma pneumoniae* in acute exacerbations of chronic bronchitis (AECB) have been reported in a number of publications. There is now a considerable weight of evidence for the pathogenic role of *C. pneumoniae* in AECB. *Legionella spp.* is not a common cause of AECB.

chronic carriage of *C. pneumoniae* in patients with chronic obstructive pulmonary disorder, is associated with a higher rate of airway microbial colonisation, more severe functional impairment, and a greater propensity for the development of acute exacerbations. *C. pneumoniae* infection has been found to be common in chronic bronchitis and could contribute to the disease progression through its toxic effect on bronchial epithelial cells, with ciliostasis and increasing chronic inflammation through pro-inflammatory cytokine production.

Keywords: Acute exacerbations of bronchitis, *Chlamydia pneumoniae*, chronic obstructive pulmonary disorder, *Mycoplasma pneumoniae*.

References

1. American Thoracic Society. Standards for the diagnosis and care of patients with chronic obstructive pulmonary disease. *Am J Respir Crit Care Med.* 1995; 152: S77–S120.
2. Fagon JY, Chastre J, Trouillet JL, *et al.* Characterization of distal bronchial microflora during acute exacerbation of chronic bronchitis. *Am Rev Respir Dis* 1990; 142: 1004–1008.
3. Ball P. Epidemiology and treatment of chronic bronchitis and its exacerbations. *Chest* 1995; 108: Suppl. 3, 43s–52s.
4. Gump DW, Philips CA, Forsyth BR, McIntosh K, Lamborn KR, Stouch WH. Role of infection in chronic bronchitis. *Am Rev Respir Dis* 1976; 113: 465–474.
5. Gump DW, Christmas WA, Forsyth BR, Philips CA, Stouch WH. Serum and secretory antibodies in patients with chronic bronchitis. *Arch Intern Med* 1973; 132: 847–851.
6. Murphy TF, Sethi S. Bacterial infection in chronic obstructive pulmonary disease. *Am Rev Respir Dis* 1992; 146: 1067–1083.
7. Wilson R. Outcome predictors in bronchits. *Chest* 1995; 198: Suppl. 2, 53s–57s.
8. Blasi F, Legnani D, Lombardo VM, *et al.* Chlamydia pneumoniae infection in acute exacerbations of COPD. *Eur Respir J* 1993; 6: 19–22.
9. Murphy TF, Sethi S. Chronic obstructive pulmonary disease: role of bacteria and guide to antibacterial selection in the older patient. *Drugs Aging* 2002; 19: 761–775.
10. Kanner RE, Anthonisen NR, Connett JE. Lower respiratory illnesses promote FEV_1 decline in current smokers but not ex-smokers with mild chronic obstructive pulmonary disease. *Am J Respir Crit Care Med* 2001; 164: 358–364.
11. Donaldson GC, Seemungal TAR, Bhowmik A, Wedzicka JA. Relationship between exacerbation frequency and lung function decline in chronic obstructive pulmonary disease. *Thorax* 2002; 57: 847–852.
12. Anthonisen NR, Manfreda J, Warren CPW, Hershfield ES, Harding GKM, Nelson NA. Antibiotic therapy in exacerbations of chronic obstructive pulmonary disease. *Ann Intern Med* 1987; 106: 196–204.
13. Stockley RA, O'Brien C, Pye A, Hill SL. Relationship of sputum colour to nature and outpatient management of acute exacerbations of COPD. *Chest* 2000; 117: 1638–1645.
14. Woolhouse I, Hill SL, Stockley RA. Symptom resolution assessed using a patient directed diary card during exacerbations of chronic bronchitis. *Thorax* 2001; 56: 947–53.
15. The Working Party on Trials of Chemotherapy in Early Chronic Bronchitis of The Medical

Research Council. Value of chemoprophylaxis and chemotherapy in early chronic bronchitis. *BMJ* 1966; 1: 317–22.

16. Davis AL, Grobow EJ, Kaminski T, Tompsett R, McClement JH. Bacterial infection and some effects of chemoprophylaxis in chronic pulmonary emphysema. II. Chemoprophylaxis with daily chloramphenicol. *Am Rev Respir Dis* 1965; 92: 900–913.

17. Priedie RB, Datta N, Massey DG, Poole GW, Schneeweiss J, Stradling P. A trial of continuous winter chemotherapy in chronic bronchitis. *Lancet* 1960; 2: 723–727.

18. Francis RS, Spicer CC. Chemotherapy in chronic bronchitis. Influence of daily penicillin and tetracycline on exacerbations and their costs. *BMJ* 1960; 1: 297–303.

19. Johnston RN, Lockart W, Smith DH, Cadman NK. A trial of phenethicillin in chronic bronchitis. *BMJ* 1961; 2: 985–986.

20. Davis AL, Grobow EJ, Tompsett R, McClement JH. Bacterial infection and some effects of chemoprophylaxis in chronic pulmonary emphysema. I. Chemoprophylaxis with intermittent tetracycline. *Am J Med* 1961; 31: 365–381.

21. Buchanan J, Buchanan WW, Melrose AG, McGuinness JB, Price AU. Long-term prophylactic administration of tetracycline to chronic bronchitis. *Lancet* 1958; 2: 719–722.

22. Pines A. Controlled trials of a sulphonamide given weekly to prevent exacerbations of chronic bronchitis. *BMJ* 1967; 3: 202–204.

23. Jonhston RN, McNeill RS, Smith DH. Five-year winter chemoprophylaxis for chronic bronchitis. *BMJ* 1969; 4: 265–269.

24. Murphy TF, Sethi S. Bacterial infection in chronic obstructive pulmonary disease. *Am Rev Respir Dis* 1992; 146: 1067–1083.

25. Elmes PC, Fletcher CM, Dutton AAC. Prophylactic use of oxytetracycline for exacerbations of chronic bronchitis. *BMJ* 1957; 2: 1272–1274.

26. Berry DG, Fry J, Hindley CP. Exacerbations of chronic bronchitis treatment with oxytetracycline. *Lancet* 1960; 1: 137–139.

27. Fear EC, Edwards G. Antibiotic regimens in chronic bronchitis. *Br J Dis Chest* 1962; 56: 153–162.

28. Elmes PC, King TKC, Langlands JHM. Value of ampicillin in the hospital treatment of exacerbations of chronic bronchitis. *BMJ* 1965; 2: 904–908.

29. Petersen ES, Esmann V, Honke P, Munkner C. A controlled study of the effect of treatment on chronic bronchitis: an evaluation using pulmonary function tests. *Acta Med Scand* 1967; 82: 293–305.

30. Pines A, Raafat H, Greenfield JSB, Linsell WD, Solari ME. Antibiotic regimens in moderately ill patients with purulent exacerbations of chronic bronchitis. *Br J Dis Chest* 1972; 66: 107–115.

31. Nicotra MB, Rivera M, Awe RJ. Antibiotic therapy of acute exacerbations of chronic bronchitis. *Ann Intern Med* 1982; 97: 18–21.

32. Anthonisen NR, Manfreda J, Warren CPW, Hershfield ES, Harding GKM, Nelson NA. Antibiotic therapy in exacerbations of chronic obstructive pulmonary disease. *Ann Intern Med* 1987; 106: 196–204.

33. Jorgensen AF, Coolidge J, Pedersen PA. Amoxicillin in treatment of acute uncomplicated exacerbations of chronic bronchitis. *Scand J Prim Health Care* 1992; 10: 7–11L.

34. Allegra F, Blasi B, de Bernardi R, Cosentini P. Tarsia. Antibiotic treatment and baseline severity of disease in acute exacerbations of chronic bronchitis: a re-evaluation of previously published data of a placebo-controlled randomized study. *Pulm Pharmacol Ther* 2001; 14: 149–155.

35. Saint S, Bent S, Vittinghoff E, Grady D. Antibiotics in chronic obstructive pulmonary disease exacerbations. A meta-analysis. *JAMA.* 1995; 273: 957–960.

36. Eller J, Ede A, Schaberg T, Neiderman MS, Mauch H, Lode H. Infective exacerbations of chronic bronchitis: relation between bacteriologic etiology and lung function. *Chest* 1998; 113: 1542–1548.

37. Miravitlles M, Espinosa C, Fernandez-Laso E, *et al.* Relationship between bacterial flora in sputum and functional impairment in patients with acute exacerbations of COPD. *Chest* 1999; 116: 40–46.

38. Ewig S, Soler N, Torres A. Severe acute exacerbations of COPD: epidemiology and antimicrobial

treatment. *In*: Allegra L, Blasi F, eds. Mechanisms and Management of COPD Exacerbations. Milan, Springer, 2000; pp. 54–62.

39.	Nouria S, Marghli S, Belghith M, Besbes L, Elatrous S, Abroug F. Once daily oral ofloxacin in chronic obstructive pulmonary disease exacerbation requiring mechanical ventilation: a randomized placebo-controlled trial. *Lancet* 2001; 358: 2020–2025.

40.	Huchon G, Woodhead M. Management of adult community-acquired lower respiratory tract infections. *Eur Respir Rev* 1998; 8: 391–426.

41.	Destache CJ, Dewan N, O'Donahue WJ, Campbell JC, Angelillo VA. Clinical and economic considerations in the treatment of acute exacerbations of chronic bronchitis. *J Antimicrob Chemother* 1994; 43: Suppl. A, 107–113.

42.	ATS. Guidelines for the management of adults with community-acquired pneumonia: diagnosis, assessment of severity, antimicrobial therapy, and prevention. *Am J Respir Crit Care Med* 2001; 163: 1730–1754.

CHAPTER 13

Cost-effective antibiotic management of community acquired pneumonia

M. Niederman

Dept of medicine, Winthrop University Hospital, Mineola, New York, US.

Correspondence: M. Niederman, 222 Station Plaza N, Suite 509, Mineola, New York, 11501, US.

Community acquired pneumonia (CAP) is a common illness in throughout the world and in the US it affects 5.6 million patients annually at a total cost-of-care of $8.4 billion [1]. Although the majority of patients (4.5 million) are treated outside of the hospital in the US, the majority of the cost ($8.0 billion) is attributed to patients that have been admitted to hospital. In order to achieve cost-effective management of CAP it is necessary to understand the factors contributing to cost, and the strategies that can reduce these influences. This chapter examines the multitude of factors that impact on the cost, which includes the decision concerning who is admitted to the hospital and the variables affecting a patient's length of stay (LOS) in the hospital. It is certainly possible to reduce costs by focusing attention at both targets. However to date the emphasis has largely been upon limiting the number of patient's admitted to hospital and not on the rapid discharge of those who have had a good clinical response to treatment.

A number of antibiotic-related decisions can impact on the cost of treating CAP. These include: the timeliness of initial antibiotic administration; the selection of appropriate (guideline-directed) therapy; the use of therapy directed at the likely aetiological pathogens; and the rapid switch from intravenous to oral therapy in appropriate hospitalised patients. Many of these antibiotic decisions can be incorporated into disease management guidelines, and the use of such guidelines has been demonstrated to lead to: improved outcomes; including reduced mortality; reduced LOS; and more cost-effective use of resources [2, 3].

The cost of treating community acquired pneumonia

Using a retrospective analysis of Medicare and insurance claims data for CAP, NIEDERMAN et al. [1] estimated that in 1995, 5.6 million US citizens were treated for CAP, in which the incidence was greatest in those aged ≥ 65 yrs or <17 yrs. The majority of patients were treated out of hospital, however a total of 1.135 million were admitted to hospital, and $>50\%$ of these patients were aged ≥ 65 yrs. The average cost of care for a hospitalised patient was $6,652 with those aged ≥ 65 yrs costing on average $7,166. Overall, the total cost of all hospitalised patients was $8,049 billion compared with a cost of $385 million for the care of 4.5 million outpatients. The cost of inpatient care was most clearly related to the cost of using the hospital. This theory is supported by the facts that the drugs costs were only 12% of the total costs spent on inpatients, and physician fees came to a total $0.48 billion. The elderly made up a disproportionate cost-of-care, as 35% of those aged ≥ 65 yrs were hospitalised, compared with 12.8% of the younger population. This finding could be attributed to the fact that comorbid illness was more

Eur Respir Mon, 2004, 28, 198–210. Printed in UK - all rights reserved. Copyright ERS Journals Ltd 2004; European Respiratory Monograph; ISSN 1025-448x. ISBN 1-904097-32-4.

prevelant in older patients (greater than three-fold more common than compared with the younger age group). In addition, the cost of care in these patients was great as they tended to stay in the hospital for longer periods of time when compared with the younger population (7.8 *versus* 5.8 days). Outpatient care, on average, was $90 per visit with costs ranging from $63 for care in the physician's office to $207 in an outpatient clinic. Among the charges for outpatients, diagnostic testing accounted for 29% of the costs and medical care for 64%, of which antibiotic costs were on average 14% of the total cost of care. These data provide a strong impetus for reducing the cost of pneumonia care by either limiting the number of patients admitted to the hospital, or by shortening LOS for those who are hospitalised, with a key target group being those aged ≥65 yrs.

Recently KAPLAN *et al.* [4] evaluated the cost of care for elderly patients with CAP in the US. Using Medicare data, they evaluated all individuals aged ≥65 yrs admitted to nonfederal hospitals in 1997. A total of 623,718 patients were admitted to the hospital, 86% of which were aged >70 yrs with the mean age being 77 yrs. An underlying illness was present in 66.6% of these patients, with congestive heart failure being the most common comorbidity present, occurring in 32% of the cases. In this population, the use of intensive care units (ICU), mechanical ventilation, or both was common, with 140,226 patients having complex courses of illness. The overall mortality rate was 10.6%, but rose higher with advancing age, nursing home residents, and comorbid illness. The majority of the deaths occurred early in the hospital course with >50% occuring within the first week of admission. The mean LOS was 7.6 days, with a mean cost of $6,949. However costs were greater for patients with complex illnesses and mechanical ventilation, and less for those with simple pneumonia. Costs generally paralleled the LOS, in the hospital although they were disproportionately high for those needing mechanical ventilation, where the mean LOS was 15.7 days and the cost $23,961. Interestingly, in general there was little extra cost for nonsurvivors compared to survivors, except in the group with complex pneumonia, but not in those requiring mechanical ventilation. In viewing the impact of CAP on the Medicare budget the authors estimated that CAP accounted for 6.2% of all Medicare admissions, 6.3% of all costs (at a total of $4.4 billion), 7% of hospital days and 12% of hospital deaths. The findings once again reinforce the high impact of CAP on costs and outcomes in the US. They also demonstrate the disproportionate increase in costs when patients are treated with mechanical ventilation, thereby raising for discussion the ethics and appropriateness of such care in the very elderly.

The studies cited above have documented that both the decision to admit a patient to the hospital and the intensity of the inpatient management have impacts on the cost of care. One other factor with an obvious influence on cost is the LOS, a parameter that is subject to reduction by the physician's input. FINE *et al.* [5] have examined the relationship between LOS and costs and have estimated the financial impact of reducing length of stay by 1 day to be $680, from a median of $5942. A total of 863 patients admitted to one of three hospitals was examined and severity of illness was similar at all three sites. Despite similar patient populations, the LOS varied among the sites from a median of 6–8 days. Interestingly, the authors demonstrated that costs were not evenly distributed throughout the hospitalisation period, with 32% of all costs being incurred on the first 2 days, and daily costs declining thereafter. This was further explained by demonstrating that while room costs were relatively constant, pharmacy costs, emergency services and radiological/laboratory tests were all greatest on the first day. Therefore, the impact of reducing LOS was primarily to reduce the dollars spent for the room costs, and there was much less of an impact on other services such as pharmacy costs or diagnostic testing. The impact of a reduction in LOS would primarily be economical as the same investigators demonstrated that in these same hospitals there was no adverse clinical outcome observed at the site that achieved the shortest duration of hospitalisation [6]. This is probably related to the fact that most patients achieve clinical stability within 2–3 days of admission, yet are often kept in hospital for several days after reaching this point [7]. This again demonstrates a realistic clinical opportunity to reduce costs without a negative impact on outcomes.

Outside of the US similar observations on the cost of CAP care have been made. Using data from1992–1993 GUEST AND MORRIS [8] estimated that there were 261,000 episoides of CAP in the UK, of which 32% (83,153) were admitted to hospital. This represents a larger percentage of hospitalised patients than in the US, but similar to the situation elsewhere. Admitted patients were found to account for the majority of the total costs for CAP treatment, 96% of the costs were spent on this population. Those aged ≥65 yrs accounted for 65% of all hospitalisations and the median LOS was 7 days, with 74% being discharged within 14 days. The cost of a hospital stay varied from £1,700–5,100 depending on LOS and the need for intensive care. When specific components of cost were examined, inpatient stay ("hotel charges") accounted for £388.7 million from a total cost of £440 million spent on the care of all pneumonia patients (inpatient and outpatient). In-hospital drugs cost £12.9 million compared with £1.5 million for drugs prescribed out of the hospital by general practioners. Inpatient diagnostic tests accounted for £12.7 million, compared with £8.4 million for outpatient testing. Similar to the US, the major driving factor for cost was hospitalisation, although the overall LOS and use of hospital admission varied between the different countries.

Factors influencing the cost of community-acquired pnuemonia

Social needs

A number of factors within the control of physicians, as well as factors outside of their immediate control, drive the use of resources for patients with CAP. One factor that is difficult to control is the safety of certain patient populations to be treated out of the hospital, particularly if the hospital fills social needs as well as providing necessary medical care. For example, in one study from Paris, 107 consecutive patients with CAP were evaluated, and 34 were identified as falling into a category of low socioeconomic status: defined as being unemployed, homeless, on government assistance, or having poor living conditions [9]. These patients were more often substance abusers than other patients, and had a higher incidence of tuberuculosis as a cause of their infection. The overall mortality rate was lower in those of lower socioeconomic status and severity of illness was similar to other patients, however their LOS was significantly longer averaging >6 days when compared with patients without this risk factor. Similar findings have emerged in other studies which have reported cost of care to be higher in urban hospitals than in rural hospitals in the US, presumably in part because of greater care needs in disadvantaged urban patients [10]. In examining the specific impact of social factors, FINE et al. [11] reported that a lack of patient homecare support increased the likelihood of admission for CAP by >50-fold, even in a population with a low risk (<5%) of death. Similarly, for patients who are hospitalised, discharge is delayed, even in clinically stable patients, in order to make arrangements for long-term care a provision which may be harder in patients of low socioeconomic status [12]. Therefore for a number of reasons the cost of care for economically disadvantaged patients is increased when CAP is present, even though severity of illness and outcomes are similar to patients without such profound social needs. Recently investigators have documented the high frequency and nature of the social needs of CAP patients admitted to the pulic hospital in the US, many of whom were homeless or substance abusers [13].

Admission to the hospital

It is clear from the preceding overview of the cost of care for CAP patients, the decision to admit a patient to hospital is the major factor effecting the amount of money spent on this illness. Although it is beyond the scope of this discussion to examine the issues surrounding the admission decision, a number of studies have pointed out that many patients at a low risk for death are admitted to the hospital with CAP. Therefore, the argument has been presented, that many of these patients could be managed out of the hospital at substantial cost savings [14]. Although this approach can save money, its impact on patients remains uncertain especially since the algorithm of reserving admission only for those at high risk of death ignores some of the broad benefits of hospitalisation, focusing only on the need for close observation and treatment of the patients who may die. In the largest prospective randomised study of the Pneumonia Severity Index (PSI), a tool that categorises patients into five risk categories for mortality, investigators found that the application of a severity score could be used to discharge more patients than if the scoring system was not used [2]. In fact in the CAP guidelines of the Infectious Disease Society of America (IDSA), the recommendation was made to consider admission only for those in PSI classes IV and V, with outpatient management for all the others, unless this would be unsafe [15]. However, in the prospective application of the PSI to guide the admission decision, clinicians admitted 30% of low risk (by PSI score) patients, despite the PSI system, indicating that clinical decisions often supercede an assessment by a specific rule [2]. The need to be able to use clinical judgment in the admission decision is quite clear. In a study of 944 patients where CAP was initially managed outside of the hospital, 71 patients were subsequently admitted within the next 30 days, 40 because of CAP related reasons. These patients required a median of 14 days to return to usual activities, and they had a 4.2% mortality [16]. These findings suggest that the incorrect decision to manage a patient out of the hospital may actually lead to a worse outcome than if such a "borderline" patient had been initially hospitalised.

Timeliness of antibiotic therapy

MEEHAN *et al.* [17] showed how the 30 day mortality of CAP can be reduced if hospitalised patients receive their first dose of antibiotic therapy within 8 h of arrival in hospital. More recently, BATTLEMAN *et al.* [18] reported that delays in initial therapy are also associated with prolonged LOS. In particular, they found that if the initial dose of antibiotics was administered in the emergency department, there was a 0.4 odds ratio (OR) of a prolonged LOS. Those initially treated in the emergency room had a mean LOS of 6.3 days, *versus* a LOS of 8.4 days if initial therapy was administered at an inpatient unit. The explanation for this association is probably due to the more timely administration of antibiotics in the emergency department (ED), compared to the inpatient floor. Those treated in the ED received therapy at a mean of 3.5 h, compared with 9.5 h in those treated outside of the ED. While site of initial therapy was important, probably due to the reflection of timely therapy, timing itself was relevant, with the OR of a prolonged LOS increasing by 1.75 for every 8 h of delay in therapy. In another study, a number of clinical factors were associated with delay in initial antibiotic therapy and these included: non-White race, treatment in a major teaching hospital, and treatment in a hospital with ≥250 beds [19]. In this study, administration of antibiotics within 8 h of arrival to the hospital was more likely if patients arrived in the ED between 15.00–23.00 h, a less busy time than earlier in the day and the findings may reflect variations in care that parallel varying demands on the medical staff.

Antibiotic choices

A number of studies have shown that the use of appropriate antibiotic therapy for CAP, often dictated by guidelines, can reduce mortality. Some studies have also shown that appropriate therapy can reduce LOS thereby reducing the cost of care for CAP [2, 3]. In one study appropriate therapy was defined as antibiotics consistent with published guidelines and the use of appropriate therapy was associated with a significant reduction in LOS but only after adjusting for severity of illness, and in patients with comorbid illness [18]. These findings suggest that complicated patients are more sensitive to specific antibiotic choices and are the ones most likely to benefit from the accurate choice of initial therapy. A more detailed discussion of antibiotic choices and the potential benefit of guidelines will be discussed later on in this chapter.

Timing of switch to oral therapy and discharge

One clear way to reduce the costs of CAP care is to discharge patients from the hospital as soon as they are clinically stable and able to be treated with oral antibiotics. The decision to switch to oral therapy, and the timing of discharge are therefore important in the cost-effective management of CAP and will be discussed in more detail later. However, the opportunity to reduce costs by focusing on these issues was recently demonstrated in a study by Rifkin et al. [20]. The study evaluated the management of 455 CAP patients. The outcomes and LOS were compared for those treated by hospital physicians with those treated by primary care physicians. In general, both types of physicians treated similarly ill patients and treatment by either type of doctor achieved clinical stability at the same time, at a median of 3 days. Despite these findings the hospital physicians switched to oral antibiotics at a mean of 0.7 days sooner than the primary care physicians. This led to a significantly shorter LOS (by 1 day) and a reduction in mean hospital costs by $600. Hospital physicians managed patients by similar processes of care as other physicians, however 14% of the patients that they discharged had one unstable clinical feature compared with only 7% with an unstable feature on discharge by a primary care physician. In addition the readmission rates were similar for patients treated by either physician group and mortality was lower for the hospital-treated patients. The authors concluded that the LOS and cost benefits occurred because hospital phycisians were more able to recognise clinical stability at an early time point and moved more aggressively to oral therapy than the other phycisans. In doing so they maximised cost–reducing opportunities without adversely impacting on outcome.

The impact of antibiotic selection and guidelines on the costs of care

As mentioned previously the use of antibiotic therapy consistent with published guidelines has been associated with reduced LOS for CAP patients. A number of studies have examined the impact of guideline-directed therapy, primarily for inpatients with CAP and have documented benefits ranging from reduced LOS to fewer days of intravenous (IV) antibiotics, and even reduced mortality [2]

The benefits of guideline-consistent antibiotic therapy

Gleason et al. [21] have examined the impact of following the 1993 American Thoracic Society (ATS) guidelines in outpatients with CAP. They found that for patients aged

<65 yrs without comorbid illness, therapy compatible with the guidelines (generally a macrolide alone) was associated with 3-fold lower costs and otherwise similar outcomes. In more complicated outpatients, therapy according to the guidelines was associated with higher cost and worse outcomes, however by today's standards the recommendations for that population included therapies which are not optimal. For example in the study 29% received therapy with trimethoprim/sulfamethoxizole, a recommended therapy at the time, but which was probably not always effective for the likely aetiological pathogens. In addition, unlike current recommendations, in 1993 routine coverage of atypical pathogens was not recommended. Most patients in the study treated in a way not compatible with guidelines did receive coverage for atypical pathogens (67% got a macrolide), and this may have also contributed to their better outcome.

Data from inpatients with CAP have shown that if therapy was administered with agents directed against pneumococcus and atypical pathogens, the patient's outcome was improved [22–24]. These specific antibiotic choices are consistent with current recommendations by both the ATS and the IDSA [15, 25]. Each of these groups recommends therapy with either an anti-pneumococcal quinolone alone, or the combination of a β-lactam (selected penicillin or cephalosporin) with a macrolide or tetracycline. In addition, the ATS guideline does allow for monotherapy with a macrolide for admitted patients who have no comorbid illness and no risk factors for drug-resistant organisms [25]. In a large study of ~13,000 Medicare patients, investigators found that compared with monotherapy, involving a third generation cephalosporin, mortality in CAP was reduced if a macrolide was added to either a second or third generation cephalosporin, or if a quinolone was used alone [22]. These findings have been interpreted to mean that routine therapy of atypical pathogens (either as primary pathogens or as co-infecting agents), in addition to pneumococcus, is needed, even for elderly patients with CAP. In that study, there was increased mortality when the combination of a macrolide and β-lactam/β-lactamase inhibitor was used, but the explanation for this finding is unknown.

Another large Medicare study also found that the addition of a macrolide to a β-lactam was associated with reduced mortality. However, when examined over three different calendar years, the magnitude of benefit was variable, suggesting temporal variability in the frequency of atypical pathogen co-infection [23]. One retrospective study in the support of a need for routine therapy of atypical pathogens, reported lower mortality rates in patients with bacteremic pneumococcal pneumonia when a macrolide or quionlone was administered in combination with a third generation cephalosporin than when a cephalosporin was administered alone [24]. Although one interpretation of these findings is that patients need combination and not monotherapy there were a few patients who received macrolide monotherapy and these patients had a 0% mortality. This suggests that the limitation of monotherapy with a third generation cehpalosporin may have been the failure to account for the possibility of atypical pathogen co-infection, even in patients with bacteremic pneumococcal pneumonia.

Other studies examining the impact of specific antibiotic-therapy regimens on the outcomes of CAP patients have shown that guideline-compatible therapies are beneficial. Using historical controls treated without the guideline algorithm and concurrent controls treated without the guideline, Dean et al. [26] identified a group of physicians who were directed to use the ATS guidelines to guide both outpatient and inpatient therapy of CAP. They found that the patients treated by physicians using the guideline had a significantly lower mortality than patients treated concurrently by physicians not using the guideline. Among admitted patients, mortality was reduced from 14.2% to 11.0 %, giving an OR for death of 0.69 for patients treated by the guideline pathway. These findings were particularly interesting, since patients treated by both groups of physicians had identical mortality rates before the intervention of guideline-directed therapy. Using historical controls, the investigators also showed that guideline implementation led to a 0.3 day reduction in LOS. In another study, involving 330 CAP patients evaluated retrospectively, investigators found that 51 were not treated according to the ATS guidelines and these patients had a 4.4 OR of death, compared with those treated by guidelines. It was also found that the guideline–compatible group had a significantly shorter LOS [27]. In fact, in a step-wise regression model looking at LOS, nonadherence to ATS guidelines was the most significant predictor of a prolonged LOS. The benefit of guideline adherence was greatest in patients with severe CAP. Similar conclusions were reached in a Spanish study that documented a reduced mortality in CAP patients treated in accordance with the ATS guidelines. However, the benefit was greatest in patients with the most severe illness (mortality of 9.3% *versus* 19.4%, comparing guideline *versus* nonguideline therapy for severe illness) [28].

Recently, NATHWANI *et al.* [3] summarised the benefits of guideline-directed therapy for CAP patients, focusing on ways that guidelines direct the use of antibiotics and the ways that these practices improve outcomes. They have emphasised the mortality benefits of administering antibiotic therapy within 8 h of arrival at the hospital. They have cited studies that document a benefit for both mortality and LOS if a macrolide is included in initial empiric therapy, again emphasising the need for routine therapy of atypical pathogens. In addition, they summarised the studies which reported that even when a guideline and pathway for care cannot reduce mortality, it can lead to a significant reduction in LOS.

The benefits of using specific antibiotic agents

While the studies cited above report an outcomes and cost benefit for the application of certain antibiotic-therapy principles when managing CAP, there are other studies that show the cost implications of choosing one antibiotic regimen rather than another. For example, FINCH *et al.* [29] compared the use of moxifloxacin monotherapy to a combination of clarithromycin with amoxicillin/clavulanate in an open label randomised study of 622 patients with CAP. In the study, more patients treated with the quinolone were afebrile by day 2 than were afebrile when treated with the comparator regimen (59% *versus* 46%). The more rapid response observed with the quinolone may explain why more patients were switched to oral therapy by day 3 in the quinolone arm of the study as compared with the comparator (50 *versus* 18%), although the study was not blinded. Therefore, it is possible that if certain antibiotics are effective and lead to a more rapid clinical response, there could be a change in the management, which could in turn lead to reduced care costs. However, no economical analysis was directly done in this study.

Other studies have looked directly at the cost-effectiveness of specific antibiotic choices. As mentioned previously, current therapy guidelines for complex patients admitted to the hospital, but not the ICU, recommend either monotherapy with an antipneumococcal quinolone, or combination therapy with a β-lactam/macrolide regimen. In one study, the cost-effectiveness of gatifloxacin was compared with that of ceftriaxone plus a macrolide in 283 CAP patients who were managed in a randomised, double-blinded clinical trial [30]. Approximately 33.3% of the ceftriaxone patients received therapy with a macrolide, the remainder received monotherapy. There was a small, but not statistically different, higher rate of treatment failure with ceftriaxone, but this translated into a significantly greater antibiotic-related LOS and mean cost per patient. The cost-effectiveness ratio (mean cost per success) was $5,236 for gatifloxacin compared with $7,047 for ceftriaxone, making the quinolone a more cost-effective choice. However, interestingly although the quinolone was always the most cost-effective choice, the addition of a macrolide to ceftriaxone increased drug costs, but led to reduced overall cost than ceftriaxone alone. This may have occurred due to the addition of the macrolide having an advantage in covering for atypical pathogen co-infection. This could therefore, explain why the use of a regimen with a macrolide led to a shorter LOS in hospital when related to antibiotic treatment failures than did ceftriaxone monotherapy.

Although most hospitalised CAP patients should not receive monotherapy with a macrolide, the ATS does recommend this regimen for admitted patients with no cardiopulmonary disease and no risk factors for drug resistant pneumococcus or enteric Gram–negative pathogens [25]. In one study, the use of azithromycin monotherapy was shown to be more cost–effective than therapy with cefuroxime, with or without the addition of erythromycin. Therefore, there may be a value in trying to identify appropriate candidates for azithromycin monotherapy [31]. In this study, 136 patients received azithromycin monotherapy, and 130 received cefuroxime (64 also received optional erythromycin), and the overall clinical outcomes were similar. However, the cost-effectiveness ratio was lower for azithromycin monotherapy than for the comparator ($5,265 *versus* $6,145). One clear implication from these findings is even though the acquisition cost of a drug such as azithromycin may exceed that of comparator agents, as in this study, the overall impact may still be favourable from a cost-effectiveness perspective. This can be explained by the reductions in LOS and duration of therapy that can occur with azithromycin, which leads to a LOS of 5.8 days compared with 6.4 days with the comparator. Similar data have also been obtained using doxycycline monotherapy, which led to lower costs and shorter LOS than comparator regimens, but in the study, the number of moderately ill patients was small [32].

The impact of a timely switch to oral therapy on discharge and length of stay in patients with community-acquired pneumonia

Since the duration of hospitalisation is a major driving factor that influences the cost of care for CAP, efforts at early discharge can have a major impact on the economical impact of this illness. Discharge generally occurs when patients have reached clinical stability and have been switched to oral antibiotic therapy. In general, there are a number of approaches to defining when to switch to oral therapy. However, many controversies remain in this area. These include whether it is necessary to observe the patient in the hospital on oral therapy after clinical stability has been achieved and whether it is necessary for patients to have no instabilities at the time of therapy switch and discharge.

RAMIREZ *et al.* [33] and associates have defined a set of criteria for the early switch from IV to oral therapy. In a study of 200 consecutive patients the switch to oral therapy was done when the following criteria were met: 1) cough and dyspnoea improved; 2) fever <37.8°C for ≥8 h; 3) white blood cell count normalising; and 4) oral intake and intestinal functions were adequate. In the study, discharge was considered when the patient was a candidate for oral therapy and when there was no requirement to treat any comorbid illness, no need for other diagnostic testing, and no unmet social needs. In this study 67% of patients had clinical improvement and met criteria for switch in therapy within the first 3 days, and 86% were improved by day 7. The mean LOS was 4.8 days, though only 3.4 days in patients who were switched early and who had no continued need for hospitalisation for nonpneumonia reasons. Once clinical improvement and switch of therapy occurred, there was only 1 patient who had a clinical failure and this patient improved with the reinstitution of IV therapy. Therefore, in this study, as in others, there was no real clinical benefit to keeping patients under observation in the hospital once the clinical criteria for switch had been met.

The need to keep patients in the hospital once clinical stability is achieved has been questioned, even though physicians commonly choose to observe patients on oral therapy for a day or so longer. In fact even in the presence of pneumococcal bacteremia, changing to oral therapy can be safely done once clinical stability is achieved and prolonged IV therapy is not needed [34]. Although it is safe fore bacteremic patients with pneumococcal pneumonia (without meningitis or endocarditis) to switch to oral therapy once stable, they do generally take longer (~0.5 day) to become clinically stable compared with nonbacteremic patients [34]. The benefits of in-hospital observation after changing to oral therapy were examined by RHEW et al. [35]. They found that this practice was not associated with the need for any medical intervention and therefore did not provide any clinical benefit. However, it did add to LOS by ~1 day and it added ~$550 to the cost of care.

While it is clear that clinically stable patients can be switched to oral therapy and be rapidly discharged, without a prolonged observation period in the hospital, it is uncertain if it is even necessary to wait for all the features of clinical stability to be present before a patient is moved onto oral therapy and sent home. As discussed previously, RIFKIN et al. [19] observed that a safe discharge could occur with some patients still having clinical instability and that hospital physicians (specialists in providing inpatient care) were more willing to discharge patients with instabilities than were family practioners [19]. However, not all instabilities may be the same and the definitions of stability vary among investigators. For example, RAMIREZ et al. [33] have included the white blood cell count as a parameter to monitor during CAP therapy, but HALM et al. [36] have not included this feature. The criteria used by HALM et al. [36] for clinical stability include: 1) fever <37.8 °C; 2) heart rate <100 min^{-1}; 3) respiratory rate <24 min^{-1}; 4) systolic blood pressure >90 mm·Hg^{-1}, 5) oxygen saturation of ≥90%; 6) ability to maintain oral intake; and 7) normal mental status. Using this definition, they found that 19.1% of 680 patients were discharged from the hospital with one or more instabilities. Death or readmission occurred in 10.5% of those with no instability on discharge, in 13.7% with one instability and in 46.2% with two or more instabilities. Overall, the risk of death or readmission was increased five-fold in patients with two or more instabilities. Interestingly, there was no correlation between LOS and the presence of instability on discharge, indicating that the discharge decision was not influenced by the presence of these features of instability. Based on their findings, the authors concluded that patients could be discharged if one instability was present, provided that patients in this category were closely followed. However, they recommended against discharge for any patient with two or more instabilities. While they did not fully evaluate whether one type of instability was more important than another, they noted that inability to eat and hypotension were the most serious single predictors of a poor outcome, if present at time of discharge.

An alternative approach in changingfrom IV to oral therapy, which may also be cost-effective, is to switch from IV to oral therapy at a pre-determined period of time, regardless of the clinical response. The first study to use this approach was by SIEGEL et al. [37] in which 75 patients were randomised to one of three approaches to 10 days of antibiotic therapy. One group received 2 days of IV therapy with cefuroxime, followed by 8 days of oral therapy. A second group was given 5 days IV and 5 days oral therapy with the same antibiotic and the third group received 10 days of IV cefuroxime. The design required some patients to switch even if they were not clinically stable, while others remained on IV therapy even though they were stable. In all three groups, the clinical responses were similar and the regimen selected did not impact on resolution of pneumonia features, with patients becoming afebrile after 2–3 days and having normal white blood cell counts by days 3–4. Discharge occurred at the discretion of the physician and LOS was directly related to the duration of IV therapy, thus early switch to oral therapy had dramatic cost benefits. The ability to achieve good outcomes, with as little as

2 days of IV therapy is interesting and suggests that many patients may be kept in hospital and on IV therapy for longer than is necessary.

This concept has recently been further expanded by a Spanish study that evaluated patients hospitalised with both mild and more severe illnesses [38]. Patients were considered either nonsevere or severe, depending on whether they had at least one severity criteria present. These criteria were: 1) arterial oxygen tension/inspiratory oxygen fraction ($Pa,O_2/FI,O_2$) ratio <286; 2) respiratory rate ≥ 30 min^{-1}, heart rate$\geq$ 125 min^{-1}; 3) systolic blood pressure <90 mm·Hg^{-1}; 4) fever >40 or <35°C, 5)altered mental status; 6) multilobar illness or progressive illness in spite of 72 h of prior therapy. The nonsevere populaton (no severity criteria present), were randomised to either oral therapy alone or IV therapy, with a switch after 72 h without fever. The severe population was randomised to either IV therapy with a switch to oral therapy after 2 days, or a full 10 day course of IV antibiotics. In all groups, therapy was with a cephalosporin or β-lactam/β-lactamase inhibitor combination, with the option of adding a macrolide. Oral switch was usually with a cephalosporin plus a macrolide. The investigators found that for the nonsevere patients, time to resolution of symptoms was similar with either regimen, and LOS and cost were similar. However, in the patients with severe illness, rapid switch to oral therapy had the same rate of treatment failures and time to resolution of symptoms as prolonged IV therapy, but the rapid switch group required fewer inpatient days (6 versus 11) and their cost of care was significantly lower (€1,247 versus €1,833). Not surprisingly, prolonged IV therapy was associated with more adverse events, including line-associated phlebitis and infection. Therefore, once again, this study demonstrated that prolonged IV therapy had no benefit, compared with a rapid switch to oral therapy and that similar outcomes were achieved with either approach, but rapid switch led to substantial cost savings.

It is beyond the scope of this discussion to examine which oral antibiotics should be used to replace IV therapy during a switch program. In general, it is acceptable to use an oral antibiotic that is either the same as the IV, or in the same drug class. The idea of switching to a highly bioavailable agent (such as a quinolone) in order to maintain high serum levels, while using oral therapy, is probably not necessary.

Conclusion

From the preceding discussion, it is clear that a number of interventions can be used to treat pneumonia in a cost–effective fashion. While many previous approaches have focused on limiting the number of patients who are admitted to the hospital, there are still a number of potent ways to reduce cost without focusing on the admission decision (table 1). These include: 1) providing initial antibiotics in a timely fashion; 2) using a highly active antimicrobial regimen that targets both common bacterial pathogens and atypical organisms; 3) rapidly addressing the social needs of patients prior to discharge; 4) using guidelines to direct initial empiric therapy; and 5) rapidly switching from IV to oral antibiotics in responding patients.

Although it may be essential to identify the responding patients as soon as possible, there are some studies that document the safety and efficacy of switch therapy after a brief course of IV therapy, regardless of the clinical response. If clinical stability is required prior to switch therapy, then it is clear that once patients meet these criteria, they can be switched and discharged without delay, provided that they have no other unmet medical or social needs. With an emphasis on these principles, pneumonia management can remain cost-effective, without denying admission to patients who may benefit from treatment and observation in the hospital.

Table 1. – Ways to achieve cost-effective management of community-acquired pneumonia

Strategy	Benefit
Limit admission to low risk	Fewer admissions, but some patients *i.e.* low risk patients need admission by clinical judgment and those incorrectly discharged may have adverse outcome
Timely antibiotic administration	Reduced mortality and LOS
Attention to unmet social needs on admission	Avoids predictable delays once patient is clinically stable
Empirical therapy according to existing guidelines	Reduced LOS and mortality
Therapy that covers atypical pathogens and bacterial pathogens	Reduced LOS and mortality
Therapy with selected antibiotics	
Macrolide monotherapy	Reduced cost, if used in appropriate patient
Quinolone monotherapy	Reduced cost, reduced LOS in appropriate patients
Rapid switch to oral therapy	Reduced cost and LOS

LOS: length of stay.

Summary

Pneumonia is a cost-intensive illness, especially if managed in the hospital rather than in the outpatient setting. In order to treat this illness in a cost–effective fashion, a variety of interventions are necessary. One approach is to reduce the number of patients admitted to the hospital, however, the optimal way to do this has not yet been defined. Alternatively, other aspects of care can be targeted. These include providing initial intravenous therapy in a timely fashion, which can reduce disease-associated mortality and the length of stay in hospital. Early attention to the social and non-pneumonia medical needs of patients can help facilitate a safe and early discharge. The use of adequate therapies that are consistent with the existing guidelines, along with the provision of adequate cover for atypical bacterial pathogens, can improve outcomes and reduce costs. For selected patients, monotherapy with a macrolide or a selected quinolone can lead to a more cost-effective outcome. Finally, a focus on rapid switch from intravenous to oral therapy, along with efforts at minimising the duration of therapy, can reduce the cost, length of stay and some of the complications of pneumonia.

Keywords: Community-acquired pneumonia, admission decision, switch therapy, antibiotic therapy, macrolides, quinolones.

References

1. Niederman MS, McCombs JS, Unger AN, Kumar A, Popovian R. The cost of treating community-acquired pneumonia. *Clin Ther* 1998; 20: 820–837.
2. Marrie TJ, Lau CY, Wheeler SL, Wong CJ, Vandervoort MK, Feagan BG. A controlled trial of a critical pathway for treatment of community-acquired pneumonia. CAPITAL Study Investigators. Community-acquired pneumonia intervention trial assessing levofloxacin. *JAMA* 2000; 283: 749–755.
3. Nathwani D, Rubinstein E, Barlow G, Davey P. Do guidelines for community-acquired pneumonia improve the cost-effectiveness of hospital care? *Clin Infect Dis* 2001; 32: 728–741.
4. Kaplan V, Angus DC, Griffin MF, Clermont G, Scott Watson R, Linde-Zwirble WT. Hospitalized community-acquired pneumonia in the elderly: age- and sex-related patterns of care and outcome in the United States. *Am J Respir Crit Care Med* 2002; 165: 766–772.

5. Fine MJ, Pratt HM, Obrosky DS, *et al.* Relation between LOS and costs of care for patients with community-acquired pneumonia. *Am J Med* 2000; 109: 378–385.

6. McCormick D, Singer DE, Coley CM, *et al.* Variation in length of hospital stay and its relation to medical outcomes in patients with community-acquired pneumonia. *Am J Med* 1999; 105: 5–12.

7. Halm EA, Fine MJ, Marrie TJ, *et al.* Time to clinical stability in patients hospitalised with community-acquired pneumonia. *JAMA* 1998; 279: 1452–1457.

8. Guest JF, Morris A. Community-acquired pneumonia: the annual cost to the National Health Service in the UK. *Eur Respir J* 1997; 10: 704–708.

9. Stelianides S, Golmard JL, Carbon C, Bantin B. Influence of socioeconomic status on features and outcome of community-acquired pneumonia. *Eur J Clin Microbiol Infect Dis* 1999; 18: 704–708.

10. Whittle J, Lin CJ, Lave Jr, Fine MJ, *et al.* Relationship of provider characteristics to outcomes, processes , and costs of care for community-acquired pneumonia. *Med Care* 1998; 36: 977–987.

11. Fine MJ, Hough LJ, Medsger AR, *et al.* The hospital admission decision for patients with community-acquired pneumonia. Results from the pneumonia Patient Outcomes Research Team cohort study. *Arch Intern Med* 1997; 157: 36–44.

12. Goss CH, Rubenfeld GD, Park DR, Sherbin VL, Goodman MS, Root RK. Cost incidence of social comorbidities in low-risk patients with community-acquired pneumonia admitted to a public hospital. *Chest* 2003; 124: 2051–2053.

13. Fine MJ, Medsger AR, Stone RA, *et al.* The hospital discharge decision for patients with community-acquired pneumonia. Results from the Pneumonia Patient Outcomes Research Team cohort study. *Arch Intern Med* 1997; 157: 47–56.

14. Fine MJ, Auble TE, Yealy Dm, *et al.* A prediction rule to identify low-risk patients with community-acquired pneumonia. *N Engl J Med* 1997; 336: 243–250.

15. Bartlett JG, Dowell SF, Mandell LA, File TM Jr, Musher DM, Fine MJ. Practice guidelines for the management of community-acquired pneumonia in adults. *Infectious Diseases Society of America Clin Infect Dis* 2000; 31: 347–382.

16. Minogue MF, Coley CM, Fine MJ, Marrie TJ, Kapoor WN, Singer DE. Patients hospitalised after intitial outpatient treatment for community-acquired pneumonia. *Ann Emerg Med* 1998; 31: 376–380.

17. Meehan TP, Fine MJ, Krumholz HM, *et al.* Quality of care, process, and outcomes in elderly patients with pneumonia. *JAMA* 1997; 278: 2080–2084.

18. Battleman DS, Callahan M, Thaler HT. Rapid antibiotic delivery and appropriate antibiotic selection reduce legth of stay of patients with community-acquired pneumonia. *Arch Intern Med* 2002; 162: 682–688.

19. Fine JM, Fine MJ, Galusha D, Petrillo M, Meehan TP. Patient and hospital characteristics associated with recommended processes of care for elderly patients hospitalised with pneumonia: results from the medicare quality indicator system pneumonia module. *Arch Intern Med* 2002; 162: 827–833.

20. Rifkin WD, Conner D, Silver A, Eichorn A. Comparison of processes and outcomes of pneumonia care between hospitalists and community-based primary care physicians. *Mayo Clin Proc* 2002; 77: 1053–1058.

21. Gleason PP, Kapoor WN, Stone RA, *et al.* Medical outcomes and antimicrobial costs with the use of the American Thoracic Society guidelines for outpatients with community-acquired pneumonia. *JAMA* 1997; 278: 32–39.

22. Gleason PP, Meehan TP, Fine JM, Galusha DH, Fine MJ. Associations between initial antimicrobial therapy and medical outcomes for hospitalized elderly patients with pneumonia. *Arch Intern Med* 1999; 159: 2562–2572.

23. Houck PM, MacLehose RF, Niederman MS, Lowery JK. Empiric antibiotic therapy and mortality among Medicare pneumonia inpatients in 10 Western states: 1993, 1995, 1997. *Chest* 2001; 119: 1420–1426.

24. Waterer GW, Somes GW, Wunderink RG. Monotherapy may be suboptimal for severe bacteremic pneumococcal pneumonia. *Arch Intern Med* 2001; 161: 1837–1842.

25. Niederman MS, Mandell LA, Anzueto A, *et al.* Guidelines for the management of adults with community-acquired pneumonia. Diagnosis, assessment of severity, antimicrobial therapy, and prevention. *Am J Respir Crit Care Med* 2001; 163: 1730–1754.

26. Dean NC, Silver MP, Bateman KA, James B, Hadlock CJ, Hale D. Decreased mortality after implementation of a treatment guideline for community- acquired pneumonia. *Am J Med* 2001; 110: 451–457.

27. Malone DC, Shaban HM. Adherence to ATS guidelines for hospitalized patients with community-acquired pneumonia. *Ann Pharmacother* 2001; 35: 1180–1185.

28. Mendendez R, Ferrqando D, Valles JM, Vallterra J. Influence of deviation from guidelines on the outcome of community-acquired pneumonia. *Chest* 2002; 122: 612–617.

29. Finch R, Schurmann D, Collins O, *et al.* Randomized controlled trial of sequential intravenous (i.v.) and oral moxifloxacin compared with sequential i.v. and oral co-amoxiclav with or without clarithromycin in patients with community-acquired pneumonia requiring initial parenteral treatment. *Antimicrob Agents Chemother* 2002; 46: 1746–1754.

30. Dresser LD, Niederman MS, Paladino JA. Cost-effectiveness of gatifloxacin vs. ceftriaxone with a macrolide for the treatment of community-acquired pneumonia. *Chest* 2001; 119: 1439–1448.

31. Paladino JA, Gudgel LD, Forrest A, Niederman MS. Cost-effectiveness of IV-to-Oral switch therapy: Azithromycin vs cefuroxime with or without erythromycin for the treatment of community-acquired pneumonia. *Chest* 2002; 122: 1271–1279.

32. Ailani RK, Agastya G, Alilani RK, Mukunda BN, Shekar R. Doxycycline is a cost-effective therapy for hospitalized patients with community-acquired pneumonia. *Arch Intern Med* 1999; 159: 266–270.

33. Ramirez JA, Vargas S, Ritter GW, *et al.* Early switch from intravenous to oral antibiotics and early hospital discharge: A prospective observational study of 200 consecutive patients with community-acquired pneumonia. *Arch Intern Med* 1999; 159: 2449–2454.

34. Ramirez JA, Bordon J. Early switch from intravenous to oral antibiotics in hospitalized patients with bacteremic community-acquired Streptococcus pneumoniae pneumonia. *Arch Intern Med* 2001; 161: 848–850.

35. Rhew DC, Hackner D, Henderson L, Ellrodt AG, Weingarten SR. The clinical benefit of in-hospital observation in "low risk" pneumonia patients after conversion from parenteral to oral antimicrobial therapy. *Chest* 1998; 113: 142–146.

36. Halm EA, Fine MJ, Kapoor WN, Singer DE, Marrie TJ, Siu AL. Instability on hospital discharge and the risk of adverse outcomes in patients with pneumonia. *Arch Intern Med* 2002; 162: 1278–1284.

37. Siegel RE, Halpern NA, Almenoff PL, Lee A, Cashin R, Greene JG. A prospective randomized study of inpatient IV antibiotics for community-acquired pneumonia. *Chest* 1996; 110: 965–971.

38. Castro-Guardiola A, Viejo-Rodriguez AL, Soler-Simon A, *et al.* Efficacy and safety of oral and early-switch therapy for community-acquired pneumonia: a randomised controlled trial. *Am J Med* 2001; 111: 367–374.

CHAPTER 14

Antibiotic treatment for nosocomial pneumonia

A. de Roux*, H. Lode*, A. Torres#

*Pneumologie I, Dept of Chest and Infectious Diseases, City Hospital, Emil von Behring affiliation, Free University of Berlin, Berlin, Germany, #Hospital Clinic of Barcelona, Barcelona, Spain.

Correspondence: A. de Roux, Pneumologie I, Dept of Infectious Diseases and Immunology, Chest City Hospital Heckeshorn, Zentralklinikum Emil von Behring, Zum Heckeshorn 33, 14109 Berlin, Germany.

The management of nosocomial pneumonia has been an object of intensive investigation during the previous two decades. Up to now some important aspects have been clarified. Firstly the recognition that early and late onset pneumonia represent two separate entities with important differences in epidemiology, risk factors, and prognosis has been established. Secondly, the role of antibiotics has been re-evaluated. Today there is strong evidence that early antibiotic treatment is crucial for a favourable outcome. However, risks associated with prolonged treatment with antimicrobial agents have been recognised. Besides the increasing costs of antibiotics it is apparent that the selection of potentially drug resistant microorganisms, associated with excess mortality, is also important. Although better treatment options, like new broad spectrum antibiotics are available, antimicrobial resistance is increasing.

Many studies have focused on the diagnostic and therapeutic strategies to improve the outcome. While some issues are clear others still remain controversial. Maybe the time has come to leave the individual diagnostic approach and turn to a more epidemiological point of view.

Previously the American Thoracic Society (ATS) made recommendations which emphasised the following aspects: 1) initial antimicrobial therapy for hospital-acquired pneumonia (HAP) must always be empirical; 2) any antibiotic regimen must be guided by the severity of the pneumonia, the time point of the pneumonia occurrence and specific risk factors; and 3) the selection of antimicrobial agents has to consider local microbial and resistance patterns. This framework can be used as a guide for the selection of appropriate antimicrobial agents.

This chapter will review the current present knowledge of antimicrobial treatment in nosocomial pneumonia. Furthermore, several issues of particular interest leading to new perspectives of antibiotic treatment will be addressed.

Aetiology of nosocomial pneumonia

Microorganisms associated with hospital-acquired pneumonia (HAP) differ from those isolated in community-acquired pneumonia (CAP). Responsible pathogens and their epidemiology have been investigated in numerous studies [1–7]. In general a high rate of Gram-negative bacteria like Gram-negative rods (mostly *Escherichia coli, Klebsiella spp., Enterobacter spp., Serratia spp. Proteus spp.*) and potentially multiresistant pathogens like *Pseudomonas aeruginosa, Acinetobacter spp.* and

Eur Respir Mon, 2004, 28, 211–228. Printed in UK - all rights reserved. Copyright ERS Journals Ltd 2004; European Respiratory Monograph; ISSN 1025-448x. ISBN 1-904097-32-4.

Stenotrophomonas spp. have been repeatedly reported [1, 3–11]. These strains are responsible for 55–85% of HAP cases. As regards Gram-positive bacteria *Staphylococcus aureus* has increasingly gained importance and it is estimated that it is now involved in 20–30% of HAP events [1, 3–7]. An important proportion of HAP events are polymicrobial, rates ranging between 13–60% [1, 12]. More uncommon microorganisms may appear, as *Legionella spp.* [13], anaeronbes [14], fungi [15] and respiratory viruses [16]. An overview of the different microorganisms responsible for HAP isolated in different series is depicted in table 1.

All reported series, dealing with the aetiology of HAP are heavily influenced by the type of patients selected and the diagnostic methods employed. However some issues are considered to have an important influence in the aetiology of HAP.

Orotracheal intubation. Orotracheal intubation favours a specific pathogenesis of infection associated with a different spectrum of microorganisms [2]. Although data are scarce there seems to be evidence that in spontaneous breathing patients multiresistant pathogens are less common and microorganisms as enteric Gram-negative bacilli, *Streptococcus pneumoniae* and methicillin sensitive *S. aureus* are more frequent.

Differentiation of the subgroups. The differentiation of the subgroups early and late onset pneumonia has been proven to be of paramount importance [7]. Early onset pneumonia is regarded as a consequence of the aspiration of the endogeneous community-acquired pathogens such as *S. aureus*, *S. pneumoniae*, and *Haemophilus influenzae*, with intubation and any type of impaired consciousness being the main risk factors [4, 17, 19]. Late onset pneumonia results from the aspiration of the oropharyngeal and gastric secretions, thereby including potentially drug-resistant nosocomial pathogens.

Previous antibiotic therapy. Previous antibiotic therapy is associated with an increased risk of infection with resistant pathogens. There is good evidence that the distribution of microorganisms responsible is markedly influenced by prior antibiotic use [7]. It is known that patients with a prolonged hospital stay and previous antibiotic treatment have the highest risk of infection by multiresistant pathogens such as *P. aeruginosa*, *Acinetobacter baumanii* and methicillin resistant *S. aureus* (MRSA) [7, 10].

Specific risk factors. Specific risk factors can modify the spectrum of potentially infecting microorganisms. *S. aureus* seems to be a common pathogen in patients suffering head injuries, coma incidences, chronic renal failure or diabetes mellitus [4, 18]. Patients with structural lung disease, bronchiectasis and advanced stages of chronic obstructive pulmonary disease (COPD) are prone to infections by *P. aeruginosa* [20]. A prolonged use

Table 1. – Bacteriology of hospital-acquired pneumonia

Early onset pneumonia	Late onset pneumonia	Other
Streptococcus pneumoniae	Psuedomonas aeruginosa	Anaerobic bacteria
Haemophilus influenzae	Enterobacter sp.	Legionella pneumophilia
Moraxella catarrhalis	Acinetobacter sp.	Influenza A and B
Staphylococcus aureus	Klebsiella. pneumoniae	Respiratory syncitial virus
Aerobic GNB[#]	Serratia marcescens	Fungi
	Escherichia coli	
	Other GNB	
	S. aureus[¶]	

GNB: Gram-negative baccilli; [#]: in patients with risk factors; [¶]: including methicillin resistant *S. aureus*. Adapted from FRANCIOLI *et al* [17].

of corticosteroids predisposes to infections caused by *Legionella spp.*, *P. aeruginosa* and *Aspergillus spp.*[20, 21]. The association of nonepidemic HAP caused by *Legionella spp.* and systemic steroid therapy was clearly shown in one study where further risk factors were malignancy, renal failure, neutropoenia and cytotoxic chemotherapy [22]. Aspiration will lead to infections, most frequently polymicrobial including anaerobes and Gram-negative bacilli [23].

Prevalence of infecting microorganisms. The prevalence of infecting microorganisms shows considerable local differences. Past antimicrobial treatment policies and the dominant patients characteristics (*e.g.* transplant patients, polytrauma patients or severe respiratory diseases) lead to specific, locally differing microbial and resistance patterns. Therefore each institution varies in its microbiological and susceptibility status [24, 25].

Aetiology in subsets of patients according to the American Thoracic Society guidelines

Based on the guidelines released by the ATS patients with an episode of HAP should be stratified into different groups, thereby allowing the most probable infecting agents to be identified. Guidance by the use of three criteria has been suggested, these include: 1) severity of pneumonia; 2) specific risk factors; and 3) the time point of the pneumonia occurrence. According to this determination patients will fall into one of three groups, each with its own set of microorganisms. A detailed description is given in table 2.

Patients without unusual risk factors. In patients without unusual risk factors or comorbid diseases, who present with mild-to-moderate HAP with onset at any time during hospitalisation or severe HAP of early onset the following core organisms should be considered: 1) community endogenous pathogens (*S. aureus*, *S. pneumoniae*, and *H. influenzae*); and 2) nonresistant Gram-negative Enterobacteriaceae (GNEB: including *E. coli*, *K. pneumoniae*, *Enterobacter spp.*, *Serratia spp.*, *Proteus spp.*)

Patients with specific risk factors. Patients with specific risk factors and/or comorbid diseases who present with mild-to-moderate HAP occurring at any time during hospitalisation or severe HAP of early onset have both core organisms and more specific microorganisms.

In addition to the previously mentioned core organisms the microbiological spectrum is influenced by specific risk factors and the time of onset. Potentially drug-resistant microorganisms must be taken into account. The role of specific risk factors has been commented on previously. According to the ATS guidelines those factors include risks for anaerobes (recent abdominal surgery), *S. aureus* (coma, head trauma, diabetes mellitus, renal failure), *Legionella spp.* (high-dose steroids) and *P. aeruginosa* (prolonged intensive care unit (ICU) stay, steroids, previous antibiotic treatment and structural lung disease). Furthermore if pneumonia develops after a prolonged hospital stay and/or the previous use of antibiotics, the risk of infections with multiresistant microorganisms is increased (MRSA, *P. aeruginosa*, *Acinetobacter spp.*, *Enterobacter spp.* and *Stenotrophomonas maltophilia*).

Patients with severe hospitalised-aquired pneumonia either of early onset with specific risk factors or of late onset. Crucial in this patient group is the severity of the disease in addition to the time of onset. The severity criteria suggested by the ATS are as follows: 1) admission to the ICU, respiratory failure (mechanical ventilation or >35%

Table 2. – Risk factors for infections by specific microorganisms according to severity, time of onset and specific risk factors, applicable to nonimmunocompromised patients

Group	Group patient characteristics	Core organisms (plus)
Group I	Patients with mild to moderate HAP No unusual risk factors Onset any time or Patients with severe disease and early onset	Enteric GNB (non-pseudomonal) Enterobacter spp. Escherichia coli Klebsiella spp. Proteus spp. Serratia marcescens Haemophilus influenzae MRSA Streptococcus pneumoniae
	Specific comments Early onset VAP in patients with previous antibiotic therapy (within the previos 15 days)	Risk of multiresistant pathogens Pseudomonas aeruginosa, Acinetobacter sp., Stenotrophomonas maltophilia (30%) MRSA (5–18%) TROUILLET et al [7] and IBRAHIM et al [10]
	Late onset, nonventilated	Risk of resistant GNB possible
Group II	Patients with mild to moderate HAP With risk factors, Onset any time	Anaerobes Recent abdominal surgery Witnessed aspiration Staphylococcus aureus Coma, head trauma, diabetes, mellitus, renal failure Legionella spp. High dose steroids Pseudomonas aeruginosa Prolonged ICU stay, steroids Antibiotics, structural lung disease, COPD
	Specific comments In case of previous antibiotic treatment Contact with children, >65 yrs, comorbid	Risk of multiresistant pathogens Resistant S. pneumoniae possibly
Group III	Patients with severe HAP With risk factors Early onset or patients with severe HAP with late onset Consider local epidemiology and resistance patterns	P. aeruginosa Acinetobacter spp. S. maltophilia MRSA

HAP: hospital-acquired pneumonia; GNB: Gram-negative bacilli; VAP: ventilator-associated pneumonia; MRSA: methicillin resistanct S. aureus; ICU: intensive care unit; COPD: chronic obstructive pulmonary disease. Data adapted from TROUILLET et al. [7], AMERICAN THORACIC SOCIETY [8], IBRAHIM et al. [10], LODE et al. [26] and EWIG et al. [27].

oxygen to maintain the saturation >90%); and 2) radiographical progression and severe sepsis with hypotension.

Cases of severe HAP with no risk factors, with early onset would rather belong to the first group. Hereby the main microorganisms responsible for infection would be *H. influenza* and Methicillin-sensitive *S. aureus* but further potentially resistant microorganisms must be considered. These include multiresistant MRSAs, GNEB, and *P. aeruginosa*, *Acinetobacter spp.*, as well as *S. maltophilia*. This is particularly true in cases of prolonged mechanical ventilation for >7 days and broad spectrum antimicrobial pretreatment [7].

The ATS guidelines do not make specific recommendations for nonventilated patients with nosocomial pneumonia. As a consequence patients with HAP, without severity criteria as well as pneumonia not occurring in the ICU are categorised as nonsevere pneumonia. They are treated as early onset HAP, with modifications in cases of additional risk factors. Although the data is scarce, it seems quite probable that the time point of pneumonia does also play a role in nonintubated patients [2].

As regards the concept of early and late onset ventilator-associated pneumonia some issues have not yet been satisfactorily resolved. A crucial factor is the starting point for the definition of early onset pneumonia, the use of hospital admission time, ICU admission time or intubation time are all possible. If the time of ICU admission is used as the starting point, patients may already have been extensively colonised during their previous hospital stay, and consequently, differences between early and late onset pneumonia are no longer evident [28]. In accordance with the ATS guidelines the use of the time of hospital admission as starting point appears reasonable. The cut-off time separating early and late onset ventilator-associated pneumonia (VAP) has been the subject of many controversies. The ATS suggested the use of the fifth day after hospital admission [8]. In a study investigating patients with central nervous system injury it was shown that colonisation patterns markedly changed within 3–4 days. Initially the oropharynx, nose and tracheobronchial tree were colonised with endogenous community-acquired pathogens, this pattern was subsequently replaced by an increasing amount of typical nosocomial pathogens [4]. TROUILLET et al. [7] could demonstrate that the length of intubation and previous antimicrobial treatment can reasonably predict the relation of core and potentially drug-resistant microorganisms. In this study, the cut-off differentiating early and late onset VAP was seven days. This prospective investigation in which the microorganisms responsible for infections in 135 consecutive episodes of VAP was documented lead to the differentiation of four groups. These were early and late onset pneumonia (>7 days) either with or without previous antibiotic therapy. As regards early and late onset pneumonia the risk for multiresistant bacteria was significantly increased by the use of previous antibiotics. Although the conclusions drawn from the study can only be applied to ventilated patients the results allowed the authors to suggest a decision tree for selecting initial antimicrobial treatment. However, a different study study demonstrated that in an ICU setting, even in early onset nosocomial pneumonia, resistant pathogens were frequent. The authors concluded that probable reasons were prior antibiotic therapy, severe basic disease and hospital stay [10]. Overall the importance of prior antimicrobial therapy is not sufficiently reflected in the ATS guidelines.

Further, emphasis on previously mentioned local differences in resistance patterns and microbiology should be made. The aetiology of nosocomial pneumonia varies from institution to institution and the kind of patients admitted [29, 30]. Further national differences have been described e.g. Enterobacter spp. was found to be more frequent in the US whilst Acinetobacter spp. is more prevalent in Europe [1, 31].

Different patient risk factors predispose them to infections by specific pathogens which may play an important role in early onset HAP. This applies especially to medical patients. Recent guidelines for the treatment of CAP have stressed that underlying medical conditions predispose to certain pathogens [32]. As community-acquired pathogens play an important role in early onset HAP, specific risk factors, present in the ambulatory setting, do not cease to exist after admission to the hospital. This might be of particular interest in patients with advanced stages of COPD and/or structural lung disease which are prone to infections by difficult to treat Gram-negative bacteria i.e. P. aeruginosa [33]. The role of antibiotic resistant strains of S. pneumoniae in HAP is not known. Risk factors such as advanced age, alcoholism, multiple medical comorbidities, living in a nursing home or exposure to children in a day care centre, identified for CAP, can also be of importance in the nosocomial setting.

The ATS guidelines and the classification of VAP suggested by TROUILLET et al. [7] has been validated the focus on microbiological data and the potential adequacy of selected antimicrobial regimens in a recently published study [34]. A total of 124 patients with HAP in a French ICU were retrospectively categorised according to the ATS guidelines [8] and the classification of TROUILLET et al. [7]. With the ATS classification patients were included into classes (1 and 3) with an increasing frequency of resistant pathogens (0–30.3%). The subsequently recommended antibiotic treatment appeared valid but proposed combinations including vancomycin for 72.5% of patients. TROUILLET et al. [7] classification categorised patients into four groups with a frequency of resistant pathogens from 4.9–35.6%. Vancomycin was proposed for 48.5% of patients. Although the ATS classification was more specific than the one by TROUILLET et al. [7] for predicting the absence of resistant causative pathogens in HAP, it lead to a greater use of vancomycin. The authors finally concluded that a stratification combining the two classifications could be an interesting alternative.

In conclusion an alternative option would be to amend the severity-based approach of the ATS guidelines to an algorithm that separates pneumonia in the nonintubated and intubated patient, further differentiates between early and late onset, and allows modifications according to the presence of risk factors allows. The recently established German guidelines for the treatment and prevention of nosocomial pneumonia suggest such an approach [27].

Current recommendations of empirical antimicrobial treatment based on the American Thoracic Society guidelines

Despite intensive investigational activity so far no consensus has been reached in basic issues as the optimal antibiotic treatment or the duration of therapy. Whereas appropriate antimicrobial treatment improves the outcome of HAP, inappropriate therapy is associated with an increased risk of death from pneumonia [29, 35]. Moreover, even if the initially inappropriate antimicrobial treatment is corrected according to diagnostic results, there remains an excess mortality compared with patients treated appropriately from the beginning [36].

Conversely, antimicrobial treatment is not without risk. Various epidemiological investigations have shown a clear relationship between increasing resistance rates and the use of antimicrobial agents [37, 38]. In a study by RELLO et al. [20] antimicrobial pretreatment was the only adverse prognostic factor in a multivariate model. However if pneumonia, due to high-risk organisms (P. aeruginosa, Acinobacter calcoaceticus, Serratia marcescens, Proteus mirabilis and fungi) was included in the model, the presence of these high risk organisms was the only independent predictor and antimicrobial pre-treatment entirely dropped out [29]. Furthermore recommendations for initial empirical antimicrobial treatment must accommodate local variations in infecting organisms and their resistance patterns [25, 39].

Limitations of diagnostic criteria for the diagnosis of HAP in the individual patient have fundamental consequences for any antimicrobial treatment strategy. As a consequence the following issues must be taken into account, partly already described by the American ATS guidelines [8]. These include: 1) the empirical character of any initial antimicrobial treatment; 2) empirical initial antimicrobial treatment can be guided by three criteria, including severity of pneumonia, time point of pneumonia occurrence, and specific risk factors; 3) the selection of particular antimicrobial agents and regimens must be adopted to regional or even local peculiarities of microbial and resistance patterns; and 4) microbiological results of diagnostic measurements may offer additional clues which must be interpreted in the context of the clinical condition of the patient.

Such information (obtained by bronchoalveolar lavage or protected specimen brush: PSB) may be particularly relevant in case of nonresponse to empirical initial antimicrobial treatment.

Based on the ATS guidelines, the following general recommendations for an empirical initial antimicrobial treatment of suspected HAP can be made:

Patients with early onset hospital acquired pneumonia and no risk factors. In these patients, core organisms such as community endogeneous pathogens (*S. aureus, S. pneumoniae,* and *H. influenzae*) and nonresistant GNEB, including *E. coli, K. pneumoniae, Enterobacter spp., Serratia spp., Proteus spp.*) should be appropriately covered. This can be afforded by a monotherapy consisting of a second-generation cephalosporin, third generation cephalosporin (cefotaxime or ceftriaxone) or an aminopenicillin plus β-lactamase inhibitor. Fluorquinolones or a combination of clindamycin and aztreonam are alternatives.

Patients with late onset hospital-acquired pneumonia and no risk factors. In addition to these core organisms, potentially drug resistant microorganisms must be taken into account. This is particularly true in cases of prolonged mechanical ventilation for more than 7 days and broad spectrum antimicrobial pretreatment [7]. These include multiresistant MRSA, GNEB, and *P. aeruginosa, Acinetobacter spp.,* as well as *S. maltophilia.* Although not proven by randomised studies, it seems prudent to administer a combination treatment, including an antipseudomonal penicillin (+β-lactamase inhibitor) or cephalosporin, a carbapenem together with a quinolone (ciprofloxacin) or an aminoglycoside. Vancomycin may be added where MRSA is a concern, especially in patients with head injury or in a coma.

Patients with early or late onset hospital-aquired pneumonia and risk factors. These patients are at risk of peculiar pathogens and should be treated according to the specific risk factors. Virtually always this treatment is identical to late onset HAP without risk factors, except in the presence of risk factors for *Legionella spp.* In that instance, these pathogens must be covered additionally. A summary of the drugs and dosage regimens are given in table 3.

Specific considerations

The principal dilemma of potential over treatment at the cost of increased microbial selection pressure could be addressed more satisfactorily if future approaches could succeed in increasing the pretest probability of the presence of pneumonia according to clinical criteria. This could be afforded by the following investigational tools:

Clinical criteria for the diagnosis of HAP currently in use (a new and persistant infiltrate in chest radiograph in addition with one to three of the following: fever or hypothermia; leucocytosis or leucopenia; and purulent tracheobronchial secretions) are outdated. It is inappropriate to ignore changes in oxygenation, the criteria for severe sepsis and/or septic shock. As regards VAP, PUGIN *et al.* [40] has suggested a scoring system, including the following six weighted clinical and microbiological variables: temperature, white blood cell count, nature and average of tracheobronchial aspirate volume, gas exchange ratio and chest radiograph infiltrates. Although this score is tedious to calculate and includes microbiological criteria it achieved a sensitivity of 72% and a specificity of 85% in a post mortem study [41]. More specific criteria for the diagnosis of VAP might significantly improve the predictive value of clinical judgment.

Table 3. – General framework for empirical initial antimicrobial treatment of ventilated-acquired pneumonia

Patient	Class of antimicrobial agents	Agents and dose regimen
Ventilated patient		
Early onset, no risk factors	Cephalosporin II	Cefuroxime 3×1.5 g
	Or	
	Cephalosporin III	Cefotaxim 3×2 g
	Or	Ceftriaxone 2×1 g
	Aminopenicillin/β-lacatamase inhibitor	Amoxicillin/clavulanic acid 3×2,2 g
	Or	
	Second-line quinolone	Levofloxacin 2×500 mg
	Or	
	Clindamycin/aztreonam	Clindamycin 3×600 mg
		aztreonam 3×2 g
Late onset, no risk factors	Quinolone	Ciprofloxacin 3×400 mg
	Or	
	Aminoglycoside	Gentamicin 5–7 mg·kg^{-1}
		Tobramycin 5–7 mg·kg^{-1}
	Plus	Amikacin 1×15 mg·kg^{-1}
	Antipseudomonal β-lactam/	Piperacillin/tazobactam 3×4.5 g
	β-lactamase-inhibitor	
	Or	
	Ceftazidime	Ceftazidime 3×2 g
	Or	
	Carbapenems	Imipenem/cilastatin 3×1 g
		Meropenem 3×1 g
	Plus/minus	
	Vancomycin	Vancomycin 2× g
Early or late onset, risk factors	Risk factors for *Pseudomonas aeruginosa*	
	Refer to late onset	
	Risk factors for *MRSA*:	
	+Vancomycin	Vancomycin 2×1 g
	Risk factor for *Legionella spp.*	
	Macrolide	Erythromycin 4×1 g
		Or
		Azithromycin 1×500 mg
		Or
		Clarithromycin 2×500 mg
		Or
		Levofloxacin 2×500 mg
		Or
		Moxifloxacin 1×400 mg
Nonventilated patient		
Early onset, no risk factors	Refer to ventilated patients	
Late onset, no risk factors	Refer to ventilated patients	
	Possibly monotherapy in the	
	absence of severe pneumonia	
Early or late onset, risk factors	Refer to ventilated patient	

Furthermore the comprehension of markers of the inflammatory response associated with HAP in particular, could be of help in guiding antimcrobial treatment decisions.

In addition it would be helpful if a validated scoring system could be used to guide the decision as to when an antimicrobial treatment could be safely withheld or stopped. A crucial question of any empirical antimicrobial treatment concept is whether treatment maybe withheld or whether it may even be stopped in the presence of bacterial counts below the threshold.

Firstly, it has generally been agreed that in patients exhibiting signs of severe sepsis or septic shock empirical antimicrobial treatment must be given. Secondly, it could be shown that patients with clinically suspected VAP yielding borderline colony counts ($\geq 10^2$ though $<10^3$ cfu·mL^{-1} in PSB) who were left untreated had an excess mortality if they developed significant colony counts in a repeated investigation within 72 h as compared to those who did not [42]. Thus, it is argued that stable patients with suspected VAP according to judicious clinical judgment but without an established pathogen and without an alternative diagnosis, compatible with these symptoms, should continue to receive empirical antimicrobial treatment. The main reason for this attitude is that in this situation the potential short-term consequences for the individual patient, if left untreated, outweighs concerns regarding over treatment, resulting in microbial resistance. In contrast to CAP, severity assessment of VAP has not received much attention [43]. However, it is evident that valid severity criteria may be of great help in deciding when antimicrobial treatment can be safely withheld or stopped.

Issues of particular interest

Monotherapy versus *combination therapy*

Until only a few years ago, most intensive care specialists and infectious disease consultants used combination therapy consisting of β-lactam antibiotics and an aminoglycoside to treat nosocomial pneumonia. The rationale was that such treatment would provide a broad spectrum antimicrobial activity, which would delay the onset of bacterial resistance and work synergistically. However, arguments have arisen which lay claim to combination therapy being too expensive and in danger of exposing patients to multiple toxicities and thereby increasing the risk of antibiotic-associated complications. The addition of an aminoglycoside has particularly been associated with drug-related toxicities. Further, new broad spectrum and highly bactericidal antibiotics, including carbapenems, penicillins with β-lactamase inhibitors, and fluoroquinolones are available [44].

Therefore, a major clinical question is whether the use of a single antibiotic is sufficient for the treatment of nosocomial infections (table 4).

Studies favouring combination therapy

As previously described resistant microorganisms *e.g. P. aeruginosa* are a serious problem in HAP. Several studies have shown that monotherapy for pseudomonal HAP is associated with an elevated rate of clinical failures, relapses, mortality and the development of resistance in 30–50% of the patients [45–46]. HILF *et al.* [47] performed a prospective clinical study of 200 patients with bacteremic *P. aeruginosa* infections. The

Table 4. – Antibiotic Therapy in Nosocomial Pneumonia: monotherapy *versus* combination therapy

Monotherapy	Antibiotic combination
Lower cost	Higher cost
Lower risk of side effects	Possible lower risk of emergence of resistance
No antagonistic effect of antibiotics	Synergistic effect
No pharmacological interactions	Wider spectrum
Equal efficacy	Lower antibiotic dose

Adapted from LODE [44].

main results showed that the mortality rate of patients receiving combination therapy was significantly lower than for monotherapy (27 *versus* 47%, p<0.02) [47].

A different study investigated the effects of combination therapy *versus* monotherapy against *Klebsiella spp.* bacteremia in 230 patients. The results showed that the 14-day mortalities in the two groups were similar (20 and 18%). However, within the subgroup of patients who experienced hypotension within 72 h prior to, or on the day of the positive blood culture, the patients who received combination therapy experienced significantly lower mortality (24%) when compared with those on monotherapy (50%) [48]. It has to be stated here that the β-lactam agents used in these studies had less potent activity than the modern antibiotics used today. A controlled multicentre, randomised European trial of 129 patients with cancer, granulocytopenia and Gram-negative bacteremia supported a benefit of adjunctive aminoglycoside treatment [49]. Ceftazidime plus either a short course (3 days) or a long (9 days) course of treatment were compared. Clinical response rates were highest with ceftazidime plus a long (9 days) course of treatment with amikacin. In addition the benefit of the aminoglycoside was pronounced when *P. aeruginosa* was implicated, resulting in 89% response for the long course *versus* 38% for the short course.

Studies favouring monotherapy. LA FORCE *et al.* [50] compared the efficacy of monotherapy and combination therapy in the management of nosocomial pneumonia. This study demonstrated that monotherapy with new antibiotics such as ceftazidime, aztreonam, cefoperazone, achieved a superior clinical success rate of 88% when compared with combination therapy which had a rate of only 76%. Furthermore the rate of superinfections was lower in the group treated with monotherapy (12 *versus* 18%). The effectiveness of the newer carbapenems for monotherapy of HAP was supported by a further study by SIEGER *et al.* [51]. In this study meropenem was compared with a combination of ceftazidime/tobramycin in patients with hospital-acquired lower respiratory tract infections. The analysis of efficacy was based on the clinical and bacteriological responses at the end of treatment. A total of 121 patients were evaluated. The clinical response was found to be superior in the meropenem-treated patients (89%) compared with 72% in the combination therapy group (p=0.04). Further, bacteriological response rates were significantly higher in the meropenem group (89 *versus* 67%; p=0.006). However both treatment groups tolerated the antibiotics well and additional toxicity caused by the aminoglycosides was not observed.

Monotherapy with imipenem has also been compared with a combination of imipenem plus netilmicin for the empirical treatment of nosocomial pneumonia, nosocomial sepsis, and severe diffuse peritonitis. Monotherapy was successful in 80% of the cases and combination therapy in 86%. Emergence of *P. aeruginosa* resistant to imipenem occurred in 6% of the patients treated with monotherapy and in 9% of those treated with the combination therapy. The authors concluded that the addition of netilmicin increased nephrotoxicity and did not prevent the emergence of resistant *P. aeruginosa* strains [52].

Previously two studies were conducted to compare different regimens of monotherapy treatment. One involved a prospective multicentre study which compared the efficacy of intravenous (IV) ciprofloxacin or imipenem in the treatment of severe nosocomial pneumonia requiring mechanical ventilation [53]. Only patients with a significant growth for potentially pathogenic microorganisms in quantitative bacterial cultures were included in the study. The success rates were satisfactory, however neither the clinical success rate (ciprofloxacin 71%; imipenem 79%) nor the bacteriological response rate (ciprofloxacin 49%; imipenem 50%) were significantly different between the study arms. In the subgroup of patients with *P. aeruginosa* (35%) both study medications showed nonsignificantly different clinical (ciprofloxacin: 71%; imipenem: 67%) or bacteriological response rates (ciprofloxacin: 50%; imipenem: 25%). Resistance by *P. aeruginosa* developed in 7% cases to ciprofloxacin and 33% cases to imipenem (p=0.147). In addition the mortality did not differ between both treatment arms. The authors finally concluded that treatment with both substances was equally effective. However, smaller differences between the treatment-arms of the study may have been missed due to sample-size limitations, especially as regards the development of resistance to *P. aeruginosa* [53].

A different multicentre, randomised double-blind trial compared intravenous ciprofloxacin with imipenem/cilastatin in 405 patients with severe pneumonia. A total of 79% of the patients required mechanical ventilation. The primary and secondary efficacy endpoints in this study were bacteriological and clinical responses at 3–7 days after the completion of therapy. The patients who received ciprofloxacin demonstrated a higher bacteriological eradication rate than those in the imipenem group (69 *versus* 59%; p=NS). Clinical response rates were also significantly higher in the ciprofloxacine group (69 *versus* 56%; p=0.02). Ciprofloxacin resulted more effective in the eradication of *Enterobacteriaceae* (93 *versus* 65%; p=0.009). However, when *P. aeruginosa* was recovered from initial respiratory tract cultures, only 41% responded to imipenem and 33% to ciprofloxacin. Resistance developed in 33% of the patients treated with ciprofloxacin and in 53% of the patients receiving imipenem. The authors concluded that in patients with severe pneumonia, monotherapy with ciprofloxacin was as least as effective as monotherapy with imipenem in terms of bacteriological eradication and clinical response. Although equally effective the authors suggest that monotherapy either with imipenem or ciprofloxacin can not be recommended for pneumonia when *P. aeruginosa* is suspected [46].

The majority of monotherapy studies addressed patients with an Acute Physiology, Age and Chronic Health Evaluation (APACHE) II score <20, consequently no evidence based data are available for the more severe patient population suffering from nosocomial pneumonias. In accordance to the guidelines published by the ATS all seriously ill patients should receive empirical combination therapy, targeting *P. aeruginosa* until culture results are available. Furthermore patients with an increased risk for *P. aeruginosa* e.g. those with prolonged steroid treatment, COPD or structural lung disease would benefit from combination therapy. However, more data are needed to support this as studies targeting other multiresistant Gram-negative bacteria i.e. *Acinetobacter spp.* or *S. maltophilia* are scarce.

The role of aminoglycosides

Aminoglycosides have been used for ~30 yrs for the treatment of nosocomial pneumonia. However, few data exist on the optimisation of dosing regimens. Today the role of aminoglycosides deserves further comment as the data accumulated are controversial. While the synergistic bactericidal activity against *P. aeruginosa* of a β-lactam in combination with an aminoglycoside is clearly shown *in vitro*, there is some doubt about a synergistic advantage *in vivo* [48, 54]. Aminoglycosides are the cheapest available antibiotics active against *P. aeruginosa*. In addition to this they are bactericidal in a concentration-dependent manner and show a prolonged postantibiotic effect enhancing bacterial growth even after serum levels are below the minimal inhibitory concentration (MIC) of the target organisms [55]. Drawbacks however are the narrow therapeutic range, the poor penetration into the lung parenchyma and a decreased activity in the presence of a low pH of the infected airways. While the bronchial secretion to serum ratio of fluoroquinolones is 0.8–2.0, higher than those in plasma, aminoglycosides only reach 0.2–0.6.

KASHUBA *et al.* analysed 78 patients with nosocomial pneumonia caused by Gram-negative bacteria treated with aminoglycosides, mostly in combination with a β-lactam antibiotic. Logistic regression predicted a 90% probability for resolution of the endpoints of temperature and leukocyte count resolution by day 7 if a C_{max}/MIC ratio of ≥ 10 was achieved within the first 48 h of therapy. The results of the study emphasise early, aggressive aminoglycoside dosing immediately followed by individualised pharmacokinetic monitoring to ensure optimal C_{max}/MIC ratios.

This pharmacocinetic consideration, lead to specific dosing regimens, in particular the administration of aminoglycosides once daily. Administration in this manner leads to peak concentrations that decline rapidly, thereby taking advantage of the concentration-dependent killing manner and the prolonged postantibiotic effect, minimising the toxicity.

Local application of aminoglycosides

To avoid systemic toxicity a direct instillation of aminoglycosides into the respiratory tract appears to make sense. A double-blind randomised trial including patients with endobronchial tubes or tracheostomies and documented Gram-negative bacilli infection (GNB) compared the clinical efficacy of intratracheal instillation of tobramycin (40 mg·8 h^{-1}) *versus* saline solution. All patients received concomitant, systemic therapy with a β-lactam antibiotic and an aminoglycoside. GNB were eradicated from sputum more frequently in the tobramycin group (68 *versus* 31% in the controls). However, clinical improvement was identical in both groups (81 *versus* 80%) [56]. Other studies have come to similar conclusions [57]. The local application of aminoglycosides appears to be an interesting option but more data are needed before this procedure can be generally recommended.

Duration of treatment

The duration of antibiotic treatment for HAP has never been defined clearly. In general, carefully controlled studies documenting duration of therapy have not been reported. In VAP, most series show a duration of ~10 days [46, 52]. The main arguments against a prolonged duration of treatment include the selection of resistant microorganisms, the increased risk of adverse events and elevated antibiotic costs. However, short courses may lead to treatment failure or a relapse, particularly in the presence of resistant microorganisms. The recommendations of the ATS are to adapt the duration of treatment according to the severity of the case, the time to clinical response and the responsible microorganism [8]. A short course lasting 7–10 days is recommended in the presence of *H. influenzae* and methicilline-sensitive *S. aureus*. A long course of treatment is suggested when microorganisms with a high risk of treatment failure are implicated, *i.e.* *P. aeruginosa* or *Acineobacter spp.* Furthermore, multilobar involvement, malnutrition, severe debilitation, cavitation, or necrotising pneumonia may be associated with delayed and often incomplete resolution. Therefore therapy lasting 14–21 days is recommended in these patients.

In an elegant study, SINGH *et al.* [58] randomised patients with suspected nosocomial pneumonia (58% VAP) and a Pugin score <6 (*i.e.* low clinical probability of pneumonia) into patients who received a standard antimicrobial treatment at the discretion of the attending physician *versus* those who received a 3 day course with ciprofloxacin. After 3 days, patients were revaluated and antimicrobial treatment was stopped in those with a persistent Pugin score <6, whereas those with a higher score received a full course of standard antimicrobial treatment. The duration of hospitalisations and mortality were not different between both randomisation groups, however resistance and superinfection rates were higher in the control group (15 *versus* 39%).

In order to reduce the microbial selection pressure imposed by empirical antimcirobial treatment a reduction in treatment duration is very important. The main challenge in such a concept would be to identify the low risk groups and to treat patients with potentially drug resistant microorganisms *i.e. P. aeruginosa* and *Acinetobacter spp.* as a separate group. Because clinical criteria are unspecific and radiological resolution might last, it is not known when empirical therapy can be withheld or withdrawn safely. It can take as long as 6 days for fever and other clinical signs of pneumonia to improve under appropriate antibiotic treatment [59, 60]. In the ICU-setting some studies show that it may be safe to withdraw therapy when quantitative cultures of the lower respiratory tract are sterile or show a bacterial concentration under the threshold of infection [61, 62]. However, it must be emphasised that these studies were not designed to address the issue of withdrawing therapy. The decision to stop antibiotic therapy was made by the physician based on culture results and clinical status. The results from the study published by SINGH *et al.* [58] shifted the perspective away from conflictive diagnostic issues. Instead a strategy was implemented which allowed, at the same time, to reduce the risk of individual undertreatment and general overtreatment with its inherent consequences.

New antibiotics

New antimicrobial drugs

In view of the growing microbial resistance rates worldwide, particularly those of Gram-positive microrganisms, the evaluation of new antimicrobial drugs becomes an emergent issue. The glycopeptides (vancomycin and teicoplanin) have been one of the last therapeutic options for infections due to multiresistant Gram-positive microorganisms, including MRSA. Despite this vancomycin has some clear disadvantages, it is only slowly bactericidal against staphylococci, furthermore it does not penetrate well into cerebrospinal fluid. Glycopeptides are potentially nephrotoxic and rapid infusion might lead to histamine release [63]. There are two promising drugs which have been investigated in nosocomial pneumonia associated with Gram-positive pathogens, these are quinopristin/dalfopristin and linezolid.

Quinopristin/dalfopristin. This is the first injectable streptogramin antibiotic. It is composed of two semisynthetic streptogramin molecules derived from *Streptomyces pristinaespirali.* Quinopristin/dalfopristin is active against a wide range of Gram-positive microorganisms including MRSA.

In a prospective, randomised, open-label multicentre study quinopristin/dalfopristin (7.5 mg·kg^{-1}·per 8 h) was compared to vancomycin (1 g per 12 h) in patients with nosocomial pneumonia. Aztreonam and tobramycin could be added in both groups as required. In total 208 patients were included in the study. In the bacteriologicaly evaluable population, cure or improvement could be achieved in 56.3% and 58.3%, respectively. Likewise, the clinical success rates for defined Gram-positive microorganisms were equivalent. Adverse effects were frequent in both groups; antimicrobial treatment was discontinued because of adverse reactions in 15.3% and 9.5% respectively. Therefore, quinopristin/dalfopristin and vancomycin were equivalent in the treatment of nosocomial pneumonia caused by Gram-positive organisms [64].

Linezolid. This is the first of a new class of antibacterial drugs, the oxazolidinones. It inhibits bacterial protein synthesis, though unlike other protein synthesis inhibitors, Linezolid acts early in translation, thereby preventing the formation of a functional initiation complex [65]. A clear advantage of this mechanism is that cross-resistance with other antibacterial drugs is not expected. Linezolid is effective against a broad range of bacteria including MRSA, glycopeptide-intermediate *S. aureus*, vancomycin resistant enterococci, and penicillin resistant *S. pneumoniae*. The drug also shows activity against certain anaerobes including *Clostridium perfingens*, *Clostridium difficile*, *Peptostreptococcus spp.* and *Bacteroides fragilis.* Linezolid has only moderate *in vitro* activity against *H. influenzae* and *Moraxella catarrhalis. P. aeruginosa* and Enterobacteriaceae are not susceptible.

In a randomised, double-blind, multicentre study, Linezolid, (600 mg *b.i.d.*) was compared with vancomycin (1 g *b.i.d.*) in patients with nosocomial pneumonia in terms of efficacy, safety and tolerability. Clinical and microbiological success rates were equivalent for both groups (66.4 *versus* 68.1% and 67.9 *versus* 71.8%, respectively). This was also true for patients with pneumonia due to MRSA. Resistance to either treatment was not detected. However, concomitant surveillance cultures for appearance of vancomycin-resistant enetrococci in stool could demonstrate the emergence of 4% vancomycin-resistant enterococci in patients treated with vancomycin, whereas no such resistance could be demonstrated in the group treated with linezolid [66].

Conclusion

Antimicrobial treatment exhibits a specific selection pressure. As a consequence past antimicrobial treatment policies lead to specific, locally differing microbial and resistance patterns. It is evident that recommendations for initial empirical antimicrobial treatment must be flexible enough to get modified according to local findings [1, 25, 39]. The change of microbial patterns and rates of microbial resistance must be recognised at the local level in order to modify general antimicrobial treatment policies [39]. Data obtained by surveillance cultures based on local epidemiological studies provide valuable information on potential pathogens and their susceptibility patterns. Regular updates of data on potential pathogens of HAP indicating trends in microbial and resistance patterns are mandatory. Investigation of each case of treatment failure is highly recommended. These data are particularly useful in order to identify patient related risk factors and microorganisms typically associated with treatment failure in the individual setting. The distribution of pathogens responsible for the majority of antimicrobial treatment failures is widely divergent and depends on local peculiarities [36, 67].

In the meantime, it is the physicians bias to judge the condition of the patient in view of all available clinical, laboratory, and radiographical information in order to increase the pretest probability for the presence or absence of HAP as much as possible.

Summary

In view of the emerging antibiotic resistance of microorganisms responsible for nosocomial pneumonia the choice of the appropriate antibiotic is a crucial issue. Although better treatment options, like new broad spectrum antibiotics are available, antimicrobial resistance is increasing worlwide. Therefore the clinician depends on guidelines to choose the appropriate antibiotic substance, as early antibiotic treatment is crucial for favourable outcome and the initial antimicrobial therapy for hospital acquired pneumonia (HAP) must always be empirical. The following aspects should be considered: 1) severity of the pneumonia; 2) time point of occurrence; and 3) specific risk factors. Further to this the selection of antimicrobial agents has to consider local microbial and resistance patterns. As regards the aetiology of HAP in general a high rate of Gram-negative bacteria like Gram-negative rods (mostly *Escherichia coli, Klebsiella spp., Enterobacter spp., Serratia spp. Proteus spp.*), as well as potentially multiresistant pathogens like *Pseudomonas aeruginosa, Acinetobacter spp.* and *Stenotrophomonas spp.* have been repeatedly reported and are responsible for 55–85% of HAP cases. Gram-positive bacteria as *Staphylococcus aureus* have increasingly gained importance being involved in 20–30% of HAP events. Two promising drugs have been investigated in nosocomial pneumonia due to Gram-positive pathogens, quinopristin/dalfopristin and linezolid. Linezolid offers some clear advantages compared to glycopeptides that have been one of the last therapeutic options for infections due to multiresistant Gram-positive microorganisms, including methicillin-resistant *S. aureus*.

Some aspects of antibiotic treatment are still under controversial discussion as the duration of antibiotic treatment, the status of aminoglycosides or the role of monotherapy. However any antimicrobial treatment regimen exhibits a specific selection pressure. As a consequence past antimicrobial treatment policies lead to specific, locally differing microbial and resistance patterns. Therefore it is evident that recommendations for initial empirical antimicrobial treatment must be flexible enough to get modified according to local findings.

Keywords: Antibiotic resistance, antibiotic treatment, duration of treatment, monotherapy, nosocomial pneumonia, ventilator-associated pneumonia.

References

1. Intensive care antimicrobial resistance epidemiology (ICARE) surveillance report, data summary from january 1996 through december 1997: A report from the National Nosocomial Infections Surveillance (NNIS) System. *Am J Infect Control* 1999; 27: 279–284.

2. Dorca J, Manresa F, Esteban L, *et al.* Efficacy, safety, and therapeutic relevance of tranthoracic aspiration with ultrathin needle in nonventilated nosocomial pneumonia. *Am J Respir Crit Care Med* 1995; 151: 1491–1496.

3. Chastre J, Trouillet JL, Vuagnat A. Nosocomial pneumonia in patients with acute respiratory distress syndrome. *Am J Respir Crit Care Med* 1998; 157: 1165–1172.

4. Ewig S, Torres A, El-Ebiary M, Fabregas N, Nicolas JM, Soto L. Bacterial colonization patterns in mechanically ventilated patients with traumatic and medical head injury. Incidence, risk factors, and association with ventilator-associated pneumonia. *Am J Respir Crit Care Med* 1999; 159: 188–198.

5. Rello J, Ollendorf DA, Oster G, *et al.* Epidemiology and outcomes of ventilator-associated pneumonia in a large US database. *Chest* 2002; 122: 2115–2121.

6. Torres A, El Ebiary M, Soler N, Monton C, Fabregas N, Hernandez C. Stomach as a source of colonization of the respiratory tract during mechanical ventilation: association with ventilator-associated pneumonia. *Eur Respir J* 1996; 9: 1729–1735.

7. Trouillet JL, Chastre J, Vuagnat A, *et al.* Ventilator-associated pneumonia caused by potentially drug-resistant bacteria. *Am J Respir Crit Care Med* 1998; 157: 531–539.

8. American Thoracic Society. Hospital-acquired pneumonia in adults; diagnosis, assessment, initial severity, and prevention. A consensus statement. *Am J Respir Crit Care Med* 1996; 153: 1711–1725.

9. Hanes SD, Demirkan K, Tolley E, *et al.* Risk factors for late-onset nosocomial pneumonia caused by *Stenotrophomonas maltophilia* in critically ill trauma patients. *Clin Infect Dis* 2002; 35: 228–235.

10. Ibrahim EH, Tracy L, Hill C, Fraser VJ, Kollef MH. The occurrence of ventilator-associated pneumonia in a community hospital: risk factors and clinical outcomes. *Chest* 2001; 120: 555–561.

11. Koprnova J, Svetlansky I, Babel'a R, *et al.* Prospective study of antibacterial susceptibility, risk factors and outcome of 157 episodes of Acinetobacter baumannii bacteremia in 1999 in Slovakia. *Scand J Infect Dis* 2001; 33: 891–895.

12. Bryan CS, Reynolds KL. Bacteremic nosocomial pneumonia. Analysis of 172 episodes from a single metropolitan area. *Am Rev Resp Dis* 1984; 129: 668–671.

13. Kirby BD, Harris AA. Nosocomial Legionnaires' disease. *Semin Respir Infect* 1987; 2: 255–261.

14. Dore P, Robert R, Grollier G, *et al.* Incidence of anaerobes in ventilator-associated pneumonia with use of a protected specimen brush. *Am J Respir Crit Care Med* 1996; 153: 1292–1298.

15. El Ebiary M, Torres A, Fabregas N, *et al.* Significance of the isolation of Candida species from respiratory samples in critically ill, non-neutropenic patients. An immediate postmortem histologic study. *Am J Respir Crit Care Med* 1997; 156: 583–590.

16. Papazian L, Autillo-Touati A, Thomas P, *et al.* Diagnosis of ventilator-associated pneumonia: an evaluation of direct examination and presence of intracellular organisms. *Anesthesiology* 1997; 87: 268–276.

17. Francioli P, Chastre J, Langer M, Santos JI, Shah PM, Torres A. Ventilator associated pneumonia-understanding epidemiology and pathogenesis to guide prevention and empiric therapy. *Clin Microbiol Infect* 1997; 3: Suppl. 1, 61–76.

18. Rello J, Ausina V, Castella J, Net A, Prats G. Nosocomial respiratory tract infections in multiple trauma patients. Influence of level of consciousness with implications for therapy. *Chest* 1992; 102: 525–529.

19. Sirvent JM, Torres A, Vidaur L, Armengol J, Bonet A. Tracheal colonisation within 24 h of intubation in patients with head trauma: risk factor for developing early-onset ventilator-associated pneumonia. *Intensive Care Med* 2000; 26: 1369–1372.

20. Rello J, Ausina V, Ricart M, *et al.* A. Risk factors for infection by *Pseudomonas aeruginosa* in patients with ventilator-associated pneumonia. *Intensive Care Med* 1994; 20: 193–198.

21. Rodrigues J, Niederman MS, Fein AM, Pai PB. Nonresolving pneumonia in steroid-treated patients with obstructive lung disease. *Am J Med* 1992; 93: 29–34.

22. Carratala J, Gudiol F, Pallares J, *et al.* 1994. Risk factors for nosocomial *Legionella pneumophila* pneumonia. *Am J Respir Crit Care Med* 149: 625–629.

23. Mier L, Dreyfuss D, Darchy B, *et al.* Is penicillin G an adequate initial treatment for aspiration pneumonia? A prospective evaluation using a protected specimen brush and quantitative cultures. *Intensive Care Med* 1993; 19: 279–284.

24. Ibrahim EH, Ward S, Sherman G, Schaiff R, Fraser VJ, Kollef MK. Experience with a clinical guideline for the treatment of ventilator-associated pneumonia. *Crit Care Med* 2001; 29: 1109–1115.

25. Rello J, Sa-Borges M, Correa H, Baraibar J. Variations in etiology of ventilator-associated pneumonia across four treatment sites: implications for antimicrobial prescribing practices. *Am J Respir Crit Care Med* 1999; 160: 608–613.

26. Lode H, Raffenberg M, Erbes R, Geerdes-Fenge H, Mauch H. Nosocomial pneumonia: epidemiology, pathogenesis, diagnosis, treatment and prevention. *Curr Opin Infect Dis* 2000; 13: 377–384.

27. Ewig S, Dalhoff K, Lorenz J, Schaberg T, Welte T, Wilkens H. Nosocomial pneumonia: recommendations on treatment and prevention. German Pneumology Society. *Pneumologie* 2000; 54: 525–538.

28. Akca O, Koltka K, Uzel S, *et al.* A comparative analysis of patients with early-onset *vs* late-onset nosocomial pneumonia in the ICU setting. *Chest* 2000; 117: 1434–1442.

29. Rello J, Ausina V, Ricart M, Castella J, Prats G. Impact of previous antimicrobial therapy on the etiology and outcome of ventilator-associated pneumonia. *Chest* 1993; 104: 1230–1235.

30. Torres A, Aznar R, Gatell JM, et al. Incidence, risk, and prognosis factors of nosocomial pneumonia in mechanically ventilated patients. Am Rev Respir Dis 1990; 142: 523–528.

31. Vincent JL, Bihardi DJ, Suter PM, et al. The prevalence of nosocomial infection in intensive care units in Europe: results of the European prevalence of infection in intensive care (EPIC) study. JAMA 1995; 278: 639–644.

32. Niederman MS, Mandell LA, Anzueto AJ, et al. Guidelines for the management of adults with community-acquired pneumonia. Diagnosis, assessment of severity, antimicrobial therapy, and prevention. Am J Respir Crit Care Med 2001; 163: 1730–1754.

33. Eller J, Ede A, Schaberg T, Niederman MS, Mauch H, Lode H. Infective exacerbations of chronic bronchitis:relation between bacteriologic etiology and lung function. Chest 1998; 113: 1542–1548.

34. Leroy O, Giradie P, Yazdanpanah Y, et al. microbiological data and potential adequacy of antimicrobial regimens. Eur Respir J 20: 432–439.

35. Kollef MH. Inadequate antimicrobial treatment: an important determinant of outcome for hospitalized patients. Clin Infect Dis 2002; 31: Suppl. 4, S131–S138.

36. Luna C, Vujachich P, Niederman MS, Gherardi C, Matera J, Jolly EC. Impact of BAL data on the therapy and outcome of ventilator-associated pneumonia. Chest 1997; 111: 676–687.

37. Kollef MH, Fraser VJ. Antibiotic resistance in the intensive care unit. Ann Intern Med 2001; 134: 298–314.

38. Meyer KS, Urban C, Eagan JA, Berger BJ, Rahal JJ. Nosocomial outbreak of Klebsiella infection resistant to late-generation cephalosporins. Ann Intern Med 1993; 119: 353–358.

39. Walger P, Mayershofer R, Marklein G, Vetter H. Initial antimicrobial policies in the ICU should be based on surveillance ratehr than on crop rotation. 40th Interscience Conference on Antimicorbial Agents and Chemotherapy 2000; 401.

40. Pugin J, Auckenthaler R, Mili N. Diagnosis of ventilator-associated pneumonia by bacteriologic analysis of bronchoscopic and nonbronchoscopic "blind" bronchoalveolar lavage fluid. Am Rev Respir Dis 1991; 143: 1121–1129.

41. Fabregas N, Ewig S, Torres A, et al. Clinical diagnosis of ventilator associated pneumonia revisited: comparative validation using immediate post-mortem lung biopsies. Thorax 1999; 54: 867–873.

42. Dreyfuss D, Mier L, Le Bourdelles G, et al. Clinical significance of borderline quantitative protected brush specimen culture results. Am Rev Respir Dis 1993; 147: 946–951.

43. Ewig S, Schäfer H, Torres A. Severity assessment in community-acquired pneumonia. Eur Respir J 2000; 16: 1193–1201.

44. Lode H. Monotherapy of nosocomial pneumonia. Sem Res Crit Care Med 2000; 21: 9–17.

45. Crouch BS, Wunderink RG, Jones CB, Leeper KV Jr. Ventilator-associated pneumonia due to Pseudomonas aeruginosa. Chest 1996; 109: 1019–1029.

46. Fink MP, Snydman DR, Niederman MS, et al. Treatment of severe pneumonia in hospitalized patients: results of a multicenter, randomized, double-blind trial comparing intravenous ciprofloxacin with imipenem-cilastatin. The Severe Pneumonia Study Group. Antimicrob Agents Chemother 1994; 38: 547–557.

47. Hilf M, Yu VL, Sharp J, Zuravleff JJ, Korvick JA, Muder RR. Antibiotic therapy for Pseudomonas aeruginosa bacteremia: outcome correlations in a prospective study of 200 patients. Am J Med 1989; 87: 540–546.

48. Korvick JA, Bryan CS, Farber B, et al. Prospective observational study of Klebsiella bacteremia in 230 patients: outcome for antibiotic combinations versus monotherapy. Antimicrob Agents Chemother 1992; 36: 2639–2644.

49. Ceftazidime combined with a short or long course of amikacin for empirical therapy of gram-negative bacteremia in cancer patients with granulocytopenia. The EORTC International Antimicrobial Therapy Cooperative Group. N Engl J Med 1987; 317: 1692–1698.

50. La Force FM. Systemic antimicrobial therapy of nosocomial pneumonia: monotherapy versus combination therapy. Eur J Clin Microbiol Infect Dis 1989; 8: 61–68.

51. Sieger B, Berman SJ, Geckler RW, Farkas SA. Empiric treatment of hospital-acquired lower respiratory tract infections with meropenem or ceftazidime with tobramycin: a randomized study. Meropenem Lower Respiratory Infection Group. *Crit Care Med* 1997; 25: 1663–1670.

52. Cometta A, Baumgartner JD, Lew D, *et al.* Prospective randomized comparison of imipenem monotherapy with imipenem plus netilmicin for treatment of severe infections in nonneutropenic patients. *Antimicrob Agents Chemother* 1994; 38: 1309–1313.

53. Torres A, Bauer TT, Leon-Gil C, *et al.* Treatment of severe nosocomial pneumonia: a prospective randomised comparison of intravenous ciprofloxacin with imipenem/cilastatin. *Thorax* 2000; 55: 1033–1039.

54. Chandrasekar PH, Crane LR, Bailey EJ. Comparison of the activity of antibiotic combinations *in vitro* with clinical outcome and resistance emergence in serious infections by *P. aeruginosa* in nonneutropenic patients. *Antimicrob Agents Chemother* 1987; 19: 321–329.

55. Crane LR. Pharmacodynamics of antimicrobial agents as a basis for determining dosage regiments. *Eur J Clin Microbiol Infect Dis* 1993; 12: s6–s8.

56. Brown RB, Kruse JA, Counts GW, Russel JA, Christou NV, Sands ML. Double-blind study of endotracheal tobramycin in the treatment of gram-negative bacterial pneumonia. The Endotracheal Tobramycin Study Group. *Antimicrob Agents Chemother* 1990; 34: 269–272.

57. Lode H, Hoffken G, Kemmerich B, Schaberg T. Systemic and endotracheal antibiotic prophylaxis of nosocomial pneumonia in ICU. *Intensive Care Med* 1992; 18: Suppl. 1, S24–S27.

58. Singh N, Rogers P, Atwood AW, Wagener MM, Yu L. Short-course empiric antibiotic therapy for patients with pulmonary infiltrates in the intensive care unit. *Am J Respir Crit Care Med* 200; 162: 505–511.

59. Dennesen PJ, van der Ven AJ, Kessels AG, Ramsay G, Bonten MJ. Resolution of infectious parameters after antimicrobial therapy in patients with ventilator-associated pneumonia. *Am J Respir Crit Care Med* 2001; 163: 1371–1375.

60. Lode H, Schaberg T, Raffenberg M, Mauch H. Lower respiratory tract infections in the intensive care unit: consequences of antibiotic resistance for choice of antibiotic. *Microb Drug Resist* 1995; 1: 163–167.

61. Bonten MJ, Bergmanns DC, Stobberingh EE, *et al.* Implemetation of bronchoscopic techniques in the diagnosis of ventilator-associated pneumonia to reduce antibiotic use. *Am J Respir Crit Care Med* 1997; 156: 1820–1824.

62. Croce MA, Fabian TC, Waddle-Smith L, *et al.* Utility of Grams stain and efficacy of quantitative cultures for posttraumatic pneumonia: a prospective study. *Ann Surg* 1998; 227: 743–751.

63. Pechere JC. Current and future management of infections due to methicilline-resistant staphylococci infection: the role of quinupristin/dalfopristin. *J Antimicrob Chemother* 1999; 44: 11–18.

64. Fagon , J, Patrick H, Haas DW, *et al.* Treatment of gram-positive nosocomial pneumonia. Prospective randomized comparison of quinupristin/dalfopristin *versus* vancomycin. Nosocomial Pneumonia Group. *Am J Respir Crit Care Med* 2000; 161: 753–762.

65. Perry CM, Jarvis B. Linezolid: a review of its use in the management of serious Gram-positive infections. *Drugs* 2001; 61: 525–551.

66. Rubinstein E, Cammarata S, Oliphant T, Wunderink R. Linezolid (PNU-100766) *versus* vancomycin in the treatment of hospitalized patients with nosocomial pneumonia: a randomized, double-blind, multicenter study. *Clin Infect Dis* 2001; 32: 402–412.

67. Rello J, Gallego M, Sonora R, Valles J. The value of routine microbial investigation in ventilator-associated pneumonia. *Am J Respir Crit Care Med* 1997; 156: 196–200.

CHAPTER 15

Pharmacological interactions between antibiotics and other drugs in the treatment of lower respiratory tract infections

A. Novelli, E. Mini, T. Mazzei

Dept of Preclinical Pharmacology, University of Florence, Florence, Italy.

Correspondence: T. Mazzei, Dept of Preclinical Pharmacology, University of Florence, Florence, Italy.

Antibiotics are commonly prescribed to patients who are also taking other medications, thereby creating a situation in which there is potential risk of pharmacological drug interactions [1–3].

This chapter will focus on the mechanisms and clinical relevance of the most important drug interactions that involve the major classes of antibacterial agents commonly used in the treatment of lower respiratory tract infections (LRTIs). Drug interactions can be classified as pharmacodynamic and pharmacokinetic [4].

Pharmacodynamic drug interactions may result when one drug changes the pharmacological effect of another drug, without any alteration in the pharmacokinetics of either.

There are very few examples in the literature regarding pharmacodynamic interactions involving antibiotics. They are mostly limited to the potentiation of neuromuscular blocking effects of succinylcholine by aminoglycosides, to the increase of cardiac QT interval when cisapride is combined with some fluoroquinolones or adverse drug reactions involving the central nervous system with the association of some nonsteroidal anti-inflammatory drugs and fluoroquinolones.

Pharmacokinetic drug interactions may concern all the pharmacokinetic phases, including absorption, distribution, metabolism and excretion. When treating infections, clinicians should know about two possible types of drug interactions involving antibiotics. The first one is that some anti-infective molecules may induce major changes in the pharmacokinetics of co-administered drugs. The second may be that the antimicrobial agents themselves undergo alterations due to the effect of the co-administered drugs [2, 3].

These interactions may or may not result in clinically relevant consequences *e.g.* adverse events or in measurable changes of response to therapy. These clinical consequences are in general more relevant if the therapeutic index of the involved drugs is narrow [2].

Pharmacokinetic interactions

Absorption

The absorption of many antibiotics can be altered by several mechanisms. Some drugs (anticholinergic and opiates) or food may slow the gastric motility, thus delaying and decreasing the peak concentration. On the contrary, prokinetic drugs (*e.g.* erythromycin,

Eur Respir Mon, 2004, 28, 229–254. Printed in UK - all rights reserved. Copyright ERS Journals Ltd 2004; European Respiratory Monograph; ISSN 1025-448x. ISBN 1-904097-32-4.

cisapride or metoclopramide) can accelerate gastric motility with a consequent higher and faster peak level of other drugs.

Variations in gastric pH may alter solubility or chemical stability of β-lactams or erythromycin. Metal cations (magnesium, aluminum or calcium) of antiacids or sucralfate may chelate many antibiotics including tetracyclines, fluoroquinolones and lincosamides, decreasing their absorption and altering their bioavailability [5].

Another mechanism involves metabolic enzymes (mainly cytochrome P450 (CYP) 3A4) present in enterocytes [3]. They can metabolise some antibiotics before they reach the serum level (first pass metabolism).

In addition, enterocytes also have some transporter proteins such as P-glycoprotein (P-gp) that can decrease the absorption of many drugs. These membrane enzymes can pump drugs back into the gastro-intestinal lumen.

Inhibition and induction of metabolic or transporter enzymes may cause drug interactions [6].

A final mechanism is alteration of the intestinal flora, such as in the case of growth inhibition of *Eubacterium lentum* by macrolides or tetracyclines. This microorganism is usually responsible for 40% of the inactivation of digoxin and co-administration with these antibiotics may result in prolonged digitalis toxicity [2, 5].

Distribution

Most antibiotics are reversibly bound to plasma proteins, mainly albumin or α1-acid glycoproteins. The displacement from protein binding (albumin) of warfarin by sulfonamides is an example, which is not very clinically important, of pharmacokinetic interaction involving altered distribution [7].

Metabolism

Many clinically relevant antimicrobial drug interactions depend on modifications of biotransformation of a compound [2, 3]. CYP is the major system involved in the oxidative metabolism of drugs in the liver and for interactions regarding some lipophilic antibiotics, such as macrolides, fluoroquinolones and rifampin or rifabutin.

The inhibition of the human liver CYP metabolism is a common mechanism for pharmacokinetic drug interactions, since generally drugs undergo a Phase 1 reaction (oxidation) followed by conjugation (Phase 2) in order to generate or increase water solubility for renal excretion. The CYP mixed function oxidase system consists of >100 different isoenzymes responsible for the majority of oxidative biotransformations of both endogenous compounds and xenobiotics. Isoenzymes that metabolise drugs in humans have been included in three separate gene families: CYP 1, 2 and 3. Within these families, five isoforms (CYP1A2, CYP2C9, CYP2C19, CYP2D6 and CYP3A4) account for almost all the clinically important drug interactions [8, 9].

CYP3A appears to be one of the most important enzymes as it transforms, at least partially, almost 60% of drugs which undergo oxidation, and is the most predominant isoform in adults. It is highly recovered in the liver and in the apical enterocytes [8, 9]. Unlike other isoforms (CYP2D6, 2C9 and 2C19) CYP3A4 does not show genetic polymorphism, though there might be a wide interindividual variability partially related to diet, age, and small bowel or liver disease [8].

Many isoenzymes can be inhibited by several antibacterial drugs (*e.g.* macrolides, fluoroquinolones, metronidazole, sulfonamides) with a consequent decrease in the metabolism of other drugs, rise in their serum concentrations and perhaps adverse clinical effects.

Alternatively rifampin or rifabutin may induce metabolic enzymes with a reduction in serum concentration and in the pharmacological effect of the interacted drug [2, 3].

Table 1 lists the most important inhibitors and inducers of CYP enzymes, including antibacterial agents.

Excretion

Interaction-drug reactions may occur due to an alteration in renal elimination of hydrophilic antibiotics (aminoglycosides, β-lactams, glycopeptides), as a result of changes or competition in glomerular filtration, tubular secretion or tubular reabsorption caused by other drugs [3, 4]. For example probenecid competitively inhibits the renal clearance of some penicillins and cephalosporins, prolonging their elimination half-life.

Cilastatin is also associated with imipenem to increase its clearance. Sulfonamides, trimethoprim and some penicillins are competitors for methotrexate excretion (glomerular filtration and tubular secretion) and have been associated with dose-related methotrexate toxicity [5].

However, in general, excretion interactions are not common causes of important clinical-interaction adverse effects [3, 4].

More recently a new mechanism of excretion and of possible interaction among drugs has been described. This is correlated to a P-gp membrane pump present in different cells, recognised to promote the excretion of different xenobiotics, including digoxin and cyclosporin from renal, biliary and intestinal cells. Some antimicrobial drugs can interact with P-gp mediated transport and may inhibit P-gp expression. At present, however, it is not possible to describe a definitive role for this interaction.

Common significant interactions involving antibacterial agents

Macrolide antibiotics

The macrolide group of antibiotics includes several natural and semisynthetic members. Erythromycin is the prototype and in recent years new subclasses have been added these

Table 1. – The most important inhibitors and inducers of P450 enzymes

Inhibitors	Inducers
Amiodarone	Barbiturates
Azole antifungals	Carbamazepine
Cimetidine	Dexamethasone
Diltiazem	Ethanol (chronic)
Fluoroquinolones	Phenytoin
Grapefruit juice	Rifampin/rifabutin
Haloperidol	Troglitazone
Macrolides	
Metronidazole	
Propranolol	
Sulfonamides	
Trimethoprim	
Protease inhibitors	
Quinidine	
SSRIs	
Verapamil	
Zafirlukast	

SSRIs: selective serotonin re-uptake inhibitors.

are azalides with azithromycin as the prototype and ketolides with telithromycin as the first member [10, 11].

Macrolides are generally well tolerated and are considered amongst the safest of the available antibiotics. Nevertheless it is well known that these antibiotics may interact with several compounds with possible effects on their pharmacokinetics, and during the last 30 yrs they have been recognised as a potential source of clinically severe drug interactions [12–14].

Following the initial report of acute ergotism due to the co-administration of troleandomycin, several authors have demonstrated drug interactions between macrolides and different drugs, from alfentanil to warfarin (table 2) [2, 12–17].

A relevant number of published studies indicate that pharmacokinetic drug interactions of macrolide antibiotics concurrently administered with several compounds, occur because of their inhibitory activity on the CYP system. Information on macrolide interactions arises from different sources. Some data have been obtained from *in vitro* studies, performed during the development of new derivatives. Unfortunately, the interaction observed *in vitro* is often not completely predictable of what is happening *in vivo*, though it may be used as an indication for clinical studies. Other sources include the investigational controlled studies performed often in healthy volunteers. However, relevant drug interactions have been based on clinical practice reports, which, in some cases have been confirmed in clinical trials. In fact, though both *in vitro* and *in vivo* investigational studies illustrate the pharmacological basis of drug interactions among different compounds, the most accurate description of this interaction comes from clinical reports or studies conducted in patient populations which were administered the combination and were receiving one of these drugs as long-term therapy, since there are also patient- and administration-related factors which may be relevant in determining potency and incidence [2, 12–17].

However, some differences were found between the different macrolide derivatives in the incidence and magnitude of these effects and not all the members of this class are potential sources of drug interaction: troleandomycin, erythromycin, and to a relatively lesser extent clarithromycin have proven to be the most commonly implicated compounds, while other semi-synthetic derivatives such as roxithromycin, dirithromycin, flurithromycin, some 16-membererd molecules *e.g.* josamycin, midecamycin, miocamycin and the azalide, azithromycin, were seldom involved. Spiramycin and rokitamycin have not so far been considered as potentially hazardous in this respect, while some drug interactions have been identified for the new ketolide derivative, telithromycin.

Therefore, based on their CYP binding and potential for inducing clinically relevant drug interactions, the different macrolide derivatives can be subdivided into four groups: Group I includes erythromycin and troleandomycin which have a high degree; Group 2 includes clarithromycin and telithromycin with an intermediate degree; Group 3 includes both 14-membered (roxithromycin, dirithromycin, flurithromycin) and 16-membered molecules (josamycin, midecamycin and miocamycin), and azithromycin, that are unable to form iron-metabolite complexes, though they can exert an effect on CYP34A and probably in some cases also on P-gp; and Group 4 includes spiramycin and rokitamycin, that have not been associated with drug interactions to date [2, 13, 14, 16, 18].

Mechanisms of macrolide interactions. There are several mechanisms by which macrolides interact with other drugs. One might be complexation, commonly associated with food and antacids, which may lead to a decreased bioavailability of these antimicrobial agents, with the exclusion of clarithromycin, enteric-coated erythromycins and dirithromycin. On the contrary, the latter compound shows increased absorption in the presence of food (table 2). [2, 13, 14]

Table 2. – Drug interactions involving macrolide antibiotics

Interacting drug	Macrolide	Mechanism of interaction	Effect	Clinical significance and management
Alfentanil	Erythromycin Troleandomycin	CYP3A4 inhibition	↓ Alfentanil clearance	Prolonged alfentanil effect Possibly avoid concomitant administration or reduce alfentanil dosage
Antacids	Azithromycin	Complexation	↓ Azithromycin C_{max}	Not established Administer the two agents at least 1–2 h apart
Anti-HIV drugs NRTI Zidovudine	Clarithromycin	Unknown	↓ Zidovudine absorption and AUC	Not established. Administer the two agents at least 2 h apart
NNRTI Delavirdine Efavirenz Nevirapine	Clarithromycin[#,¶]	CYP3A4 inhibition	↑ NNRTI AUC	Possible alternative antimicrobial therapy
PI Indinavir Ritonavir Saquinavir	Clarithromycin[¶]	CYP3A4 inhibition	↑ PI AUC and plasma concentrations	No dosage adjustment, probably clinically irrelevant
Astemizole	Erythromycin Clarithromycin Dirithromycin	CYP3A4 inhibition	↑ Astemizole serum levels and $t_{1/2}\,\beta$	Possible QT prolongation, risk for torsades de pointes Monitor QT interval Avoid concomitant administration
Benzodiazepines Alprazolam Diazepam Flunitrazepam Midazolam Triazolam	Erythromycin Troleandomycin Clarithromycin Roxithromycin[+] Telithromycin	CYP3A4 inhibition	↑ Benzodiazepine levels and AUC	Possible enhanced effects Sedation Ataxia Monitor effects Possibly avoid concomitant administration or reduce benzodiazepine dosage
Bromocriptine	Erythromycin	CYP3A4 inhibition (decreased metabolism)	↑ Bromocriptine levels and AUC	Increased gastrointestinal side effects? Risk of psychosis?
Calcium antagonists Felodipine Verapamil	Erythromycin Clarithromycin	CYP3A4 inhibition	↑ Calcium antagonist AUC and C_{max}	Severe hypotension (felodipine, arrhythmia verapamil) Monitor blood presure and heart rate
Carbamazepine	Erythromycin Troleandomycin Clarithromycin Josamycin Miocamycin Flurithromycin	CYP3A4 inhibition	↑ AUC, ↑ Css, ↑ C_{min} 11-epoxide metabolite ↓ C_{max}, ↓ AUC, ↓ $t_{1/2}\,\beta$	Excess sedation, carbamazepine toxicity, reduce dosage by 25–50%
Cimetidine	Clarithromycin	Unknown	Clarit prolonged absorption, ↓ C_{max} and ↑ $t_{1/2}$ ↑ for Clarit and 14-OHC	Unknown Possible reduced antimicrobial efficacy
Cisapride	Erythromycin Troleandomycin Clarithromycin Telithromycin	CYP3A4 inhibition	↑ Cisapride AUC, ↑ Css, ↑ C_{max}	Possible QT prolongation, risk of torsades de pointes Monitor QT interval Avoid concomitant administration
Clozapine	Erythromycin	CYP3A4 inhibition (decreased metabolism)	↑ Clozapine levels	Leukocytosis, somnolence, disorientation, seizure Usually avoid concomitant administration

233

Table 2. Continued

Interacting drug	Macrolide	Mechanism of interaction	Effect	Clinical significance and management
Cyclosporin	Erythromycin Clarithromycin Azithromycin Dirithromycin Miocamycin	CYP3A4 inhibition P-gp interference	↑ Cy A C_{min} levels and AUC, ↓ clearance	Monitor Cy A levels and toxicity
Digoxin	Erythromycin Clarithromycin Azithromycin[§] Roxithromycin Telithromycin	Decreased gastrointestinal metabolism or reduced P-gp mediated renal secretion	↑ Digoxin levels	Avoid concomitant administration or monitor digoxin levels
Disopyramide	Erythromycin Clarithromycin	CYP3A4 inhibition?	↑ Disopyramide $t_{1/2}$ β	Cardiac arrhythmia, risk for torsades de pointes and major hypoglycaemia Avoid concomitant administration, monitor closely ECG
Ergot alkaloids	Erythromycin Troleandomycin Troleandomycin Clarithromycin	CYP3A4 inhibition (decreased metabolism)	↑ Ergotamine serum levels	Clinical ergotism Avoid concomitant administration
HMG-CoA inhibitors[f] Lovastatin Simvastatin	Erythromycin Clarithromycin Azithromycin Telithromycin	CYP3A4 inhibition	↑ Statin concentrations and AUC	Possible rhabdomyolysis. Monitor serum creatinine kinase
Hypnosedatives and anxiolytics[##]: Zopiclone Zolpidem Zaleplon Buspirone	Erythromycin	CYP3A4 inhibition	↑ Sedative levels	Enhanced sedative effects. Reduce sedative doses
Methylprednisolone	Erythromycin Troleandomycin Clarithromycin	CYP3A4 inhibition	↑ Methylprednisolone serum levels, ↓ clearance	Increased risk for steroid-induced adverse effects
Pimozide	Clarithromycin	CYP3A4 inhibition	↑ Pimozide serum levels and AUC	Possible arrhythmias, QT prolongation, risk for torsades de pointes Monitor QT interval Avoid concomitant administration
PPI Lansoprazole Omeprazole	Clarithromycin[¶¶]	CYP3A4 inhibition (decreased metabolism)	↑ PPI AUC and $t_{1/2}$ β	No therapeutic influence, dosage adjustment unnecessary
Quinidine	Erythromycin	CYP3A4 inhibition	↓ Quinidine total clearance	Possible arrhythmias, QT prolongation, risk for torsades de pointes Monitor QT interval Avoid concomitant administration
Rifabutin	Erythromycin Clarithromycin	CYP3A4 inhibition	↑ Rifabutin AUC	Increased risk of rifabutin side effects, neutropenia Use with caution, monitor closely
Rifabutin	Azithromycin	Unknown		Neutropenia Use with caution, monitor closely

Table 2. Continued

Interacting drug	Macrolide	Mechanism of interaction	Effect	Clinical significance and management
Rifabutin	Clarithromycin Azithromycin	Induction of macrolide metabolism	↑ Macrolide AUC	Possible reduced macrolide efficacy Avoid concomitant administration
Rifampicin	Erythromycin Clarithromycin	Induction of macrolide metabolism. Intestinal P-gp induction.	Possible low concentrations	Possible reduced macrolide efficacy
Sildenafil	Erythromycin Clarithromycin	CYP3A4 inhibition	↑ Sildenafil serum levels.	Risk of cardiotoxicity and priapism Reduce sildenafil doses
Tacrolimus	Erythromycin Clarithromycin	CYP3A4 inhibition	↑ Tacrolimus serum levels.	Possible hyperazotemia, monitor renal function
Terfenadine[++]	Erythromycin Troleandomycin Clarithromycin	CYP3A4 inhibition	↑ Terfenadine AUC and C_{max}	QT prolongation, risk for torsades de pointes Monitor QT interval Avoid concomitant administration
Theophylline	Erythromycin Troleandomycin Clarithromycin Roxithromycin Josamycin Telithromycin	CYP1A2 and CYP3A4 inhibition	↑ Theophylline AUC, ↓ clearance	Possible theophylline toxicity Monitor serum theophylline concentrations
Vinblastine	Erythromycin	CYP3A4 inhibition (decreased metabolism)?	↑ Vinblastine levels	Increased toxicity Avoid concomitant administration?
Warfarin	Erythromycin Troleandomycin Clarithromycin Azithromycin	CYP1A2 and CYP3A4 inhibition	↑ Warfarin clearance (mainly R eniantomer)	Risk of increased INR and PT Monitor both INR PT

CYP: cytochrome P450; C_{max}: peak concentration; NRTI: nucleoside reverse transcriptase inhibitors; AUC: area under the concentration-time curve; NNRTI: non-nucleoside reverse transcriptase inhibitors; PI: protease inhibitor; $t\frac{1}{2}$ β: elimination half-life; Css: steady state concentration; C_{min}: trough concentration; P-gp: P-glycoprotein; Cy A: cyclosporine; ECG: electro cardiograph; HMG-CoA: hydroxy-methyl-glutaryl-CoA; PPI: proton pump inhibitors; INR: international normalised ratio; PT: prothrombin time; ↑: increase; ↓: decrease; [#]: reduced clarithromycin AUC; [¶]: increased clarithromycin AUC and C_{max}; [+]: weaker effect, limited clinical significance; [§]: with digitoxin; [f]: hydroxymethylglutaryl coenzyme-A inhibitors; [##]: newer compounds, other than benzodiazepines; [¶¶]: increased clarithromycin and/or 14-OH clarithromycin AUC and C_{max}; [++]: same observations with loratidine which is not cardiotoxic.

Ethanol decreases the absorption of erythromycin ethyl succinate, while cimetidine has been associated with a prolonged absorption of clarithromycin with a decrease in serum peak concentration (C_{max}) of both clarithromycin and the 14-OH metabolite. The mechanism of this interaction is unknown, though there might be the possibility of a decreased production of 14-OHC which is effective against *Haemophilus influenzae* strains [2, 16, 17].

Alteration of intestinal flora is another mechanism of drug interactions. For example, macrolides, azalides and ketolides, by eliminating *Eubacterium lentum* from the intestinal tract, may decrease the gastrointestinal metabolism of digoxin or digitoxin, at least in some patients, thereby increasing serum levels [2, 11–13, 16–19].

However, the higher bioavailability of digoxin might also be due to the inhibition of

P-gp with a reduction in mediated renal secretion. Among antimicrobial drugs, macrolides can interact with P-gp-mediated transport and may inhibit P-gp expression. At present it is not possible to draw a definitive role for this interaction. Nevertheless, since macrolides are metabolised by the CYP system and may potently inhibit its activity, which is the main mechanism for their clinically important drug interactions, simultaneous inhibition of P-gp might contribute to individual variations in the extent of this effect as there is an overlap in drugs that are substrates for both proteins [17, 19].

Erythromycin is metabolised by CYP3A and CYP1A and causes an initial induction followed by a significant (reversible) inhibition with the possible formation of an inactive CYP-iron-nitrosoalkane metabolite complex. In general macrolides primarily, competitively inhibit the CYP3A4 isoform, whilst having a weaker effect on CYP1A2 enzyme [8, 13, 14, 17]. Telithromycin also inhibits CYP2D6 isoform [18].

However, as previously mentioned, not all the macrolides share the same inhibitory potency, which is mainly related to two major structural features: the presence of an accessible, unhindered N-methylamino group and the hydrophobic grade of the molecule [13, 14].

Psychotropic agents. *Benzodiazepines.* The effect of different macrolides on the pharmacokinetics of various benzodiazepines has been assessed in many studies, both *in vitro* and *in vivo*. Erythromycin induces increased serum concentrations, significantly higher area under the concentration-time curve (AUC) and reduced clearance of triazolam (as well as troleandomycin), midazolam (as well as clarithromycin and telithromycin) and alprazolam, with possible enhanced effects, sedation and even ataxia. Erythromycin exerts lesser effects also on diazepam and flunitrazepam. Roxithromycin shows a weaker interaction with midazolam. Therefore, co-administration of these benzodiazepines and macrolide derivatives should be avoided, if possible, or at least the benzodiazepine dosage should be reduced [8, 9, 11–13, 16–18, 20].

Hypnosedatives and anxiolytics. Erythromycin, as other CYP inhibitors, enhances the sedative effects of new hypnosedative derivatives such as zopiclone and zolpidem, zaleplon and of buspirone, an anxiolytic with minimal sedative effects, which undergoes extensive first-pass metabolism, by inhibiting their hepatic metabolism and consequently increasing serum levels. Based on these findings, if co-administration cannot be avoided, sedative dosage reduction is recommended [8, 16, 21].

Neuroleptics. Clozapine is a new antipsychotic drug mainly used for the management of schizophrenia. An interaction between erythromycin and clozapine is possible and has been reported in the literature. Leukocytosis, somnolence, disorientation and seizure have been observed in relation to increased clozapine levels. Clozapine is metabolised by the liver. The main CYP enzymes involved are CYP2D6, CYP1A2 and CYP3A4, and there can be large intervariability. Since erythromycin inhibits two of these pathways, caution should be used for concurrent administration of the two drugs [2, 9, 14, 16]. At present, though no data are available, a possible interaction with telithromycin cannot be excluded since the ketolide also inhibits *in vitro* CYP2D6 isoform [18].

Pimozide is an agent used in the treatment of various psychiatric disorders. Clarithromycin inhibits CYP3A-mediated pimozide metabolism and the resulting elevation in plasma concentrations may increase the risk of pimozide cardiotoxicity with possible arrhythmias, QT prolongation and risk of torsades de pointes. Two fatal cases of ventricular dysrrhythmia have been reported as a consequence of this interaction. Therefore this association is contraindicated [2, 8, 9, 12, 16, 22, 23].

Carbamazepine. Carbamazepine is both a substrate and inducer of CYP3A4 enzyme. Therefore this anticonvulsivant induces the metabolism of many drugs metabolised by this pathway and interacts with different drugs which act as inhibitors of its own metabolism. The interaction between carbamazepine and erythromycin is well known and its extent is directly related to the erythromycin dose. In case of co-administration, serum carbamazepine concentrations should be carefully monitored to avoid toxicity and the anticonvulsivant dosage may be reduced by 25–50%. This interaction has been reported also for troleandomycin, clarithromycin, josamycin, miocamycin and flurithromycin [8, 9, 12–14, 16, 22].

CYP3A4 substrate drugs. Several compounds which are CYP3A4 substrates can prolong the QT interval and might be associated with torsades de pointes, which is a life-threatening ventricular arrhythmia. QT prolongation is probably due in part to a concentration-dependent block of the potassium rectifier current in cardiac conduction. These drugs are: the antipsychotic molecule pimozide, the gastrointestinal prokinetic drug cisapride and the nonsedating antihistamines astemizole and terfenadine. All these drugs can interact with different macrolide derivatives (troleandomycin, erythromycin, clarithromycin, dirithromycin, telithromycin) with the risk of a torsade de pointes occurrence (table 2). Therefore, it is prudent to avoid co-administration of these drugs with macrolides because of the seriousness of the possible adverse effects [2, 8–14, 16, 18].

Antiarrhythmic drugs. Quinidine undergoes extensive oxidative metabolism in the liver and approximately one half of its metabolism depends on CYP3A4. Disopyramide has a concentration-dependent binding and is eliminated by both hepatic metabolism and renal excretion (unchanged drug). Among macrolide derivatives, erythromycin has proven to interact with both drugs, either by increasing the elimination half-life or reducing the clearance. Another possible mechanism of drug interaction of quinidine might be P-glycoprotein inhibition by erythromycin. Cases of severe cardiac arrhythmia and major hypoglycemia have also occurred in patients receiving disopyramide simultaneously with clarithromycin. There is also a risk for prolongation of the QT interval and/or torsades de pointes and co-administration should be avoided [9, 12–14, 17].

Calcium antagonists. CYP3A4 and P-gp have a high impact on both metabolism and transport of different calcium channel blockers. Therefore, a drug interaction has been observed between erythromycin and felodipine with severe hypotension and between clarithromycin and verapamil with hypotension and bradycardia [14, 16, 17].

Hydroxy-methyl-glutaryl-CoA reductase inhibitors. These agents, with the exclusion of pravastatin, are primarily metabolised by CYP3A4, though cerivastatin is also metabolised by CYP2C8 and fluvastatin is mostly metabolised by CYP2C9 [24]. Statins have dose-related toxic effects on muscles such as myopathy and rhabdomyolysis. The concomitant administration of a macrolide derivative can increase statin concentrations. There are reports regarding erythromycin, clarithromycin, azithromycin and telithromycin interactions with different hydroxy-methyl-glutaryl-CoA reductase inhibitors. Therefore, co-administration should be avoided and at least creatinine kinase should be carefully monitored [9, 11–14, 16–18].

Immunosuppressive agents. Cyclosporin is also primarily metabolised by the CYP3A isoform so there is a reasonable potential for interaction with macrolide derivatives. There are numerous reports of a significant increase in AUC and decrease in cyclosporin clearance with concurrent administration of erythromycin. However P-gp is involved in cyclosporin kinetics and the interaction with erythromycin might not only be due to inhibition of CYP3A4 both in liver and intestine, but also to an inhibition of P-gp in the intestine. This aspect might be important since an interaction with cyclosporin has been reported not only for erythromycin but also for clarithromycin (capable of inhibiting both CYP3A4 and P-gp) and dirithromycin, miocamycin and azithromycin, which have a low effect on CYP3A.

Tacrolimus, which has been noticed later than cyclosporin, is extensively metabolised by CYP3A4 and transported by P-gp. Significant interactions of this immunosuppressive agent with both erythromycin and clarithromycin have been reported, similarly to cyclosporin. Consequently, concomitant administration of these immunosuppressive drugs and macrolides, including telithromycin, should be avoided, though at present there are no data for a possible interaction [2, 9, 12, 13, 16, 17].

Theophylline. Theophylline is metabolised by *N*-demethylation and 8-hydroxylation. It is generally recognised that the primarily involved isoform is CYP1A2, in addition both CYP2E1 and CYP3A4 play a role. It seems that the well-known interaction of macrolides with theophylline might be related to both CYP3A4 and CYP1A2 inhibition, though the effect on the latter pathway is relatively weak. The interaction with macrolides may be enhanced in subjects who have low CYP1A2 activity and a proportionally higher CYP3A4 activity, acting as a substitute metabolic pathway. This hypothesis may support the observation that interaction occurs mainly in patients receiving high doses of erythromycin or prolonged therapy. An interaction with theophylline has been reported also for troleandomycin, clarithromycin, roxithromycin, josamycin and telithromycin. From a clinical point of view, in the presence of antimicrobial treatment with macrolides, it is important to monitor theophylline serum concentrations to avoid risk of toxicity related to an unpredictable extent of the interaction [2, 9, 11, 13, 14, 16–18, 22].

Ergot alkaloids. Ergotamine is metabolised by the liver and unchanged drug can be found in faeces and urine only in traces. The drug has a low bioavailability and is an apparently substrate of CYP3A4 enzyme.

Ergotism has been recognised in patients concomitantly treated with CYP3A4 inhibitors, including erythromycin, troleandomycin and clarithromycin. Accordingly, CYP3A4 inhibitors should not be given in patients under ergot-derivative treatment. Erythromycin is also capable of increasing bromocriptine levels and AUC, possibly leading to increased gastrointestinal side-effects [2, 9, 13, 14, 17].

Warfarin. The commercial preparation of warfarin is a racemic mixture of S- and R- enantiomers, which differ in anticoagulant potency, metabolism, elimination and drug interactions. In addition warfarin is almost completely bound to plasma-proteins. S-warfarin is metabolised primarily by CYP2C9, while CYP1A2 and CYP3A4 metabolise the R-enantiomer which is two- to five-fold less potent. Erythromycin induces limited kinetic modifications of warfarin in healthy volunteers and mainly for R-enantiomer. Similar observations have been made with troleandomycin, and a potential interaction has been reported for clarithromycin and azithromycin. Nevertheless the disease state and the presence of pulmonary infection may substantially reduce the catalytic activity of CYP system and interactions with macrolides may become unpredictable with the risk of an increased hypoprothrombinemic effect. Thus, in patients receiving both drugs a careful monitoring of the prothrombin time (PT) and the international normalised ratio (INR) is recommended [2, 9, 12, 13, 17, 22].

Miscellaneous drugs. CYP3A4 inhibition, mainly exerted by erythromycin, may lead to interactions with other drugs with alternative clinical significance. Alfentanil clearance is reduced by both erythromycin and troleandomycin and caution should be used when co-administering this analgesic in patients treated with macrolides because of the risk of prolonged respiratory depression [13, 14, 17].

Erythromycin, troleandomycin and clarithromycin can affect methylprednisolone clearance. This effect is not observed with prednisolone and the clinical implication is not completely clear [13, 14, 16, 17].

Cholestatic jaundice in women receiving troleandomycin and oral contraceptives (OC) has been described in numerous reports, dirithromycin seems capable of increasing the apparent oral clearance of ethinylestradiol, without a significantly higher risk of ovulation. However, other authors demonstrated no interference by roxithromycin with OC effectiveness [13, 14, 25].

Erythromycin raises sildenafil serum levels with the resulting risk of cardiotoxicity and priapism. The dose of this phosphodiesterase type-5 inhibitor should be reduced [8, 26].

Vinca alkaloids, mainly vinblastine, might have increased serum concentrations when concomitantly administered with erythromycin, resulting in severe neutropoenia and myalgias [9, 16, 27].

Erythromycin, clarithromycin and azithromycin can increase the rifabutin AUC with risk of neutropoenia. Conversely, rifabutin and rifampicin can induce macrolide metabolism and induce also intestinal P-gp, resulting in low macrolide concentrations and reduced AUC with possible impaired antimicrobial efficacy [14, 16, 17, 19, 22].

Clarithromycin may increase both the AUC and elimination half-life of the proton pump inhibitors omeprazole and lansoprazole, though without clinical significance, while the latter drugs can enhance AUC and peak concentration of the macrolide derivative [22].

Finally, different interactions have been observed between clarithromycin and anti-HIV compounds, ranging from reduced zidovudine absorption due to an unknown mechanism to increased concentrations of either some protease inhibitors (indinavir, ritonavir and saquinavir) or non-nucleoside reverse transcriptase inhibitors (delavirdine, efavirenz, nevirapine), which require a better evaluation in order to establish the clinical significance [14, 16, 17, 20, 22].

At present it may be concluded that Group 1 and, to a lesser extent, Group 2 macrolides produce frequent drug interactions and consequently co-administration with other compounds whose metabolism is known to be affected or that could potentially be impaired should be avoided or done with caution, since alternative therapeutic strategies are available in most or all of these cases. Group 3 members are unable to form iron-metabolite complexes, though they can exert an effect on CYP34A and probably in some cases also on P-gp. These derivatives are seldom involved in drug interactions. Group 4 macrolides have not been associated with drug interactions to date. However, caution is suggested in using Group 3 and 4 macrolides in patients concurrently treated with drugs implicated in important adverse interactions such as torsades de pointes, hypotension, rhabdomyolysis, excessive sedation, ataxia and ergotism. Finally, at present, the possibility that additional interactions and or drugs should be added to this list cannot be ruled out.

Fluoroquinolones

Drug-to-drug interactions are a relevant issue with the fluoroquinolones, because of their extensive use, and the fact that they are often administered with other drugs.

Several types of interactions between fluoroquinolones and other drugs have been described that can be of either pharmacokinetic or pharmacodynamic nature.

Pharmacokinetic interactions occur either during the absorption phase of quinolones, since they are usually administered orally, leading to opposition of the quinolone antimicrobial effects, or during the renal excretion of some quinolones, leading to potentiation of their effects. These interactions involve fluoroquinolones as object drugs.

In addition, some quinolones are potent inhibitors of the CYP isoenzyme CYP1A2 and are thus capable of inhibiting the metabolism of other concomitantly administered drugs which are substrates of the same isoenzyme, resulting in drug accumulation and toxicity. These interactions involve fluoroquinolones as precipitant drugs. Because this inhibition seems to be rather specific, significant interactions between fluoroquinolones and other drugs that are metabolised by other hepatic CYP enzymes are not very likely.

Pharmacodynamic interactions, such as increased central nervous system and cardiac toxicity, may as well occur when quinolones are given with other drugs with similar toxic organotropic effects.

Several outstanding reviews address the topic of drug-to-drug interactions with fluoroquinolones [3, 17, 28–32]. Table 3 lists the most significant quinolone-drug interactions. This paragraph focuses on currently clinically used fluoroquinolones and new fluoroquinolones under clinical development. Data on older fluoroquinolones are also cited when they are considered clinically relevant and for a more general comprehension of interaction phenomena within this class of antimicrobial agents.

Metal cation-containing drugs. Divalent and trivalent cations significantly reduce the absorption and bioavailability of fluoroquinolones when these drugs are given together [33] and clinical failures resulting from this interaction have been reported [34]. The probable cause of the interaction is the formation of unadsorbable chelate complexes between the cation and the 4-oxo and 3-carboxyl groups of the quinolone [35]. The reduction in bioavailability is more striking for derivatives with fewer substitutions on the essential structure and on the piperazinyl group, such as norfloxacin, ciprofloxacin and enoxacin. Substitution at the 5 position diminishes the interaction [36]. The magnitude of the effect depends not only on the specific quinolone but also on the specific cation, its dose and dosage form, and the timing of administration.

Magnesium or aluminum-containing antacids and sucralfate, have the greatest effects and decrease the AUC for enoxacin, norfloxacin and ciprofloxacin from ~70% to >90% [30]. Absorption remains decreased when the cation is given 2 h before the quinolone, though the effect is less pronounced than with simultaneous administration. The newer agents are also affected by this interaction but typically to a lesser degree [28, 37].

Co-administration with oral calcium, iron preparations or multivitamins with minerals such as zinc can also decrease the absorption of ciprofloxacin and newer agents such as levofloxacin, gatifloxacin, gemifloxacin and moxifloxacin though the magnitude of the effect is less than that seen with magnesium and aluminum [28, 30].

The clinical importance of the interaction will depend on the location of the infection, the *in vitro* susceptibility of the pathogen, and the magnitude of the effect. Concomitant use of quinolones with magnesium-, aluminum-, or calcium-containing antacids, sucralfate, or iron/vitamin-mineral preparations should be avoided, unless the quinolone is administered at least 2 h before the cation.

Didanosine tablet formulations

Didanosine tablet formulations contain magnesium and aluminum buffers to prevent it from acid-mediated degradation. When didanosine buffering agents are given

Table 3. – Drug interactions involving quinolone antibiotics

Interacting drug	Quinolone	Mechanism of interaction	Effect	Clinical significance and management
Antacids	Enoxacin, norfloxacin, ciprofloxacin, sparfloxacin, moxifloxacin, gatifloxacin, gemifloxacin	Cation-quinolone chelation complex formation	↓ Absorption of all quinolones ↓ F% or ↓ AUC	Clinically relevant. Avoid combination, or separate doses by 2 h, give quinolone first
Sucralfate	Enoxacin, norfloxacin, ciprofloxacin	Cation-quinolone chelation complex formation	↓ Absorption of most quinolones, ↓ F%	Clinically relevant Avoid combination, or give quinolone 2 h before sucralfate
Iron	Enoxacin, norfloxacin, ciprofloxacin, levofloxacin, moxifloxacin, gatifloxacin, gemifloxacin	Cation-quinolone chelation complex formation	↓ Absorption of all quinolones, ↓ F% or ↓ AUC	Clinically relevant Avoid combination, or separate doses by 2 h, give quinolones first
Calcium	Enoxacin, norfloxacin, ciprofloxacin, gemifloxacin	Cation-quinolone chelation complex formation	↓ Absorption of most quinolones, ↓ F%	Clinically relevant Avoid combination, or separate doses by 2 h, give quinolones first
Multivitamins with zinc	Enoxacin, norfloxacin, ciprofloxacin,	Cation-quinolone chelation complex formation	Small ↓ absorption	Clinically relevant Avoid combination, or separate doses by 2 h, give quinolones first
Didanosine, standard tablet formulations	Ciprofloxacin	Buffer cation-quinolone chelation complex formation	↓ Absorption, ↓ C_{max} and ↓ AUC	Clinically relevant Avoid combination, or separate doses by 2 h, give quinolones first, or use enteric-coated didanosine
Probenecid	Enoxacin, norfloxacin, ciprofloxacin, levofloxacin, gatifloxacin	Inhibition of the renal anionic transport system	↓ Renal excretion of certain quinolones, ↓ Cl_R	Unlikely to be clinically relevant
Ranitidine	Enoxacin	Increase of the gastric pH	↓ quinolone absorption, ↓ F and ↓ C_{max}	Unclear clinical significance
Cimetidine	Enoxacin, norfloxacin, ciprofloxacin	Inhibition of the renal cationic transport system	↓ renal excretion of certain quinolones, ↓ Cl_R	Unclear clinical significance
Theophylline	Enoxacin, ciprofloxacin	Inhibition of the CYP1A2 isoenzyme by quinolones	↑ Theophylline levels with certain quinolones ↑ C_{max} and ↑ AUC	Clinically relevant Enoxacin and ciprofloxacin are most likely to result in an interaction; most other quinolones safe
Caffeine	Enoxacin, ciprofloxacin	Inhibition of the CYP1A2 by quinolones	↑ Caffeine levels with certain quinolones	Unclear clinical significance

Table 3. continued

Interacting drug	Quinolone	Mechanism of interaction	Effect	Clinical significance and management
Warfarin	Enoxacin, ciprofloxacin	Disputed	Conflicting data on increased warfarin PD effects, no significant PK effects $\uparrow t_{1/2}$ (R)-warfarin, NE on (L)-warfarin, slight $\uparrow$ on PT	Unclear clinical significance Monitor INR and PT when a quinolone is administered to patients receiving warfarin
Cyclosporin	Enoxacin, norfloxacin, ciprofloxacin	Metabolic, disputed	$\uparrow$ cyclosporin levels with ciprofloxacin and norfloxacin (case report), possible $\uparrow$ nephrotoxic effects; no significant PK effects	Unlikely to be clinically important
NSAIDs	Enoxacin, norfloxacin, ciprofloxacin	Enhancement of the inhibitory effects on GABA receptor	Early reports of seizures with fenbufen and enoxacin	Interaction appears to be of little clinical relevance with current quinolones and NSAIDs
Antiarrhythmics Class IA and III quinidine, disopyramide, sotalol, amiodarone	Fluoroquinolones (class effect)	Potential enhancement on QTc prolongation	Theoretical potential for QTc prolongation if used with quinolones with similar effects	Uncertain clinical significance Caution if used with quinolones that increase QTc interval
Cholinegic agents Cisapride	Fluoroquinolones (class effect)	Potential enhancement on QTc prolongation	Theoretical potential for QTc prolongation if used with quinolones with similar	Uncertain clinical significance Caution if used with quinolones that increase QTc interval
Macrolides Clarithromycin/ erythromycin	Fluoroquinolones (class effect)	Potential enhancement on QTc prolongation	Theoretical potential for QTc prolongation if used with quinolones with similar	Uncertain clinical significance Caution if used with quinolones that increase QTc interval
Tricyclic antidepressants, (imipramine, amitryptiline)	Fluoroquinolones (class effect)	Potential enhancement on QTc prolongation	Theoretical potential for QTc prolongation if used with quinolones with similar	Uncertain clinical significance Caution if used with quinolones that increase QTc interval.

F%: bioavailability percentage; AUC: area under the concentration-time-curve; Cmax: peak concentration reached in the plasma/serum; ClR: renal clearance; CYP: cytochrome P450; PD: pharmacodynamic; PK: pharmacokinetics; $t_{1/2}$: half-life; NE: no effect; PT: prothrombin time; INR: international normalisation ratio; NSAIDs: nonsteroidal anti-inflammatory drugs; GABA: gamma-aminobutyric acid; QTc: corrected QT interval; $\uparrow$: increase; $\downarrow$: decrease.

concomitantly with ciprofloxacin, absorption of the quinolone is significantly reduced [38, 39]. Enteric coated formulations of didanosine are instead unlikely to cause such drug interactions because they lack antacids [40].

The simultaneous administration of ciprofloxacin and didanosine tablets should therefore, be avoided. The dose of ciprofloxacin should be taken at least 2 h prior to didanosine.

Dairy products and enteral feedings. Ciprofloxacin and norfloxacin bioavailability are decreased when concomitantly administered with milk or yogurt. The effect of dairy products is most likely caused by calcium ions contained in milk. In contrast, absorption of other quinolones appears unaffected.

The concomitant administration of quinolones and enteral feeding can result in decreased absorption of quinolones. Data from several studies investigating the effects of different enteral feeding supplements on the bioavailability of ciprofloxacin demonstrate mixed results. Three studies have shown that various enteral products can decrease ciprofloxacin Cmax and AUC [28]. However, one study found no statistically significant changes in AUC, Cmax and *t*max when ciprofloxacin was administered with enteral feeding [28]. The apparent discrepancy in results may be due to differing cation concentrations in the various enteral formulations. The potential interaction between enteral feeds and the newer fluoroquinolone agents has not been well studied.

Probenecid. Probenecid is a competitive inhibitor of the renal tubular secretory pathway of anionic compounds [41]. Quinolones are generally excreted in the urine, with tubular secretion being a prominent excretory pathway. Since they are zwitterions at physiological pH, they may be secreted in the renal tubules generally through either the anionic or the cationic transport systems or both. Probenecid significantly decreases the renal elimination of fluoroquinolones primarily excreted in urine by active tubular secretion. This results in decreased clearance and potentially increased half-life and bioavailability of several fluoroquinolones such as ciprofloxacin, enoxacin, norfloxacin, levofloxacin, gatifloxacin, but not moxifloxacin [28, 42].

This is not likely to be a clinically important interaction, unless there is concurrent renal impairment. Monitoring signs of toxicity is recommended, if this is an issue.

H₂-receptor antagonists. Treatment with H_2-receptor antagonists increases the gastric pH to a range in which the solubility of fluoroquinolones is considerable reduced.

Ranitidine does not significantly inhibit the CYP enzyme system and exhibits few interactions with other drugs. Intravenous (IV) ranitidine administered 2 h prior to oral intake of enoxacin led to a 40% reduction in enoxacin bioavailability [43]. The mechanism of this interaction is due to the increase in the gastric pH, leading to a decrease in enoxacin absorption [44].

NIX *et al.* [45] and HOFFKEN *et al.* [46] found no significant effects of ranitidine on the pharmacokinetics of ciprofloxacin and ofloxacin. Also ranitidine does not affect the absorption of newer fluoroquinolones [28].

In contrast, cimetidine is a nonselective inhibitor of the CYP enzyme system and alters the pharmacokinetics of a variety of drugs undergoing hepatic biotransformation. Cimetidine also interacts with the renal cationic transport system [47]. This is the putative mechanism by which it significantly increases AUC and clearance of some quinolones, such as pefloxacin, enoxacin, ciprofloxacin and levofloxacin [30, 48, 49].

Methylxanthines. The interaction between quinolones and methylxanthines (*i.e.* theophylline and caffeine) is well known and has been thoroughly investigated. This interaction was initially reported for enoxacin, which is the most potent inhibitor of theophylline biotransformation when a number of patients receiving theophylline had toxic reactions including seizures [50, 51]. This is associated with a strong decrease in the total body clearance of theophylline [52, 53].

On the basis of pharmacokinetic and clinical data, fluoroquinolones have been classified into three groups according to the degree of their theophylline interaction [54].

Group I includes quinolones (*e.g.* pipemidic acid, enoxacin) that induce a >40% increase in C_{max} and/or AUC values for theophylline, associated with a very high risk of inducing toxic effects.

Group II agents induce a 15–40% increase in plasma theophylline levels, causing a lower incidence of side effects. Ciprofloxacin, which is included in this group, has been shown to precipitate seizures in the susceptible patient at high doses (>500 mg) [30].

Group III quinolones which include ofloxacin, levofloxacin, sparfloxacin, gatifloxacin, gemifloxacin and moxifloxacin have negligible or no effect on theophylline metabolism [28, 54]. Data on the interactions between methylxanthines and sitafloxacin are currently unknown.

Monitoring of theophylline levels and dose adjustment, when necessary, is recommended during ciprofloxacin administration. Monitoring for clinical signs of theophylline toxicity should be performed for the newer fluoroquinolones.

Patients who are prescribed quinolones should also be advised on possible interactions with caffeine.

Warfarin. There are conflicting opinions in the literature about interactions of fluoroquinolones with the anticoagulant drug warfarin. Several case reports describe increased anticoagulant effect of warfarin in patients previously stabilised on warfarin therapy who also began to receive concomitant quinolones such as ciprofloxacin [55], norfloxacin, or ofloxacin [17], and more recently levofloxacin [56] suggesting a risk of bleeding complications during co-treatment, especially in the elderly and during a polypharmacologic treatment.

However, multiple studies in healthy volunteers and anticoagulated patients have shown no significant effect on either warfarin pharmacokinetics or measures of anticoagulation (PT and INR) when various quinolones were given. A pharmacokinetic study conducted in adult patients showed that ciprofloxacin 750 mg *b.i.d.* for 12 days caused a significant increase in concentrations of R-enantiomer of warfarin, while the concentrations of the most potent enantiomer S-warfarin (endowed with 2–5× more anticoagulant activity than the R-warfarin) remained unchanged [57]. A slight, however nonclinically relevant (*i.e.* <30%), increase in PT was observed. Similar results were obtained in trials investigating enoxacin and norfloxacin interactions with warfarin [58, 59]. Administration of levofloxacin, gatifloxacin, gemifloxacin or moxifloxacin have not shown alterations in the pharmacokinetic or pharmacodynamic effects of warfarin [28, 32]. Although specific drug interaction studies of gatifloxacin and warfarin were not identified, pooled data from over 3,000 patients who received gatifloxacin have not demonstrated interactions with hepatic enzymes [60].

In retrospect, the lack of a warfarin interaction in prospective investigations is consistent with the known effects of the quinolones on drug metabolising enzymes. The S-enantiomer of warfarin is mainly metabolised by CYP2C9. This enzyme is not inhibited by the available quinolones, thus decreasing the probability of significant pharmacokinetic interactions.

Due to the low plasma protein binding of fluoroquinolones (20–60%), displacement of warfarin from the binding sites is very unlikely. One prospective investigation did report statistically significant increases in INR in healthy volunteers receiving warfarin who received a 2-week course of clinafloxacin [61]. There was no significant effect on warfarin pharmacokinetics, and the increase in INR was attributed to a reduction in gut flora producing vitamin K by the quinolone. Although this local effect on gastrointestinal microorganisms may explain the enhancement of the warfarin response, this phenomenon remains poorly investigated and understood.

It may be concluded that the clinical significance of this interaction is variable. Patients receiving warfarin for whom a quinolone is indicated can probably be treated safely, although it would be prudent to monitor PT/INR.

Cyclosporin. Case reports suggest an interaction between quinolones and cyclosporin, resulting in changes in cyclosporin concentrations and consequently in nephrotoxicity [62–64]. Patients treated with ciprofloxacin required reduction in cyclosporin dosage to maintain cyclosporin concentrations within the therapeutic range. These observations have, however, not been confirmed by prospective trials showing that quinolones such as pefloxacin, ciprofloxacin and levofloxacin do not alter cyclosporin pharmacokinetics or increase its adverse effects [17]. These negative findings are consistent with the contention that quinolones inhibit primarily CYP1A2 but not the rate-limiting cyclosporin metabolising enzyme CYP3A4.

Consistent with clinical results, PICHARD *et al.* [65] found that norfloxacin did not inhibit cyclosporin metabolism in human liver microsomes *in vitro*. Quinolones have threfore, been recommended for the treatment of *Legionella pneumophila* infections in transplant patients instead of macrolides and rifampicin because the latter treatments significantly alter cyclosporin pharmacokinetics.

In conclusion, no cyclosporin dosage modifications are needed during co-treatment with fluoroquinolones.

Glibenclamide (Glyburide). Case reports suggest that some individuals receiving glibenclamide experience hypoglycemia and subsequent symptoms when ciprofloxacin is taken concomitantly [29]. In contrast, a clinical study found no significant effect of ciprofloxacin on glibenclamide metabolism [66]. Therefore, monitoring of blood glucose is recommended when this agent is co-administered with ciprofloxacin. No clinically significant interactions have been observed with newer fluoroquinolones.

Digoxin. Interactions with the use of digoxin and fluoroquinolones have not been documented. However, since digoxin has a narrow therapeutic index, it has been studied with most of the new fluoroquinolones for interactions. No significant interactions have been shown between digoxin and levofloxacin, gemifloxacin and moxifloxacin [32].

Gatifloxin treatment caused instead a slight increase in the steady state C_{max} and AUC of digoxin (12 and 19%, respectively) [32]. This was not associated with any adverse event or significant changes in laboratory tests. Therefore, no recommendations for dosage adjustment are warranted.

Nonsteroidal anti-inflammatory drugs. Fluoroquinolones have been associated with adverse drug reactions on the central nervous system (CNS) either minor, *e.g.* dizziness and headache, or severe, *e.g.* convulsions [67]. They can occur as a result of either direct action of quinolones on CNS receptors or as a result of interaction between quinolones and other agents, such as nonsteroidal anti-inflammatory drugs (NSAIDs). The clinical observation that several patients receiving the combination of enoxacin and fenbufen, an NSAID available in Japan, prompted the Japanese Welfare Ministry to issue a warning to avoid prescribing this combination.

Studies in healthy volunteers did not show any significant change in the pharmacokinetics of some fluoroquinolones (ofloxacin and pefloxacin) when combined with NSAIDs [68, 69].

Based on data from several studies in experimental *in vitro* models and in animals, it appears that this interaction is predominantly pharmacodynamic in nature.

Excitatory CNS effects of fluoroquinolones are thought in part to be related to a dose-dependent inhibition of the binding of gamma-aminobutyric acid (GABA), an inhibitory neurotransmitter, to its brain receptors [70]. Recent studies have suggested that the convulsive potency of fluoroquinolones may relate more directly to primary stimulation of the N-methyl-D-aspartate receptor [71]. Some of the newer fluoroquinolones, notably trovafloxacin, demonstrated particularly high excitatory potency. The effects on GABA receptor probably explain the interaction between fluoroquinolones and NSAIDs, since they are enhanced markedly by NSAIDs in experimental systems, most notably with biphenyl acetic acid (BPAA), the active metabolite of fenbufen [72].

Considerable differences exist between the various fluoroquinolones with regards to their activity as GABA antagonists. The rank order of potency in inhibiting GABA receptor binding is norfloxacin >enoxacin >ofloxacin >ciprofloxacin [73]. Sparfloxacin and levofloxacin have less epileptogenical effect than other fluoroquinolones in experimental models. Also, in the presence of BPAA, drug concentrations necessary to inhibit 50% of GABA receptor binding for both sparfloxacin and levofloxacin remain high, well above clinically relevant levels. These phenomena may relate to intermolecular interactions between the different fluoroquinolones and BPAA.

It is believed that the piperazine ring at position seven of quinolones is responsible for GABA receptor binding antagonism since this structure closely mimics GABA. The substituent at the C7 position is an important predictor of GABA binding. Quinolones that possess piperazine substituted with one or more methyl groups at position seven exhibited lower inhibition of GABA binding [35, 74]. This may be relevant for new agents, such as levofloxacin and sparfloxacin.

Clearly the concomitant use of fenbufen and enoxacin should be avoided. However, quinolones and NSAIDS are commonly prescribed together and CNS effects appear to be very uncommon, suggesting that this interaction is unlikely to be clinically important with current quinolones.

Quinolone-induced QT prolongation. Certain fluoroquinolones have a demonstrated potential for the development of ventricular arrhythmias-torsades de pointes and, more rarely, sudden cardiac deaths in susceptible individuals by causing prolongation of the rate-corrected electrocardiographic QT (QTc) interval [67].

The quinolone-induced QTc prolongation phenomenon and associated cardiotoxic effects have originally been described for sparfloxacin [75], but they were highlighted as a class-effect by the grepafloxacin withdrawal from the world market in November 1999 [76].

Analysis of the structure-side effect relationship has revealed that cardiotoxicity is dependent upon the substituent added to position five of the fluorine ring. In this situation, an amino group possessed by sparfloxacin and a methyl group by grepafloxacin increase toxicity, while the hydrogen possessed by other major fluoroquinolones is less likely to cause QTc prolongation (*e.g.* moxifloxacin, levofloxacin, gemifloxacin).

Evidence supporting the relationship between QTc interval length and risk of sudden death from arrhythmia has been published, showing that the risk of sudden cardiac death with a QTc interval of 440 msec is 1.0. However, this rises to 1.4 with a QTc of 500 msec and to 1.8 at a QTc of 640 msec [77].

The risk of prolonged QTc increases as higher doses of drug are used, as these produce higher AUC levels. Females are also at greater risk than males, as are the elderly. Ranking the fluoroquinolones in terms of their risk of prolonging QTc shows sparfloxacin to be worse than grepafloxacin, followed by gatifloxacin, moxifloxacin, ciprofloxacin and gemifloxacin. Much less risk is associated with sitafloxacin, trovafloxacin and levofloxacin.

It was also possible to directly correlate the strength of the fluoquinolone QTc prolongation effect with their potassium antagonist action [78]. This revealed that sparfloxacin and grepafloxacin have a high affinity for potassium current antagonists potentially causing ventricular tachycardia.

A number of other drugs have been recognised as causing prolonged QTc interval and torsade de pointes. These include anaesthetics (halothane), class IA or class III antiarrhythmics (quinidine, disopyramide, sotalol, amiodarone), tricyclic antidepressants (imipramine, amitryptiline), antihistaminics (terfenadine), antipsychotics (thioridazine, haloperidol), cholinergic agents (cisapride) and antibiotics, notably macrolides, but also cotrimoxazole, imidazoles and certain quinolone-related antimalarial agents [79].

When quinolones that increase the QTc interval are given with these drugs, a theoretical potential pharmacodynamic interaction consisting in increased QTc interval may occur. Although the clinical significance of this interaction is yet uncertain, quinolones that have been associated with QT prolongation should be avoided in certain patients [80, 81] These include people with known prolongation of the QT interval, patients with uncorrected hypokalaemia, and patients receiving other drugs interfering with the QT interval.

Other drugs. The possible interactions between fluoroquinolones and other drugs have been investigated. As a result of a considerable number of studies, no other information on clinically relevant interactions has emerged. For example, no significant interaction was detected between ciprofloxacin and diazepam, phenytoin, omeprazole and metoprolol [30, 31].

Rifampicin

Rifampicin is the most potent inducer of several CYP isoenzymes (mainly CYP3A, CYP2C9 and CYP2C19) as well as of P-gp [82]. The clinical consequence is that the co-administration of rifampicin with highly metabolised drugs may significantly increase their intestinal and hepatic clearance with an important decrease in efficacy and therapeutic failure.

The most important drug interactions involving rifampicin are summarised in table 4. They include benzodiazepines, immunosuppressive agents, antiarrhythmics, oral contraceptives, corticosteroids, digoxin, theophylline and warfarin [83, 84].

No less important are the interactions with most protease inhibitors. Rifampicin is contraindicated with most protease inhibitors and non-nucleoside reverse transcriptase inhibitors, because it can reduce their AUC by ~80% [85, 86].

Other interacting drugs are antifungals (itraconazole and fluconazole), methadone and clarithromycin [82]. All patients receiving the above mentioned combinations must be carefully monitored and dosing adjustments should be considered.

Trimethoprim-sulfamethoxazole

Trimethoprim-sulfamethoxazole is the cause of several types of interactions with other drugs mediated by metabolic or pharmacodynamic effects and by competitive tubular secretion [2]. Trimethoprim-sulfamethoxazole can decrease the clearance of phenytoin, cyclosporin and warfarin, mainly by inhibition of hepatic metabolism with enhanced effects of these drugs. Therefore patients should be monitored for drug levels or for an increase in PT/INR [2, 3, 87, 88].

Trimethoprim may inhibit renal tubular secretion of the NRTIs (lamivudine, zidovudine and zalcitabine), amantadine, dapsone, digoxin, methotrexate procainamide. This can enhance the toxicity of these object drugs. Hypoglycemia has also been reported when sulfonylurea hypoglycemics are co-administered with trimethoprim-sulfamethoxazole. Trimethoprim has caused hyperkalemia in combination with potassium-sparing

Table 4. – Main drug interactions involving rifampicin

Interacting drug	Mechanism of interaction	Effect	Clinical significance and management
Benzodiazepines Midazolam Triazolam	CYP3A4 induction	↓ Benzodiazepine levels, AUC and $t\frac{1}{2}$	Great decrease in hypnotic effect
Immunosuppressive agents Cyclosporin Tacrolimus	CYP3A4 and P-glycoprotein induction	↓ Cyclosporin and tacrolimus levels ↓ Bioavailability ↑ Clearance	Monitor drug levels for both drugs and increase the dosage, if required
Calcium antagonists Verapamil Nifedipine Diltiazem	Hepatic and intestinal enzymes induction	↓ Calcium antagonist levels ↓ Bioavailability	Decrease cardiovascular effect Increase the calcium antagonist dose
Beta blockers Propanolol Metoprolol Bisoprolol	Hepatic enzymes induction	↓ β-blocker levels	Decrease effects. Increase the β blocker dose
Oral contraceptives	Hepatic enzyme induction	↓ Ethylylestradiol AUC ↓ Norethindrone AUC	Increased risk of pregnancy Use additional (barrier) contraceptive methods
Digoxin	P-glycoprotein induction	↓ Digoxin AUC ↓ Bioavailability	Monitor digoxin levels and increase the dose, if required
Theophylline	Hepatic enzyme induction	↓ Theophylline levels ↑ Theophylline clearance	Monitor theophylline levels and for clinical response; increase the dose, if necessary
Warfarin	Hepatic enzyme induction	↓ Warfarin levels ↑ Warfarin clearance	Monitor INR and PT
Corticosteroids	CYP3A4 induction	↓ Prednisolone AUC ↑ Prednisolone clearance	Monitor for clinical response. Increase prednisolone dose

CYP: cytochrome P450; AUC: area under the time-concentration curve; $t1/2$: half-life; INR: international normalisation ratio; PT: prothrombin time; ↑: increase; ↓: decrease.

diuretics (inhibition of sodium channels in renal distal tubules) or hyponatremia with thiazide diuretics [87, 88].

Patients should be monitored for serum potassium and sodium levels.

β-lactams

β-lactam agents are rarely a cause of drug interactions. However, they may occur during co-administration with drugs which competitively inhibit their tubular secretion (*e.g.* probenecid, salicylate and methotrexate) [89].

Conflicting data have been published about the effect of furosemide on β-lactams. Some authors suggest an inhibition on tubular secretion and others demonstrated a significant increase in renal excretion [17]. The oral absorption of some cephalosporins (cefpodoxime proxetil and cefuroxime axetil) is pH dependent and can be modified by antiacids, H_2 blockers and proton pump inhibitors [3].

Metronidazole

Metronidazole, an inhibitor of hepatic metabolism, may significantly interact with warfarin and 5-fluorouracil, resulting in enhanced effects of these drugs [4, 5]. Patients receiving warfarin should be monitored for INR and PT.

Patients taking metronidazole should also avoid ingesting alcohol, oral tinctures or IV drugs containing ethanol (*e.g.* diasepam, nitroglycezin, phenobarbital and trimethoprim-sulfamethoxazole), because of the risk of a disulfiram-like reaction [4].

Quinopristin-dalfopristin

Quinopristin-dalfopristin may significantly inhibit the CYP3A4-mediated metabolism of several drugs such as antihistamines (astemizole, terfenadine), antihuman immuno-deficiency virus (HIV) drugs, benzodiazepines (midazolam, diazepam), calcium channel blockers (nifedipine, verapamil, diltiazem), statins, immunosuppressive agents (cyclosporin, tacrolimus) and steroids.

The co-administration with these drugs may result in higher serum levels which could increase therapeutic or adverse effects. However, only in a few cases (*e.g.* cyclosporin) should monitoring be performed [3, 90].

Finally, concomitant administration of drugs metabolised by CYP3A4 that may cause QTc prolongation should be avoided [90].

Linezolid

Linezolid is not metabolised by CYP enzymes. Moreover, both in *in vitro* and *in vivo* systems, linezolid does not induce or inhibit CYP activity. Therefore, no CYP-mediated drug interactions are possible.

Linezolid is a reversible inhibitor of human monoamine oxidase with the potential to interact with adrenergic and serotoninergic drugs and to induce an increase in systolic blood pressure and serotonin syndrome (*e.g.* confusion, delirium, tremors and hyperpyrexia). Patients receiving linezolid should be advised to avoid food or beverages containing tyramide [91].

Conclusions

Antibiotic interactions are an important aspect of the safety profile of these drugs, but are often forgotten or underestimated by physicians. The most important step in avoiding adverse clinical consequences is knowledge of the potential toxicity of drug combinations so that a rational prescription can be made. For example, the clinician may administer the antibiotic if the interaction is unlikely to be important, or can choose an alternative antibiotic that does not have the potential for drug interaction. In some cases which are well defined in this article, a dose reduction or increase of the interacting drug may be necessary. Sometimes it is only necessary to alter the administration time by 2 or 3 h, as with the fluoroquinolones and some other antibiotics. Finally, the physician may administer the antibiotic in question but should monitor serum concentrations of the interacting drug, as in the case of digoxin, cyclosporin and theophylline.

Summary

Antibacterial drug interactions are an important aspect of the safety profile of these drugs, though they are often forgotten or underestimated by physicians. Different antibiotics may have a potential risk of pharmacological drug interactions, which can be classified as either pharmacodynamic or pharmacokinetic. The former are rare and are mostly limited to the potentiation of neuromuscular blocking effects by aminoglycosides and to either central nervous system adverse drug reactions or cardiac QT interval prolongation, due to the combination of fluoroquinolones either with some nonsteroidal anti-inflammatory drugs or cisapride. On the contrary, the pharmacokinetic drug interactions are relatively common, may concern all the different kinetic phases, and may result in clinically relevant consequences. Drug interactions involving antibiotics may impair their pharmacokinetics or may induce major changes in the kinetic parameters of co-administered drugs. Many clinically relevant interactions of macrolides, fluoroquinolones, rifampin or rifabutin depend on modifications of the biotransformation of different compounds, involving the cytochrome P450 system. This chapter will focus on the mechanisms and clinical relevance of the most important drug interactions that involve the major classes of antibacterial agents commonly used in the treatment of lower respiratory tract infections.

Keywords: Antibiotics, clinical relevance, drug interactions, lower respiratory tract infections treatment, pharmacodynamics pharmacokinetics.

References

1. Piscitelli JH, Rodvold K eds. Drug Interaction in Infectious Diseases. Totowa, Humana Press, 2000.
2. Gregg CR. Drug interactions and anti-infective therapies. *Am J Med* 1999; 106: 227–237.
3. Polk R, Qaqish RB. Drug interactions involving antimicrobial agents. *In*: Finch RG, Greenwood D, Norrby SR, Whitley RJ, eds. Antibiotic and Chemotherapy. Anti-Infective Agents and Their Use in Therapy, 8th Edn. Edinburgh, Churchill Livingstone, UK, 2003: 67–100.
4. Kashuba ADM, Bertino JS. Mechanisms of drug interactions. *In*: Piscitelli JH, Rodvold KA, Masur H, eds. Drug Interaction In Infectious Disease. Totowa, Humana Press, 2000: 13–38.
5. Tatro DS. Drug interaction facts, 5th Edn. St. Louis, Facts and Comparisons, 1996.
6. Zhang Y, Benet LZ. The gut as a barrier to drug absorption: combined role of cytochrome P_{450} 3A and P-glycoprotein. *Clin Pharmacokinet* 2001; 40: 159–168.
7. Sansom LN, Evans AM. What is the true clinical significance of plasma protein binding displacement interactions? *Drug Safety* 1995; 12: 227–233.
8. Dresser GK, Spence JD, Bailey DG. Pharmacokinetic-pharmacodynamic consequences and clinical relevance of cytochrome P450 3A4 inhibition. *Clin Pharmacokinet* 2000; 38: 41–57.
9. Westphal JF. Macrolide - induced clinically relevant drug interactions with cytochrome P-450A (CYP) 3A4: an update focused on clarithromycin, azithromycin and dirithromycin. *Br J Clin Pharmacol* 2000; 50: 285–295.
10. Mazzei T, Mini E, Novelli A, Periti P. Chemistry and mode of action of macrolides. *J Antimicrob Chemother* 1993; 31: Suppl. C, 1–9.
11. Zhanel GG, Walters M, Noreddin A, *et al.* The ketolides: a critical review. *Drugs* 2002; 62: 1771–804.
12. Rubinstein E. Comparative safety of the different macrolides. *Int J Antimicrob Agents* 2001; 18: Suppl. 1, S71–S76.
13. Periti P, Mazzei T, Mini E, Novelli A. Pharmacokinetic drug interactions of macrolides. *Clin Pharmacokinet* 1992; 23: 106–31.
14. Von Rosensteil NA, Adam D. Macrolide antibacterials. Drug interactions of clinical significance. *Drug Safety* 1995; 13: 105–122.
15. Hayton AC. Precipitation of acute ergotism by triacetyloleandomycin. *N Z Med J* 1969; 69: 42.
16. Pai MP, Graci DM, Amsden GW. Macrolide drug interactions: an update. *Ann Pharmacother* 2000; 34: 495–513.

17. Pea F, Furlanut M. Pharmacokinetic aspects of treating infections in the intensive care unit: focus on drug interactions. *Clin Pharmacokinet* 2001; 40: 833–868.

18. Shain CS, Amsden GW. Telithromycin: the first of the ketolides. *Ann Pharmacother* 2002; 36: 452–464.

19. Paine MF, Wagner DA, Hoffmaster KA, Watkins PB. Cytochrome P450 3A4 and P–glycoprotein mediate the interaction between an oral erythromycin breath test and rifampin. *Clin Pharmacol Ther* 2002; 72: 524–535.

20. Malaty LI, Kuper JJ. Drug interactions of HIV protease inhibitors. *Drug Safety* 1999; 20: 147–169.

21. Hesse LM, von Moltke LL, Greenblatt DJ. Clinically important drug interactions with zopiclone, zolpidem and zaleplon. *CNS Drugs* 2003; 17: 513–532.

22. Rodvold KA. Clinical pharmacokinetics of clarithromycin. *Clin Pharmacokinet* 1999; 37: 385–398.

23. Flockhart DA, Drici MD, Kerbusch T, *et al.* Studies on the mechanism of a fatal clarithromycin-pimozide interaction in a patient with Tourette syndrome. *J Clin Psychopharmacol* 2000; 20: 317–324.

24. Paoletti R, Corsini A, Bellosta S. Pharmacological interactions of statins. *Atheroscler* 2002; 3: 35–40.

25. Wermeling DP, Chandler MH, Sides GD, Collins D, Muse KN. Dirithromycin increases ethinyl estradiol clearance without allowing ovulation. *Obstet Gynecol* 1995; 86: 78–84.

26. Muirhead GJ, Faulkner S, Harness JA, Taubel J. The effects of steady-state erythromycin and azithromycin on the pharmacokinetics of sildenafil in healthy volunteers. *Br J Clin Pharmacol* 2002; 53: Suppl. 1, 37S–43S.

27. Tobe SW, Siu LL, Jamal SA, Skorecki KL, Murphy GF, Warner E. Vinblastine and erythromycin: an unrecognized serious drug interaction. *Cancer Chemother Pharmacol* 1995; 35: 188–190.

28. Aminimanizani A, Beringer P, Jelliffe R. Comparative pharmacokinetics and pharmacodynamics of the newer fluoroquinolone antibacterials. *Clin Pharmacokinet* 2001; 40: 169–187.

29. Gillum JG, Israel DS, Polk RE. Pharmacokinetic drug interactions with antimicrobial agents. *Clin Pharmacokinet* 1993; 25: 450–482.

30. Kuhlmann J, Schaefer H-G, Beermann D. Clinical pharmacology. *In*: Kuhlmann J, Dalhoff A, Zeiler H-J, eds. Handbook Experimental Pharmacology, Quinolone Antibacterials. Berlin, Springer. 1998: pp. 339–406.

31. Stahlmann R, Lode H. Safety review. Toxicity, adverse effects, and drug interactions. *In*: Andriole VT, ed. The Quinolones, 2nd Edn. Academic Press, 1998: pp. 369–415.

32. Zhanel GG, Ennis K, Vercaigne L, *et al.* A critical review of the fluoroquinolones: focus on respiratory infections. *Drugs* 2002; 62: 13–59.

33. Lomaestro BM, Bailie GR. Quinolone-cation interactions: a review. *DICP* 1991; 25: 1249–1258.

34. Spivey JM, Cummings DM, Pierson NR. Failure of prostatitis treatment secondary to probable ciprofloxacin-sucralfate drug interaction. *Pharmacotherapy* 1996; 16: 314–316.

35. Structure-activity, structure-side-effect relationships for the quinolone antibacterials. *J Antimicrob Chemother* 1994; 33: 685–706.

36. Mizuki Y, Fujiwara I, Yamaguchi T. Pharmacokinetic interactions related to the chemical structures of fluoroquinolones. *J Antimicrob Chemother* 1996; 37: Suppl. A, 41–55.

37. Stass H, Kubitza D. Profile of moxifloxacin drug interactions. *Clin Infect Dis* 2001; 32: Suppl. 1, S47–S50.

38. Knupp CA, Barbhaiya RH. A multiple-dose pharmacokinetic interaction study between didanosine (Videx) and ciprofloxacin (Cipro) in male subjects seropositive for HIV but asymptomatic. *Biopharm Drug Dispos* 1997; 18: 65–77.

39. Sahai J, Gallicano K, Oliveras L, Khaliq S, Hawley-Foss N, Garber G. Cations in the didanosine tablet reduce ciprofloxacin bioavailability. *Clin Pharmacol Ther* 1993; 53: 292–297.

40. Damle BD, Mummaneni V, Kaul S, Knupp C. Lack of effect of simultaneously administered didanosine encapsulated enteric bead formulation (Videx EC) on oral absorption of indinavir, ketoconazole, or ciprofloxacin. *Antimicrob Agents Chemother* 2002; 46: 385–391.

41. Bonate PL, Reith K, Weir S. Drug interactions at the renal level. Implications for drug development. *Clin Pharmacokinet* 1998; 34: 375–404.

42. Stass H, Sachse R. Effect of probenecid on the kinetics of a single oral 400 mg dose of moxifloxacin in healthy male volunteers. *Clin Pharmacokinet* 2001; 40: Suppl. 1, 71–76.

43. Grasela TH Jr, Schentag JJ, Sedman AJ, *et al.* Inhibition of enoxacin absorption by antacids or ranitidine. *Antimicrob Agents Chemother* 1989; 33: 615–617.

44. Lebsack ME, Nix D, Ryerson B, *et al.* Effect of gastric acidity on enoxacin absorption. *Clin Pharmacol Ther* 1992; 52: 252–256.

45. Nix DE, Watson WA, Lener ME, *et al.* Effects of aluminum and magnesium antacids and ranitidine on the absorption of ciprofloxacin. *Clin Pharmacol Ther* 1989; 46: 700–705.

46. Höffken G, Lode H, Wiley R, Glatzel P, Sievens D, *et al.* Pharmacokinetics and bioavailability of ciprofloxacin and ofloxacin: effect of food and antacid intake. *Rev Infect Dis* 1988; 10: Suppl. 1, 138–139.

47. Besseghir K, Roch-Ramel F. Renal excretion of drugs and other xenobiotics. *Ren Physiol* 1987; 10: 221–241.

48. Misiak PM, Eldon MA, Toothaker RD, Sedman AJ. Effects of oral cimetidine or ranitidine on the pharmacokinetics of intravenous enoxacin. *J Clin Pharmacol* 1993; 33: 53–56.

49. Gaitonde MD, Fowler CA, Palmer M, *et al.* The effects of cimetidine and probenecid on the pharmacokinetics of levofloxacin (LVFX). San Francisco, 35th Interscience Conference on Antimicrobial Agents and Chemotherapy, 1995; A41.

50. Wijnands WJA, van Herwaarden CLA, Vree TB. Enoxacin raises plasma theophylline concentrations. *Lancet* 1984; 2: 108–109.

51. Maesen FPV, Teengs JP, Baur C, Davies BI. Quinolones and raised plasma concentrations of theophylline. *Lancet* 1984; 2: 530.

52. Wijnands WJ, Vree TB, Van Herwaarden CL. Enoxacin decreases the clearance of theophylline in man. *Br J Clin Pharmacol* 1985; 20: 583–588.

53. Wijnands WJ, Vree TB, van Herwaarden CL. The influence of quinolone derivatives on theophylline clearance. *Br J Clin Pharmacol* 1986; 22: 677–683.

54. Niki Y, Hashiguchi K, Okimoto N, Soejima R. Quinolone antimicrobial agents and theophylline. *Chest* 1992; 101: 881.

55. Ellis RJ, Mayo MS, Bodensteiner DM. Ciprofloxacin-warfarin coagulopathy: a case series. *Am J Hematol* 2000; 63: 28–31.

56. Jones CB, Fugate SE. Levofloxacin and warfarin interaction. *Ann Pharmacother* 2002; 36: 1554–1557.

57. Israel DS, Stotka J, Rock W, *et al.* Effect of ciprofloxacin on the pharmacokinetics and pharmacodynamics of warfarin. *Clin Infect Dis* 1996; 22: 251–256.

58. Toon S, Hopkins KJ, Garstang FM, Aarons L, Sedman A, Rowland M. Enoxacin-warfarin interaction: pharmacokinetic and stereochemical aspects. *Clin Pharmacol Ther* 1987; 42: 33–41.

59. Rocci ML Jr, Vlasses PH, Distlerath LM, *et al.* Norfloxacin does not alter warfarin's disposition or anticoagulant effect. *J Clin Pharmacol* 1990; 30: 728–732.

60. Breen J, Skuba K, Grasela D. Sagety and tolerability of oral gatifloxacin, a new 8-methoxy fluoroquinolone: overview of clinical data. San Francisco, 39th Interscience Conference on Antimicrobial Agents and Chemotherapy, 1999; 200.

61. Randinitis EJ, Alvey CW, Koup JR, *et al.* Drug interactions with clinafloxacin. *Antimicrob Agents Chemother* 2001; 45: 2543–2552.

62. Avent CK, Krinsky D, Kirklin JK, Bourge RC, Figg WD. Synergistic nephrotoxicity due to ciprofloxacin and cyclosporine. *Am J Med* 1988; 85: 452–453.

63. Elston RA, Taylor J. Possible interaction of ciprofloxacin with cyclosporin A. *J Antimicrob Chemother* 1988; 21: 679–680.

64. McLellan RA, Drobitch RK, McLellan H, Acott PD, Crocker JF, Renton KW. Norfloxacin interferes with cyclosporine disposition in pediatric patients undergoing renal transplantation. *Clin Pharmacol Ther* 1995; 58: 322–327.

65. Pichard L, Fabre I, Fabre G, *et al.* Cyclosporin A drug interactions. Screening for inducers and inhibitors of cytochrome P-450 (cyclosporin A oxidase) in primary cultures of human hepatocytes and in liver microsomes. *Drug Metab Dispos* 1990; 18: 595–606.

66. Ludwig E, Szekely E, Graber H, Csiba A. Study of interaction between oral ciprofloxacin and glibenclamide. *Eur J Clin Microbiol Infect Dis* 1999; 10: 378–379.

67. Mandell LA, Ball P, Tillotson G. Antimicrobial safety and tolerability: differences and dilemmas. *Clin Infect Dis* 2001; 32: Suppl. 1, S72–S79.

68. Fillastre JP, Leroy A, Borsa-Lebas F, Etienne I, Gy C, Humbert G. Effects of ketoprofen (NSAID) on the pharmacokinetics of pefloxacin and ofloxacin in healthy volunteers. *Drugs Exp Clin Res* 1992; 18: 487–492.

69. Leroy A, Fillastre JP, Borsa-Lebas F, Etienne I, Gy C, Humbert G. Effect of ketoprofen on the pharmacokinetics of two fluoroquinolones in males. *Pathol Biol* 1993; 41: 379–384.

70. Nozaki M. Safety and side effects of ofloxacin: central nervous system effects. *Penetration* 1996: 32–35.

71. Schmuck G, Schurmann A, Schluter G. Determination of the excitatory potencies of fluoroquinolones in the central nervous system by an in vitro model. *Antimicrob Agents Chemother* 1998; 42: 1831–1836.

72. Akahane K, Kimura Y, Tsutomi Y. Hayakawa I. Possible intermolecular interaction between quinolones and biphenylacetic acid inhibits gamma-aminobutyric acid receptor site. *Antimicrob Agents Chemother* 1994; 38: 2323–2329.

73. Hori S, Shimada J, Saito A, *et al.* Comparison of inhibitory effect of new quinolones on gamma-aminobutyric acid receptor binding in the presence of anti-inflammatory drugs. *Rev Infect Dis* 1989; 11: Suppl. 5, S1397–S1398.

74. Akahane K, Sekiguchi M, Une T, Osada Y. Structure-epileptogenicity relationship of quinolones with special reference to their interaction with gamma-aminobutyric acid receptor sites. *Antimicrob Agents Chemother* 1989; 33: 1704–1708.

75. Anderson ME, Mazur A, Yang T, Roden DM. Potassium current antagonist properties and proarrhythmic consequences of quinolone antibiotics. *J Antimicrob Chemother* 1996; 37: Suppl. A, 161–167.

76. Glaxo Wellcome. Withdrawal of product: RAXAR (grepafloxacin HCl) 600 mg tablets, 400 mg tablets, and 200 mg tablets. (1999) www.fda.gov/medwatch/SAFETY/1999/raxhcp.html. Novemner 1999.

77. Viskin S. Long QT syndromes and torsade de pointes. *Lancet* 1999; 354: 1625–1633.

78. Anderson ME, Mazur A, Yang T, Roden DM. Potassium current antagonist properties and proarrhythmic consequences of quinolone antibiotics. *J Pharmacol Exp Ther* 2001; 296: 806–810.

79. Owens RC Jr. Risk assessment for antimicrobial agent-induced QTc interval prolongation and torsades de pointes. *Pharmacotherapy* 2001; 21: 301–319.

80. Ball P. Quinolone-induced QT interval prolongation: a not-so-unexpected class effect. *J Antimicrob Chemother* 2000; 45: 557–559.

81. Kahn JB. Quinolone-induced QT interval prolongation: a not-so-unexpected class effect. *J Antimicrob Chemother* 2000; 46: 847–848.

82. Burman WJ, Gallicano K, Peloquin C. Comparative pharmacokinetics and pharmacodynamics of the rifamycin antibacterials. *Clin Pharmacokinet* 2000; 40: 327–341.

83. Kuper JI, D'Aprile M. Drug-drug interactions of clinical significance in the treatment of patients with *Mycobacterium avium* complex disease. *Clin Pharmacokinet* 2000; 39: 203–214.

84. Finch CK, Crisman CR, Baciewicz AM, Self TH. Rifampin and rifabutin drug interactions: an update. *Arch Int Med* 2002; 162: 985–992.

85. Centers for Disease Control and Prevention. Updated guidelines for the use of rifabutin or rifampin for the treatment and prevention of tuberculosis among HIV-infected patient taking protease inhibitors or nonnucleoside reverse transcriptase inhibitors. *Morbidity and Mortality Weekly Report* 2000; 49: 185–189.

86. Tseng A. AIDS/HIV drugs for opportunistic infections. *In*: Piscitelli JH, Rodvold KA, Masur H, eds. Drug Interaction in Infectious Disease. Totowa, Humana Press, 2000: pp. 61–107.

87. Hansten PD, Horn JR. Drug Interactions. Philadelphia Lea and Febiger and Vancouver, Applied Therapeutics, 1997.

88. Rizack M, Gardner D. Handbook of adverse drug interactions. New Rochelle, The medical Letter Inc., 1998.

89. Overbosch D, Van Gulpen C, Hermans J, *et al.* The effect of probenecid on the renal tubular excretion of benzylpenicillin. *Br J Clin Pharmacol* 1988; 25: 51–58.

90. Rubinstein E, Prokocimer P, Talbot GH. Safety and tolerability of quinupristin/dalfopristin: administration guidelines. *J Antimicrob Chemother* 1999; 44: Topic, A 37–46.

91. Bain KT, Wittbrodt ET. Linezolid for the treatment of resistant Gram-positive Cocci. *Ann Pharmacother* 2001; 35: 566–575.

CHAPTER 16

Future antibiotics and current practices for treating respiratory tract infections

D. Ben avid, G. Rahav, E. Rubinstein

The Infectious Diseases Unit, Sheba medical Center, Tell Aviv University School of Medicine, Tel Hashomer, Israel.

Correspondence: E Rubinstein, Infectious diseases Unit, Sheba Medical center, Tel Hashomer 52621, Israel.

Pneumonia

Community-acquired pneumonia (CAP) is one of the most common reasons for antibiotic therapy and for hospitalisation. It has been estimated that four million cases of CAP occur annually in the US and three million annually throughout Europe. In the US alone some 600,000 of these cases will require hospitalisation, and a total of 10 million physician visits will occur an annual cost of ~$23 million [1]. It is believed that in Europe these proportions are similar. In the US pneumonia is ranked sixth amongst the leading causes of death and may reach 30% in patients with severe disease and up-to 50% of those that need artificial respiration assistance. The elderly constitute >90% of all pneumonia deaths [2]. The overall prevalence of CAP is ~12 per 1,000 of the population of all ages and rises to a rate of 36 per 1,000 in children aged 2–5 yrs and is 30 per 1,000 in those aged >65 yrs rising to a further 34 per 1,000 in those >70 yrs. Therefore pneumonia is one of the most common causes for hospitalisation in medical, paediatric, geriatric and pulmonary hospital services From a total of 2,500 individuals diagnosed with "chest infections" and treated with antibiotics in the UK, there will be 100 patients with a "true" pneumonia, from these 20 will need hospitalisation for an average period of 3.5–6.9 days, of those one patient will need hospitalisation in the intensive care unit with a high risk (>50%) of dying [3]. Evidently, respiratory tract in general and CAP in particular are large consumers of antibiotics, old and new and are of a major interest to the pharmaceutical companies. Despite all recent achievements in vaccine production, patient care, reduction of smoking and improved living conditions the incidence of pneumonia and of respiratory tract infections (RTI) is increasing with an aging population and the relative under utilisation of respiratory vaccines in the elderly.

During the last decade, both the epidemiology and treatment of CAP have undergone rapid changes, including bacteriological, epidemiological, the contribution of atypical pathogens to morbidity and mortality, increased resistance, and potent new antimicrobial agents. Despite extensive studies, there are still many controversies regarding the management of patients with CAP and the need for new agents to be introduced for this indication.

During 2000–2001 recommendations and guidelines were published by several major associations including the Infectious Disease Society of America (IDSA) [4], American Thoracic Society (ATS) [5], the Canadian Infectious Diseases Society-Canadian Thoracic Society (CIDS-CTS) [6] and CDC Drug Resistant *Streptococcus pneumoniae* Working Group [7]. Paul Ehrlich Society (The Chemotherapy and Infectious Diseases Society for

Eur Respir Mon, 2004, 28, 255–267. Printed in UK - all rights reserved. Copyright ERS Journals Ltd 2004; European Respiratory Monograph; ISSN 1025-448x. ISBN 1-904097-32-4.

German speaking countries) [8]. French speaking countries guidelines [9], European Respiratory Society guidelines [10] and other national guidelines issued by various societies, organisations and health maintanace organisations.

Most panels and guidelines agree that antimicrobial coverage must include activity against the principal pathogens involved in CAP, including *S. pneumoniae, Haemophilus influenzae*, and *Morraxella catarrhalis*, as well as against atypical organisms (*Mycoplasma pneumonia, Chlamydia pneumoniae, Coxiella burnetti* and *Legionella pneumophila*). However, antibiotic selection strategies vary among the guidelines and expert panels. Variations among the guidelines include: 1) emphasis on the importance of avoiding induction of resistance to new classes (new fluoroquinolones); and 2) the necessity to empirically cover drug-resistant *S. pneumoniae* (DRSP).

The impact of antibiotic resistance

During the 1990s, many of the common respiratory pathogens, including *S. pneumoniae* and *H. influenzae*, have become resistant to widely used antibiotics. Although the emergence of DRSP is increasingly common in the USA and elsewhere [11], controversy continues whether the presence of resistance to penicillin requires new therapeutic approaches, in view of the fact that mortality increases only when the minimal inhibitory concentration (MIC) of penicillin is >4 $\mu g \cdot mL^{-1}$ [12, 13]. Despite the fact that there is only sparse data showing that the presence of DRSP with intermediate levels of resistance to penicillin MIC <4 $\mu g \cdot mL^{-1}$) influences the outcome of pneumococcal pneumonia, most organisations have adopted an approach of using agents other than penicillin. Growing resistance to penicillin (and macrolides) have been the main driving force behind the search for new agents to treat CAP and RTIs.

Use of newer quinolones

The newer fluoroquinolones offer potential significant advantages over existing agents, these include: 1) having a broader spectrum of activity; 2) lower MICs of relevant pathogens; 3) rapid bacterial kill; 4) attractive pharmacokinetic and pharmacodynamic features; 5) improved safety; and 6) shorter courses of therapy thereby resulting in shorter periods of hospitalisation for the patient and enhanced patient compliance which all lead to cost savings [14].

The newer fluoroquinolones have demonstrated good activity against both susceptible and nonsusceptible *S. pneumoniae* [14, 15]. The ease of using a single drug once daily makes the new fluoroquinolone option very appealing and has led to their increased use. It should be stressed that only the newer fluoroquinolones with antipneumococcal activity *e.g.* levofloxacin, moxifloxacin, gatifloxacin and gernafloxacin are suitable, at the present time, for the treatment of RTIs. Older fluoroquinolones *e.g.* ciprofloxacin, ofloxacin, pefloxacin *etc.* because of their low activity against *S. pneumonia*, are not suitable for this indication.

IDSA guidelines have recommended the routine use of newer fluoroquinolones for the empirical treatment of outpatients and hospitalised patients with CAP. Alternatively the CDC approach is that the overuse of fluoroquinolones could lead to a spread of resistance amongst respiratory pathogens and thus should be avoided. Similarly, the ATS emphasises that treatment with antipneumococcal fluoroquinolones would be effective, but unnecessary for routine use among patients with no modifying factors. Routine use of fluoroquinolones for CAP could therby create selection pressure of resistant strains, and limit its use in the future.

Fluoroquinolone resistance amongst *S. pneumoniae* has remained <1% until recently, presumably because of low use of fluoroquinolones for respiratory infections. However, widespread use of fluoroquinolones has been associated with rising resistance rates to Gram-negative and Gram-positive bacteria.

Recent reports from Hong Kong, Korea, Singapore [16], Canada [17, 18] and the US [19], demonstrate the emergence of fluoroquinolone resistance among strains of *S. pneumoniae*. The report from Hong Kong has documented a marked increase in the prevalence of resistance to levofloxacin among *S. pneumoniae* over a period of 2 yrs. The prevalence of levofloxacin-resistant pneumococci has increased from 5.5% in 1998 to 13.3% in 2000. This resistance was most likely to emerge in penicillin-resistant strains (9.2% in 1998 and 28.4% in 2000). Routine use of fluoroquinolones for CAP could thus create selection pressure of resistant strains, and limit its use in the future. Recently, several reports describing development of resistance to levofloxacin during therapy and clinical failure have been published.

Risk factors for colonisation or infection with fluoroquinolone-resistant pneumococci include a history of chronic obstructive lung disease and prior fluoroquinolone exposure. As these reports were published recently, none of the guidelines have indicated that history of previous use of fluoroquinolone should be a reason to avoid use of fluoroquinolones for the empirical treatment of pneumonia. Nevertheless, the cross ability to select fluoroquinolone-resistant *S. pneumoniae* mutants and thereby the possible cross resistance between the various fluoroquinolones, casts a certain doubt on their continous suitability to treat severe pneumococcal infections. However, in several recent surveys including fluoroquinolone-resistant mutants, garenoxacin had MICs against *S. pneumoniae* in the range of 0.03–0.06 mcg·mL^{-1}, that were lower than those of moxifloxacin, gatifloxacin and levofloxacin and similar or just one dilution higher than those of gemifloxacin [20, 21]. Garenoxacin, similar to other fluoroquinolones achieves adequate concentrations in the epithelail lining fluid (ELF), alveolar macrophages and bronchial mucosa that will make it an attractive alternative to present fluoroquinolones for treating pneumococcal infections even in areas with limited susceptibility to this class of agents [22].

While all newer fluoroquinolones have been used with success in acute exacerbations of chronic obstructive pulmonary disorders (AE-COPD) and in sinusitis, their use is difficult to justify particularly in regions with low *S. pneumoniae* fluoroquinolone resistance rates. The reasons being that similar clinical success rates can be obtained with other less potent agents.

Garenoxacin (BMS 284756)

Garenoxacin (BMS 284756) is also known as T-3811 ME, it is a defluorinated (Des-F(6)-Quinolone) fluoroquinolone developed by Toyoma (Tokyo, Japan) and Bristol-Meyers-Squibb (BMS; Wallingford, CT, US). It has lower MICs (<0.0016–0.06 mcg·mL^{-1}) compared with ciprofloxacin, levofloxacin and moxifloxacin against quinolone-susceptible *S. pneumoniae* as well as against quinolone-resistant *S. pneumoniae* (MICs 0.03–1.0 mcg·mL^{-1}) [19–21, 23]. Geranoxacin also exhibited excellent *in vitro* activity against all other respiratory pathogens [23–26] and therapeutic concentrations in different lung compartments [22, 26].

Sitafloxacin

This new fluoroquinolone developed by Daiichi Pharmaceuticals (Totyo, Japan) has excellent *in vitro* activity against *S. pneumoniae* and other respiratory pathogens [18].

Initial clinical trials in patients hospitalised with pneumonia reveal 94–97% cure rate (91% in the intention-to-treat analysis) [27].

New β-lactams

Ertapenem

Ertapenem is a carbapenem antibiotic and is a new injectable β -lactam recently introduced into mediacl practice. Against 102 isolates of *S. pneumoniae*, selected to include organisms resistant to a variety of drug classes ertapenem MICs ranged from ≤0.008–4 mg·L^{-1}, MIC50=0.5 (MIC of 50% of the bacteria) mg·L^{-1}, and MIC90=2 mg·L^{-1} (MIC of 90% of the bacteria). Based on MIC90, ertapenem potency was 4-fold greater than cefuroxime, 2-fold greater than amoxycillin/clavulanate= penicillin, 2-fold less than meropenem and ceftriaxone, and 4-fold less than imipenem [28]. Ertapenem has been as efficacious as ceftriaxone in two multicentric studies where a >92% cure rate in clinically evaluable patients with CAP [29, 30]. However, ertapenem is not expected to be active against atypical pathogens including *Legionella sp.* and thus cannot be recommended as a "blind" therapy approach for patients with severe CAP. In patients with nosocomial pneumonia, particularly ventilator associated pneumonia (VAP), *Pseudomonas. aeruginosa* is a frequent pathogen. Due to its inferior antipseudomonal activity compared to imipenem and meropenem ertapenem is expected to render inferior clinical results to these two agents in cases of VAP.

RWJ-54428

This is a new cephalosporin with activity against resistant Gram-positive organisms, including penicillin-resistant *S. pneumoniae*. RWJ-54428 was more active than penicillin G and cefotaxime against penicillin-resistant, intermediate, and susceptible strains of *S. pneumoniae* (MIC90, 0.25, 0.125, and ≤0.0625 mcg mg·L^{-1}, respectively) [31]. In a mouse model of pneumonia due to a penicillin-susceptible strain of *S. pneumoniae*, RWJ-54428 displayed efficacy and potency superior to those of penicillin G and cefotaxime[32].

BAL 9141

This is a new pyrrolidinone cephalosporin with excellent activity against Gram-positive cocci including streptococci and staphylococci [33]. At the present time there are no data regarding efficacy in animal models with pneumonia but in an endocarditis methecillin resistant *S. aureus* (MRSA) model, results were encouraging [33].

Daptomycin

Daptomycin is a lipopepetide which was originally developed by Eli Lilly (Indianpolis, IN, US) pharmaceutical company and more recently by Cubist Pharmaceuticals (Boston, MA, US) is aimed at Gram-positive cocci, including those resistant to penicillin, methicillin and vancomycin. In a recent European survey, 9.4% of all *S. pneumoniae* isolates collected were resistant to penicillin with variation by country from 0% in the Netherlands to 20.7% in Portugal. Multidrug resistance, defined as concurrent resistance to three or more antimicrobials of different chemical classes, was observed in 3.6% of *S. pneumoniae* Daptomycin was more active against penicillin-resistant *S. pneumoniae* (MIC90 0.25 mg·L^{-1}) than was quinupristin-dalfopristin (MIC90 0.5 mg·L^{-1}) or linezolid (MIC90 2 mg·L^{-1}) [34]. A recent study of CAP in Europe comparing ceftriaxone to daptomycin failed to demonstrate any superiority of daptomycin. More has to be learnd about pulmonary pharmacokinetics of daptomycin before it can be safely used in pneumonia. Nevertheless, should vancomycin-resistant *S. pneumoniae* develop causing respiratory infections, daptomycin may have a role in such cirumstances.

Quinupristin/Dalfopristin (Synercid)

This new injectable streptogramin developed by Aventis (Paris, France). It is particularly active (like daptomycin) against resistant Gram-positive cocci causing severe infections, but also against atypical pathogens causing pneumonia. The MICs against *S. pneumoniae*, including penicillin-resistant and penicillin-intermediate strains is in the range of 0.5–1.0 mcg·mL^{-1}, against *H. influenzae* 4–8 mcg·mL^{-1}, against *Legionella spp.* 4–8 mcg·mL^{-1}, against *M. pneumoniae* 0.1–1.0 mcg·mL^{-1}and against *M. cattarhalis* 1.0 mcg·mL^{-1} [35]. No direct studies evaluating synercid in CAP or other RTI were performed, however isolated case reports suggest that synercid might be effective in severe pneumococcal pneumonia [36]. The need for a central line to administer this antibiotic along with the most frequently reported adverse effects with administration of quinupristin/dalfopristin which are: infusion-site inflammation, pain, and eodema; other infusion-site reactions, thrombophlebitis, arthralgia, myalgia, nausea, diarrhoea, vomiting, and a rash occurring in 2.5–4.6%, make this agent suitable for a selected group of patients with CAP [37].

Oritavancin

This is a semisynthetic glycopeptide that is active against vancomycin-resistant Gram-positive cocci. The initial development was in Eli Lilly laboratories and the further development at InterMune (Brisbane, CA, USA). Its MIC against penicillin-susceptible, penicillin- intermediate and penicillin-resistant *S. pneumoniae* strains is in the range of <0.001–0.06 mcg·mL^{-1} [38, 39]. In a pharmacodynamic model the area under the concentration curve (AUC)/MIC ratio of oritavancin against DRSP (944) as well as time >MIC (100%) were far above the therapeutic minimum [40].

Dalbavancin

This is a semisynthetic derivative of the natural glycopeptide A-40926 developed by Versicor US, and recently by Vicuron (Boston, MA, US), it is in phase II trials in the US. Both dalbavancin and MDL-63246 are dimethylaminopropyl amide derivatives of A-40926; dalbavancin differs from MDL-63246 in its acylamino sugar, which consists of glucuronic acid in dalbavancin and glucosamine in MDL-63246 (216093; 98527). The development of MDL-63246 has been discontinued (298527). The compound has better activity than vancomycin against many Gram-positive pathogens. The MICs against penicillin-susceptible and -resistant *S. pneumoniae* is <0.03–0.13 mcg·mL^{-1}. The antibiotic has a very long *t1/2* in plasma allowing for once a week administration. Little is known yet about the lung pharmacokinetics of this agent [41].

Telithromycin

Telithromycin (HMR 3647, RU 66647) is a new ketolide developed by Aventis that was launched in the US (summer 2001) and several other countries. Erythromycin-susceptible *S. pneumoniae* are inhibited at a telithromycin concentration of

≤ 0.03 mcg·mL^{-1} and erythromycin resistant strains are inhibited at a telithromycin concentration of 0.25 mcg·mL^{-1} with 99.9% killing within 24 h for both macrolide-susceptible and -resistant strains [42]. This activity was also demonstrable for *H. influenzae*. The rapid killing effect of telithromycin was demonstrable in animal studies [43]. In addition to its antibacterial activity, telithromycin may have some salutary effects in pneumonia by reducing neutrophil recruitment, decreasing pneumococcal induced release of interleukin (IL)-6, IL-1β and nitiric oxide levels in the bronchoalveolar lavage [44].

In humans, telithromycin was found to penetrate well into alveolar macrophages (AM) and ELF exceeding the MICs of common pulmonary pathogens and remaining there for prolonged periods of time [45]. Telithromycin demonstrated time-dependent killing, with no inoculum effect for *S. pneumoniae* but with an inoculum effect for *H. influenzae*. Telithromycin exhibited a postantibiotic effect against respiratory pathogens as an additional salutary therapeutic feature [46]. A randomised, double-blind study compared the efficacy and tolerability of telithromycin (800 mg once daily) with that of amoxicillin (1,000 mg *t.i.d.*) in the treatment of CAP in 404 adult patients. The clinical cure rate for telithromycin-treated patients (per protocol) post-therapy (days 17–24) was 141 from a total of 149 (94.6%) and that of amoxicillin was 137 from a total of 152 (90.1%). Subset analysis of patients (per protocol) showed high clinical cure rates for patients aged ≥ 65 yrs (telithromycin 21/24, 87.5%; amoxycillin 22/29, 75.9%), those with documented pneumococcal bacteremia (telithromycin 10/10; amoxicillin 7/9) and patients with a Fine score $\geq$ III (telithromycin 31/34, 91.2%; amoxicillin 38/47, 80.9%). Bacterial eradication rates were comparable (telithromycin 42/48, 87.5%; amoxycillin 39/45, 86.7%), with 22/23 *versus* 18/21 *S. pneumoniae* strains 9/12 *versus* 11/13 *H. influenzae* strains and all *M. catarrhalis* isolates (five and three patients, respectively) eradicated at the test-of-cure visit. [47]. In a randomised, double blinded, multicentre comparative trial in which telithromycin (800 mg once daily) for 10 days was compared with clarithromycin (500 mg *b.i.d.* for 10 days) in 448 patients. The cure rates were onserved to be similar at 88.3% and 88.5% for telithromycin and clarithromycin respectively [48]. In a multicentre randomised study of AE-COPD, in Europe, South America and Australia in which telithromycin (800 mg once daily for 5 days) was compared with amoxicillin/clavulanate (500/125 mg *t.i.d.* for 10 days), 321 patient took part. The cure rates were 86% and 82% in the telithromycin and amoxicillin/clavulanate groups respectively [49]. In a similarly conducted North American study in which 495 patients participated, telithromycin in the same dose for 5 days was compared to cefuroxime axetil 500 mg once daily for 10 days. The cure rates were 89% and 86% respectively in patients belonging to high risk groups [50].

Cethromycin

Cethromycin (ABT-773) is a ketolide developed by Abbott Laboratories (Chicago, Illinois, US) Its chemical name is 11-amino-11deoxy-3-oxo-5-O-desosaminyl-6-O-[1'-(3'-quinolyl-2'-propenyl)] erythronolide A 11,12-cyclic carbamate. It has a tighter ribosomal binding and higher intracellular penetration than erythromycin and hence is active against macrolide resistant *S. pneumoniae* [51]. ABT-773 is active against penicillin-susceptible and resistant and macrolide resistant *S .pneumonaie* with MIC in the range of <0.008–0.25 mcg·mL^{-1}, good activity against *M .cattarhalis* and mediocre activity against *H. influenzae* with MIC50 of 2 and MIC90 of 4 mcg·mL^{-1}[52]. In an animal model of pneumonia it was found that the AUC$_{free}$/MIC50 (area under the time-concentration curve divided by MIC50) or maximum concentration (Cmax),free/MIC of cethromycin results in bacteriostatic effects, while higher values (two-fold) maximise survival [53].

Linezolid

This compound belongs to the oxazolidinones, a relatively new class of antibiotics (developed initially by Pharmacia). It inhibits bacterial protein synthesis by inhibition of the formation of the 70S initation complex by binding to the 50S ribosomal subunit at the interface with the 30S subunit [54]. The MIC_{50} and MIC_{90} against penicillin-susceptible and penicillin-resistant *S. pneumoniae* are 0.5 and 1.0 mcg·mL^{-1} respectively [49]. The MICs of linezolid against other respiratory pathogens were: *H. influnzae* 4–16 mcg·mL^{-1}, *M. cattarhalis* 4–8 mcg·mL^{-1}, *Bordatella. pertusis* 4 mcg·mL^{-1}, *Legionella spp.* 4–16 mcg·mL^{-1} [55]. Thus only respiratory infections that are clearly caused by *S. pneumoniae* should be treated with linezolid as a single agent. Linezolid is rapidly and completely absorbed from the gastrointestinal tract achieving peak and trough serum levels of ~18 and 6 mcg·mL^{-1} respectively with an elimination half-life of 4.5–5.5 h [56]. In a study of outpatient CAP comparing linezolid 600 mg *b.i.d.* with cefpodoxime 200 mg *b.i.d.* for 7–14 days, clinical cure rates and microbiological eradication rates were similar (85% and 90%) [56, 57]. In another open-labelled study comparing linezolid to ceftriaxone in patients with CAP admitted to hospital similar results were found with cure rates of 80–90% in each group [56, 57]. Notably in relatively few patients with bacteremic *S. pneumoniae* infections the results with linezolid were significantly better than with the comparators (93 *versus* 70%) [57].

Empirical treatment of outpatients

Approximately 80% of patients with CAP are treated as outpatients. As the signs and symptoms of pneumonia are not specific, a chest radiograph is mandatory to confirm the diagnosis. The approach to antibiotic therapy usually will be empirical and should account for a number of clinical, epidemiological and local resistance patterns of respiratory pathogens. All patients should be treated for the possibility of atypical pneumonia, including monotherapy (macrolide or new fluroquinolone), evidently the new fluoroquinolones with low MICs against DRSP are the preferred agents. Another option is a combination of a β-lactam with a macrolide. Patients with various epidemiological or clinical risk factors (structural lung disease, alcoholism, residence in a nursing facility, *etc.*) suggest the need for intensification and expansion of bacterial coverage to include coverage against *P. aeruginosa* (ceftazidime, carbapenems or piperacillion/tazobactam) and possibly even *S. aureus* including MRSA with one of the new anti-Gram-positive compounds added to the conventional therapeutic regimen.

The recommendation of IDSA for outpatients is administration of a macrolide, doxycycline, or a fluoroquinolone with enhanced activity against *S. pneumoniae* (with no preference). The alternative approach by the ATS and the Canadian guidelines is based on patient stratification according to the presence of factors that influence the likely etiological pathogens, and initial antibiotic treatment should be selected according to the different patient subsets. The ATS committee recommends using a narrow-spectrum empirical therapy, if possible, in order to avoid spread of resistance among respiratory pathogens [17]. For outpatients without modifying factors or cardiopulmonary disease, the ATS recommended that therapy should be with an advanced generation macrolide, or with a doxycycline as a second choice because of lesser activity against *S. pneumoniae*. Due to lower incidence of side effects, favourable pharmacokinetics, and broader spectrum of activity, the advanced generation macrolides are clearly preferred over erythromycin. The ATS emphasises that treatment with antipneumococcal fluoroquinolone would be effective, but unnecessary, as the overuse of fluoroquinolone could lead to the spread of resistance amongst respiratory pathogens. Outpatients with cardio-pulmonary disease or with modifying factors and increased risk for DRSP should be treated with either a β-lactam/macrolide combination or with an antipneumococcal fluoroquinolone. Doxycycline can be used as an alternative for a macrolide. In order to avoid selection pressure causing resistance, the ATS recommends using both options for different patients.

The CIDS-CTS recommends the use of fluoroquinolones for patients with COPD and a history of antibiotic use or use of oral steroids. For outpatients without modifying factors, treatment with a macrolide is their first choice.

It is unclear whether DRSP or macrolide resistant *S. pneumoniae* are important treatment issues in outpatient CAP. The frequency of DRSP (MIC>4 mcg·mL^{-1}) causing outpatient's CAP, as estimated by the CDC, is very low (in the range of 0.14–1.9%). This analysis has prompted the CDC panel to conclude that antibiotics with activity against penicillin resistant are not essential as part of empirical treatment. Therefore, macrolides or β-lactam monotherapy is recommended by the CDC working group as initial treatment. The working group suggested that new fluoroquinolones should not be first line treatment in outpatients with CAP and should be avoided because of concerns about resistance emergence.

Empirical treatment of hospitalised patients

In several studies among hospitalised patients with CAP, in which detailed microbiological investigations were performed, a high incidence of atypical pathogens was reported (*C. pneumoniae, M. pneumoniae* and Legionella), often as a part of a mixed infection, often in elderly populations [58, 59]. The importance of mixed infections causing pneumonia is uncertain. However, some investigators report that co-infection with typical and atypical pathogens together may lead to more complicated courses and a higher mortality if not both agents are adequately treated [60] This concept has led all groups to recommend either the use of combinations of β-lactam antibiotics with macrolides or to antipneumococcal fluoroquinolones as single therapy [60, 61]. The β-lactam should be with enhanced activity against PRSP. Such agents include ampicillin, cefotaxime, ceftriaxone and ampicillin-sulbactam. In contrast, cefuroxime and ceftazidime are substantially less active *in vitro* against *S. pneumoniae* and thus are not recommended for empirical treatment of hospitalised patients with CAP [4–6].

The ATS and IDSA recommend the use of combination treatment of β-lactam/macrolide or monotherapy with fluoroquinolone without special preference. However, the CIDS-CTS recommend treatment with fluoroquinolones as the first choice, over combination treatment, due to logistical and financial advantages. The CDC suggests that fluoroquinolones should be considered only in the presence *S. pneumoniae* with high level resistance to penicillin (MIC>4 mg·dL^{-1}) or failure of other agents.

For patients with severe CAP, therapy should be with β-lactam plus macrolide or a β-lactam and a fluoroquinolone. All organisations agree that antipneumococcal fluoroquinolones not be used as monotherappy, since the published clinical studies have involved too few patients with severe CAP and their efficacy is therefore unknown.

Should treatment be pathogen-directed?

The IDSA and the CIDS-CTS recommends that an attempt should be made to achieve pathogen-directed antimicrobial treatment for hospitalised patients. Antibiotic regiments selected empirically should be changed when results of culture become available. Once infection with a copathogen has been excluded, initial empirical treatment should be modified so that the treatment is directed at the specific pathogens involved. However, with the increasing recognition that a significant proportion of patients, particularly the elderly, may have polymicrobial CAP, current approaches may need to be re-evaluated. New information suggests that even patients with bacteremic pneumococcal CAP have an improved outcome when treated with a combination of a β-lactam and a macrolide [60, 61]. Further studies are now needed to resolve whether bacteremic pneumococcal pneumonia should be treated with a single antibiotic treatment or with combination therapy.

Duration of treatment

The IDSA recommends treating pneumonia caused by *S. pneumoniae* until the patient is afebrile for 72 h. Pneumonia caused by bacteria that can cause necrosis of pulmonary parenchyma (*e.g. S. aureus* or *P. aeruginosa*) should be treated for longer than 2 weeks, and pneumonia caused by atypical pathogens (e.g, *M. pneumoniae* or *C. pneumoniae*) should be treated for at least 2 weeks. However, these recommendations are not based on randomised clinical trials and are supported by expert opinion only. A recent double-blind, randomised controlled trial has assessed the efficacy of 3-day compared with the standard 5-day course of amoxycillin in children with nonsevere pneumonia [62]. Treatment with the abbreviated treatment was equally as effective compared to the 5-day course. However, there are no controlled trials that compare short antimicrobial courses with long courses (>7 days) in adult CAP patients.

Summary

Community-acquired pneumonia (CAP) is a common disease with a substantial morbidity and mortality. It is believed that appropriate and timely antibiotic therapy can improve the outcome of pneumonia. Therefore, many professional societies have composed guidelines that take into account the various epidemiological micro-biological features of pneumonia pathogens, demographical characteristics of the patients, pharmcokinetic and pharmacodynamic characteristics of the antibiotics to be used and the associated costs of hospitalisation and treatment. Nevertheless pneumonia pathogens are acquiring new resistances and new drugs with improved therapeutic features are on the verge of being introduced into clinical practice. Linezolid, daptomycin, quinupristin/dalfopristin, oritavancin and dalbavancin are all active against Gram-positive pathogens including methicillin resistant *Staphylococcus aureus*, acquired nosocomially and penicillin resistant *Streptococcus pneumonia*, as well as other respiratory pathogens resistant and susceptible to conventional drugs. These drugs are primarily used systemically in hospitalised individuals with moderate-severe pneumonia. Telithromycin and cethromycin are both ketolides appropriate for the therapy of *S. pneumoniae* and other pathogens and are primarily oral agents and aimed for community therapy of such mild-moderate infections. As the aetiology of a patient who presents with CAP is rarely known, therapy will have to rely on the clinical presentation of the patient and the epidemiological data. The exact definition of the place of each of the agents in the management of pneumonia has not yet been defined but in future years studies and epidemiological developments are expected to outline for the appropriate use of these agents.

Keywords: Community-acquired pneumonia, drug-resistant *Streptococcus pneumoniae*, guidelines of management, resistant pathogens, therapy.

References

1. Bartlett JG, Mundy LM. Community-acquired pneumonia. *N Eng J Med* 1995; 333: 1618–162.
2. Macfarlane JT. An overview of community acquired pneumonia with lessons learned from the British Thoracis Society Study. *Semin Respir Infect* 1994; 9: 153–165.
3. Bartlett JG, Breiman RF, Mandell LA, File TM Jr. Community-acquired pneumonia in adults: guidelines for management. The Infectious Diseases Society of America. *Clin Infect Dis* 1998; 26: 811–838.
4. Bartlett JG, Dowell SF, Mandell LA, *et al.* Practice guidelines for the management of community acquired pneumonia in adults. *Clin Infect Dis* 2000; 31: 347–382.
5. Niederman MS, Mandell LA, Anzueto A, and the American Thoracic Society. Guidelines for the management of adults with community-acquired pneumonia. *Am J Respir Crit Care Med* 2001; 163: 1730–1754.
6. Mandell LA, Marrie TJ, Grossman RF, Chow AW, Hyland J. Canadian guidelines for the initial management of community-acquired pneumonia: an evidence based update by the Canadian Infectious Diseases Society and the Canadian Thoracic Society. *Clin Infect Dis* 2000; 31: 383–421.
7. Heffelfinger JD, Dowell SF, Jorgensen JH, *et al*, and the Drug-Resistant *Streptococcus Pneumoniae* Therapeutic Working Group. Management of community-acquired pneumonia in the era of pneumococcal resistance. *Arch Intern Med* 2000; 160: 1399–1408.
8. Vogel F, Worth H, Adam D, Elies W, *et al.* Rationale therapie bakterieller atemsweginfektionen. Empehlunge einer expertengruppe der Paul Ehrlich Gesellschaft fur Chemotherapie e. V. und der Deutschhen atemsswege e. V. *Chemotherapie J* 2000; 9: 3–23.
9. Huchon G, Chidiac C, Delaval P, Leophonte P, Mouton Y, Roche N, Tremolieres F. Management of community-acquired lower respiratory tract infection in the adult. Recommendations by the French Language Society of Pneumology with collaboration of the French Language Society of Infectious Pathology, from the recommendations of the European Respiratory Society. *Rev Mal Respir* 1999; 16: 224–233.
10. ERS Task Force Report. Guidelines for management of adult community-acquired lower respiratory tract infections. European Respiratory Society. *Eur Respir J* 1998; 11: 986–991.
11. Whitney CG, Farley MM, Hadler J, *et al.* Increasing prevalence of multidrug-resistant Streptococcus pneumoniae in the United States. *N Engl J Med* 2000; 343: 1917–1924.
12. Pallares R, Linares J, Vadillo M, *et al.* Resistance to penicillin and cephalosporin and mortality from severe pneumonia in Barcelona, Spain. *N Engl J Med* 1995; 333: 474–480.
13. Feikin D, Schuchat A, Kolczak M, *et al.* Mortality from invasive pneumococcal pneumonia in the era of antibiotic resistance. 1995–1997. *Am J public Health* 2000; 90: 223–229.
14. Appelbaum PG. Microbiological and pharmacodynamic considerations in the treatment of infection due to antimicrobial-resistant *Streptococcus pneumoniae. Clin Infect Dis* 2000; 31: Suppl. 2, S29–S34.
15. Jones RN, Pfaller MA. *In vitro* activity of newer fluoroquinolones for respiratory tract infection and emerging patterns of antimicrobial resistance: data from the SENTRY antimicrobial surveillance program. *Clin Infect Dis* 2000; 31: Suppl. 2, S16–S23.
16. Ho PL, Que TL, Tsang DN, *et al.* Emergence of fluoroquinolone resistance among multiply resistant strains of *Streptococcus pneumoniae* in Hong Kong. *Antimicrob Agents Chemother* 1999; 43: 1310–1313.

17. Chen DK, McGeer A, de Azavedo JC, Low DE. Decreased susceptibility of *Streptococcus pneumoniae* to fluoroquinolones in Canada. *N Engl J Med* 1999; 341: 233–239.

18. Low DE, de Azavedo J, Weiss K, *et al.* Antimicrobial resistance among clinical isolates of *Streptococcus pneumoniae* in Canada during 2000. *Antimicrob Agents Chemother* 2002; 46: 1295–1301.

19. Jones RN, Pfaller MA. Macrolide and fluoroquinolone (Levofloxacin) resistance among *Streptococcus pneumoniae* strains: significant trends from the SENTRY antimicrobial surveillance program (North America, 1997–1999). *J Clin Microbiol* 2000; 38: 4298–4299.

20. Clark CL, Nagai K, Davies TA, *et al.* Single- and multistep selection study of the antipneumococcal activity of BMS-284756 compared to ciprofloxacin, levofloxacin, trovafloxacin and moxifloxacin. *Clin Microbiol Infect* 2002; 8: 373–380.

21. Bell JM, Turnidge JD, Jones RN. The SENTRY Regional Participants Group Antimicrobial resistance trends in community-acquired respiratory tract pathogens in the Western Pacific Region and South Africa: report from the SENTRY antimicrobial surveillance program, (1998–1999) including an in vitro evaluation of BMS284756. *Int J Antimicrob Agents* 2002; 19: 125–132.

22. Andrews J, Honeybourne D, Jevons G, *et al.* Concentrations of garenoxacin in plasma, bronchial mucosa, alveolar macrophages and epithelial lining fluid following a single oral 600 mg dose in healthy adult subjects. *J Antimicrob Chemother* 2003; 51: 727–730.

23. Pankuch GA, Nagai K, Davies TA, Jacobs MR, Appelbaum PC. Antipneumococcal activity of BMS 284756 compared to those of six other agents. *Antimicrob Agents Chemother* 2002; 46: 251–254.

24. Biedenbach DJ, Jones RN, Pfaller MA, The Sentry participants group (Americas and Europe). Activity of BMS 284756 against 2,681 recent clinical isolates of *Haemophilus influenzae* and *Moraxella catarrhalis*: report from the SENTRY antimicrobial surveillance program (2000) in Europe, Canada and the United States. *Diagn Microbiol Infect Diseases* 2001; 39: 245–250.

25. Andrews J, Honeybourne D, Jevons G, *et al.* Concentrations of garenoxacin in plasma, bronchial mucosa, alveolar macrophages and epithelial lining fluid following a single oral 600 mg dose in healthy adult subjects. *J Antimicrob Chemother* 2003 Mar; 51: 727–730.

26. Zhanel GG, Ennis K, Vercaigne L, *et al.* A critical review of the fluoroquinolones: focus on respiratory infections. *Drugs* 2002; 62: 13–59.

27. Feldman C, White H, O'Grady J, Flitcroft A, Briggs A, Richards G. An open, randomized, multicentre study comparing the safety and efficacy of sitafloxacin and imipenem/cilastatin in the intravenous treatment of hospitalized patients with pneumonia. *International J Antimicrob Agents* 2001; 17: 177–188.

28. Hilliard NJ, Johnson CN, Armstrong SH, Quarles S, Waites KB. *In vitro* activity of ertapenem (MK-0826) against multi-drug resistant *Streptococcus pneumoniae* compared with 13 other antimicrobials. *Int J Antimicrob Agents* 2002; 20: 136–140.

29. Vetter N, Cambronero-Hernandez E, Rohlf J, *et al.* Protocol 020 Study Group. A prospective, randomized, double-blind multicenter comparison of parenteral ertapenem and ceftriaxone for the treatment of hospitalized adults with community-acquired pneumonia. *Clin Ther* 2002; 24: 1770–1785.

30. Ortiz-Ruiz G, Caballero-Lopez J, Friedland IR, Woods GL, Carides A, Protocol 018 Ertapenem Community-Acquired Pneumonia Study Group. A study evaluating the efficacy, safety, and tolerability of ertapenem *versus* ceftriaxone for the treatment of community-acquired pneumonia in adults. *Clin Infect Dis* 2002; 34: 1076–1083.

31. Chamberland S, Blais J, Hoang M, *et al.* *In vitro* activities of RWJ-54428 (MC-02,479) against multiresistant gram-positive bacteria. *Antimicrob Agents Chemother* 2001; 45: 1422–1430.

32. Griffith DC, Harford L, Williams R, Lee VJ, Dudley MN. *In vivo* antibacterial activity of RWJ-54428, a new cephalosporin with activity against Gram-positive bacteria. *Antimicrob Agents Chemother* 2003; 47: 43–47.

33. Entenza JM, Hohl P, Heinze-Krauss I, Glauser MP, Moreillon P. BAL9141, a novel extended-spectrum cephalosporin active against methicillin-resistant *Staphylococcus aureus* in treatment of experimental endocarditis. *Antimicrob Agents Chemother* 2002; 46: 171–177.

34. Critchley IA, Draghi DC, Sahm DF, Thornsberry C, Jones ME, Karlowsky JA. Activity of daptomycin against susceptible and multidrug-resistant Gram-positive pathogens collected in the SECURE study (Europe) during 2000–2001. *J Antimicrob Chemother* 2003; 51: 639–649.

35. Bouanchaud DH. In-vitro and in-vivo antibacterial activity of quinupristin/dalfopristin. *J Antimicrob Chemother* 1997; 39: Suppl. A, 15–21.

36. Fagon J, Patrick H, Haas DW, *et al.* Treatment of Gram-positive nosocomial pneumonia. Prospective randomized comparison of quinupristin/dalfopristin versus vancomycin. Nosocomial Pneumonia Group. *Am J Respir Crit Care Med* 2001; 163: 1759–1760.

37. Lamb HM, Figgitt DP, Faulds D. Quinupristin/dalfopristin: a review of its use in the management of serious gram-positive infections. *Drugs* 1999; 58: 1061–1097.

38. Garcia-Garrote F, Cercenado E, Alcala L, Bouza E. *In vitro* activity of the new glycopeptide LY333328 against multiply resistant Gram-positive clinical isolates. *Antimicrob Agents Chemother* 1998; 42: 2452–2455.

39. Zeckel M, Preston DA, Allen BS. *In vitro* activity of LY 33328 and comparative agents against nosocomial gram-positive pathogens collected in 1997 global surveillance study. *Antimicrob Agents Chemother* 2000; 44: 137–134.

40. Coyle EA, Ryback MJ. Activity of oritavancin (LY 33328), an investigational glycopeptide, compared to that of vancomycin against multidrug-resistant *Streptococcus pneumoniae* in an invitro pharmacodynamic model. *Antimicrob Agents Chemother* 2001; 45: 706–709.

41. Steiert M, Schmitz FJ. Dalbavancin (Biosearch Italia/Versicor). *Curr Opin Investig Drugs* 2002; 3: 229–233.

42. Pankuch GA, Visali MA, Jacobs MR, Appelbaum PC. Susceptibilities of penicillin-and erythromycin susceptible and resistant pneumococci to HMR 3647 (RU 66647), a new ketolide, compared with susceptibilities to 17 other agents. *Antimicrob Agents Chemother* 1998; 42: 624–630.

43. Agouridas C, Bonnefoy A, Chantot JF. Antibacteria activity of RU 64004 (HMR 3004), a novel ketolide derivative active against respiratory pathogens. *Antimicrob Agents Chemother* 1997; 41: 2149–2158.

44. Duong M, Simard M, Bergeron Y, Ouelet N, Cote-Richer N, Bergeron M. Immunomodulating effects of HMR 3004 on pulmonary inflammation caused by heat-killed *Streptococcus pneumoniae* in mice. *Antimicrob Agents Chemother* 1998; 42: 3309–3312.

45. Kadota J-I, Ishimatsu Y, Iwashita T, *et al.* Intrapulmonary pharmacokinetics of telithromycin, a new ketolide, in healthy Japanese volunteers. *Antimicrob Agents Chemother* 2002; 46: 917–921.

46. Odenholt I, Lowdin E, Cars O. Pharmacodynamics of telithromycin *in vitro* against respiratory tract pathogens. *Antimicrob Agents Chemother* 2001; 45: 23–29.

47. Hagberg L, Torres A, van Rensburg D, Leroy B, Rangaraju M, Ruuth E. Efficacy and tolerability of once-daily telithromycin compared with high-dose amoxicillin for treatment of community-acquired pneumonia. *Infection* 2002; 30: 378–386.

48. Teller G, Hassman J, Leroy B, Sidarous E. Oral telithromycin (HMR 3647) 800 mg once daily is well tolerated and as effective as oral clarithromycin 500 mg twice daily in community-acquired pneumonia in adults. Toronto, 40th Interscience Conference on Antimicrobial Agents and Chemotherapy, 2000; Abstract.

49. Leroy B, Rangaraju M, Bienfait-Beozon C. Telithromycin is as effective as amoxicillin/clavulante in acute exacerbations of chronic bronchitis. *Respir Med* 2002; 96: 862–871.

50. DeAbate CA, Heyder A, Leroy B, Sidarous E, *et al.* Oral telithromycin (HMR 3647) 800 mg once daily for 5 days is well tolerated and and as effective as cfuroxime axetil 500 mg twice daily for 10 days, in adults with acute exacerbation of chronic bronchitis. Toronto, 40th Interscience Conference on Antimicrobial Agents and Chemotherapy, 2000; 2228.

51. Capobianco JO, Cao Z, Shoertridge VD, Ma Z, Flamm RK, Zhong P. Studies of novel ketolide

ABT-773: transport, binding to ribosomes, and inhibition of protein synthesis in *Streptococcus pneumonaie*. *Antimicrob Agents Chemother* 2000; 44: 1562–1567.

52. Brueggemann AB, Doern GV, Huynh HK, Wingert EM, Rhomberg PR. In vitro activity of ABT-773, a new ketolide, against recent clinical isolates of Streptococcus pneumoniae, *Haemophilus influenzae*, and *Moraxella catarrhalis. Antimicrob Agents Chemother* 2000; 44: 447–449.

53. Kim MK, Zhou W, Tessier PR, Xuan D, Ye M, Nightingale CH, Nicolau DP. Bactericidal effect and pharmacodynamics of cethromycin (ABT-773) in a murine pneumococcal pneumonia model. *Antimicrob Agents Chemother* 2002; 46: 3185–3192.

54. Swaney SM, Aoki H, Clelia Ganoza M, Shinabarger DL. The oxazolidinone linezolid inhibits initiation of protein synthesis in bacteria. *Antimicrob Agents Chemother* 1998; 42: 3251–3255.

55. Diekema DJ, Jones RN. Oxazolidinone antibiotics. *Lancet* 2001; 358: 1975–1982.

56. Perry CM, Goa KL. Linezolid: a review of its use in the managemat of serious gram-positive infections. *Drugs* 2001; 61: 525–551.

57. Cammarata SK, Hempsall KA, Timm JA, Todd WM, Oliphant TH, Hafkin B. Linezolid is superior to cephalosporins in the treatment of patients with bacteremic Streptococcus pneumoniae community-acquired pneumonia. Toronto, American Thoracic society International Conference, 2000; E74.

58. Marston BJ, Plouffe JF, File TM, *et al.* For the Community-Based Pneumonia incidence Study Group. Incidence of community acquired pneumonia requiring hospitalizations: results of a population-based active surveillance study in Ohio. *Arch Intern Med* 1997; 157: 1709–1718.

59. Lieberman S, Schlaeffer F, Boldur I, *et al.* Multiple pathogens in adult patients with community-acquired pneumoniae: a one-year prospective study of 346 consecutive patients. *Thorax* 1996; 51: 179–184.

60. Waterer GW, Somes GW, Wunderink RG. Monotherapy may be suboptimal for severe bacteremic pneumococcal pneumonia. *Arch Intern Med* 2001; 161: 1837–1842.

61. Gleason PR, Meehan TP, Fine JM, *et al.* Associations between initial antimicrobial therapy and medical outcomes for hospitalized elderly patients with pneumonia. *Arch Intern Med* 1999; 159: 2562.

62. Pakistan Multicentre Amoxicillin Short Course Therapy (MASCOT) pneumonia study group. Clinical efficacy of 3 says versus 5 days of oral amoxicillin for treatment of childhood pneumonia: a multicentre double blind trial. *Lancet* 2002; 360: 835–841.